Healthcare for an Aging Population

Meeting the challenge

Jennifer R. Jamison MBBCh PhD EdD

Professor of Primary Care, Murdoch University, Australia

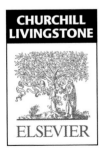

EDINBURGH   LONDON   NEW YORK   OXFORD   PHILADELPHIA   ST LOUIS   SYDNEY   TORONTO   2007

CHURCHILL LIVINGSTONE
ELSEVIER

© 2007, Elsevier Limited. All rights reserved.

First published 2007

ISBN-13: 9780443103278
ISBN-10: 0 443 10327 5

British Library Cataloguing in Publication Data
A catalogue record for this book is available from the British Library.

Library of Congress Cataloging in Publication Data
A catalog record for this book is available from the Library of Congress.

Note

Knowledge and best practice in this field are constantly changing. As new research and experience broaden our knowledge, changes in practice, treatment and drug therapy may become necessary or appropriate. Readers are advised to check the most current information provided (i) on procedures featured or (ii) by the manufacturer of each product to be administered, to verify the recommended dose or formula, the method and duration of administration, and contraindications. It is the responsibility of the practitioner, relying on their own experience and knowledge of the patient, to make diagnoses, to determine dosages and the best treatment for each individual patient, and to take all appropriate safety precautions. To the fullest extent of the law, neither the Publisher nor the Author assumes any liability for any injury and/or damage to persons or property arising out of or related to any use of the material contained in this book.

The Publisher

Printed in China
The Publisher's policy is to use paper manufactured from sustainable forests.

Healthcare for an Aging Population

For Elsevier

Commissioning Editor: Susan Young
Development Editor: Catherine Jackson
Project Manager: Morven Dean
Design Direction: Sarah Russell
Illustration Manager: Merlyn Harvey
Illustrator: Cactus

Contents

Preface

This book provides scientifically sound advice on how to increase your chances of dying healthy. While it fails to provide a template for immortality, it does hint at lifestyle choices that may increase longevity and it certainly provides guidance on which lifestyle choices have the potential to improve your health related quality of life.

The text is divided into two parts. Section 1 focuses on the aging process and explores the repercussions of advancing age on the quality of life. It considers possible explanations for the phenomenon of aging and addresses many of the challenges faced by the elderly. It looks at how reduced reserves can lead to various dysfunctions that potentially compromise wellbeing in old age. It describes how alterations to physiological processes predispose to pathological changes and emphasizes how elderly persons can minimize their personal risk. In particular, it provides suggestions on how the elderly can deal with fatigue and pain, both symptoms with enormous potential to blight the 'golden years'.

While section 1 discusses tribulations that are so widespread as to be considered inevitable consequences of aging, section 2 looks at pathologies prevalent in old age. The emphasis moves from coping with functional changes to preventing disease. It concentrates on how elderly individuals can minimize their personal risk of conditions prevalent in later life.

Applying the suggestions in this book will not stop the aging process; implementing the lifestyle tips may, however, enable one to have the biological capacity to have a more enjoyable old age.

Abbreviations

bd	twice daily
BMI	body mass index
BMR	basal metabolic rate
BP	blood pressure
CHD	coronary heart disease
GI	glycaemic index
HbA1c	glycosylated haemoglobin
HDL	high density lipoprotein
LDL	low density lipoprotein
MET	metabolic equivalent task
NSAIDs	non-steroidal anti-inflammatory drugs
PSA	prostate specific antigen
qds	four times daily
SAMe	S-adenosyl-methionine
tds	three times daily

SECTION 1 THE AGING PROCESS

SECTION CONTENTS

Chapter 1

Delaying aging: the free radical hypothesis

Jo is a 72-year-old woman. She presents complaining of backache. You notice she has a dowager's hump. She also complains of muscle weakness and says she is becoming a little unsteady and has difficulty getting out of some chairs.

She has been treated for breast cancer and has angina.

- Is aging inevitable or can it be halted or at least delayed?
- What is the mechanism underlying aging?
- Can a single process account for all the changes associated with aging?

IS AGING INEVITABLE?

It has been suggested the only two certainties in life are death and taxes. The chance of death at a given age is a measure of the physiological age i.e. the average number of aging changes accumulated by persons of that age. Aging represents the accumulation of changes that increase the risk of death. While the outcome may be a certainty, the question arises as to whether one can modify the process. The tax bill can be decreased by reducing income or employing tax minimizing schemes. Can the aging process be modified? Superficial interventions such as cosmetic surgery provide temporary psychological benefit but fail to deal with the underlying issue. A facelift can be likened to a tax evasion scheme that provides tax relief in one year but at best fails to ensure any long term benefit and at worst may later cause anguish. More fundamental changes that address the aging process are needed if aging is to be impeded. Only physiological changes that modify the aging process will increase longevity. Legitimate tax avoidance schemes can provide long term benefits. Is there a biological equivalent to delay the aging process?

Aging changes can be attributed to development, genetic defects, the environment, disease, and the inborn aging process.[1] The aging process is the major risk factor for disease and death after age 28 in the developed countries, where the actual average life expectancy at birth now ranges from 76 to 79 years. This is 6–9 years less than the anticipated 85–95 years attributed to the aging process. Today the inherent aging process appears to limit the average life expectancy at birth to around 85 years, but the maximum life span is closer to 122 years.[2] Numerous animal experiments suggest the inherent aging process can be retarded. Aging may be inevitable but it appears that the rate at which any individual ages can be modified by lifestyle choices.

THE ELIXIR OF LIFE

The most reliable way of extending both mean and maximum life span in laboratory animals appears to be to restrict energy intake. Rats introduced to a diet containing about two-thirds of the calories normally provided 2 weeks after weaning increased their median life span by 76% compared to ad libitum fed animals.[3] Maximum life span was also significantly increased. The benefits of caloric restriction have been confirmed and extended to other species.[4,5] The explanation underlying the anti-aging effects of caloric reduction remains uncertain. It has been postulated that food restriction may retard aging by slowing down the basal metabolic rate, causing either a major reorganization of energy utilization and/or by reducing the formation of free radicals.

THE FREE RADICAL THEORY OF AGING

The free radical theory proposes that aging is the cumulative result of oxidative damage to cells, primarily as a result of aerobic metabolism.[6]

There is considerable support for this hypothesis. Variation in species' life span correlates with metabolic rate and protective antioxidant activity. Enhanced expression of antioxidative enzymes significantly increases longevity in experimental animals. Cellular levels of free radical damage increase with age but caloric restriction reduces the generation of reactive oxygen species and increases life span.[6] Nonetheless, aging is a complex, multifactorial process and free radical generation is influenced both by environmental lifestyle choices and genetic composition. Life span in a nematode worm was increased following a genetic mutation that resulted in increased activities of the antioxidative enzymes Cu-Zn superoxide dismutase and catalase. In humans, persons with Down syndrome (trisomy 21) have a shortened life span and are at increased risk of free radical-related disorders. The genomic and free radical theories of aging appear inseparable.[7]

Oxygen: a two-edged sword

Oxygen is essential for survival. However oxygen is toxic to aerobic animals because it is reduced intracellularly to oxygen free radicals which are highly reactive. Around 2–3% of oxygen consumed by a cell is converted to free radicals. This natural by-product of metabolism contains an unpaired or odd number of electrons. Although not the only source of free radicals in biological systems, oxygen is the most common source. The most common site of free radical production is the mitochondrion. During the course of energy production, mitochondria reduce molecular oxygen in sequential steps to produce water. This process produces a number of short-lived intermediates including the superoxide (O_2^-), hydrogen peroxide (H_2O_2) and the hydroxyl radical ($\cdot OH$)—all of which are capable of cellular damage. The reactive oxygen species (ROS) produced in mitochondria can damage cellular proteins, lipids and genetic material.

Oxidatively modified proteins have been shown to increase as a function of age.[8] Amino acid residues of proteins are highly susceptible to oxidative attack. Free radical activity may cross-link proteins resulting in impaired enzymatic activity and connective tissue rigidity. Factors that decelerate protein oxidation increase life span and vice versa. Furthermore, a number of age-related diseases are associated with elevated levels of oxidatively modified proteins, e.g. oxidized methionine and cross-linked and glycated proteins.

Cell membranes are also susceptible to peroxidizing reactions.[6] Free radicals reacting with polyunsaturated fatty acids in cell membranes compromise function by irreversibly impairing membrane fluidity and elasticity. Furthermore, lipid peroxides may decompose to yield a cascade of reactions including known mutagens, e.g. malondialdehyde. The breakdown products of lipid peroxides also contribute to the production of lipofuscin, a structurally heterogeneous yellowish brown granular pigment that accumulates with age. In humans, further evidence of ongoing lipid peroxidation is demonstrated by the increase with age of exhaled ethane and n-pentane. Dietary restriction suppresses age-related oxidative damage by modulating the amount as well as the fatty acid composition of tissue phospholipids.[9]

Interaction between an oxygen radical and DNA can delete a base or cause a strand breakage, producing a harmful or even lethal event. It has been estimated that deoxyribonucleic acid (DNA) in an average human cell is subject to 10 000 oxidative hits each day.[10] Despite repair systems correcting much of the damage, oxidative DNA lesions nevertheless accumulate with age. It is not, however, nuclear DNA that is most at risk. The organelles that bear the brunt of the damage caused by free radicals are mitochondria. Mitochondrial DNA, unprotected by histones and located in organelles utilizing around 90% of the cell's oxygen, incurs and accumulates more nucleic acid damage than nuclear DNA. Similarly, the lipid membrane of the mitochondrion, with a number of different enzymes involved in energy production, suffers substantial oxidative exposure. The mitochondria of older animals produce significantly higher levels of ROS and yield less energy than those in younger animals. Long-lived homeothermic vertebrates consistently have lower rates of mitochondrial ROS production and lower levels of steady-state oxidative damage in their mitochondrial DNA than short-lived ones.[11] They also have lower levels of antioxidants.

A Fine Balance

Accumulation of oxidatively modified lipids, proteins and DNA is thought to reflect deficiencies in the delicate balance between the production and neutralization of free radicals, between prooxidants and antioxidants, and the repair, replacement or elimination of biologically damaged molecules.[8] Both enzymatic and non-enzyme based systems are poised ready to neutralize free radicals. Natural protective enzyme based mechanisms to prevent oxyradical-induced cellular damage include superoxide dismutase, catalase, glutathione peroxidase and glutathione reductase. Once nicotinamide adenine dinucleotide phosphate (NADPH) oxidase has reduced oxygen releasing superoxide, the enzyme system swings into action to prevent free radical damage. Superoxide dismutase rapidly converts superoxide to H_2O_2, which in turn is detoxified by catalase and the oxidative reduction of glutathione. The enzyme system is backed up by a non-enzymatic system which includes intrinsic antioxidants, such as uric acid, bilirubin, –SH proteins and glutathione, and an extrinsic system including vitamins C, E, carotenoids, flavonoids and metal chelating proteins.[7] Non enzymatic components of the antioxidant defence system can interrupt free radical initiated oxidative chain reactions and neutralize free radicals before they react with cellular components. Like the enzymatic system, there is interaction between various elements of the non-enzymatic system. Water-soluble ascorbate, glutathione and urate act in concert with lipid-soluble tocopherols and carotenoids, and intermediatory-soluble flavonoids and hydroxycinnamic acids.

The extrinsic non-enzymatic system is amenable to dietary modification. A diet rich in ascorbic acid has a sparing effect on vitamin E.[12] The amount of vitamin E required can be reduced by increased vitamin C intake; however, the requirement for vitamin E is increased by eating a diet rich in polyunsaturated fats. While a healthy diet may easily meet the recommended daily vitamin E requirement of 19 international units (IU), diet alone may not provide the 400 IU/day vitamin E required to prolong clotting times,[13] or the 800 IU/day required to stimulate immunity in the elderly.[14] This raises the issue of the desirability, even the necessity, for dietary supplementation. However, evidence suggests that while eating certain fruit and vegetables can decrease oxidative DNA damage, supplementation with vitamin C, E, or beta-carotene cannot.[15] Whole foods provide an integrated reductive environment created by plant antioxidants of differing solubility in each of the tissue, cellular and macromolecular phases.[16] While whole foods may provide the appropriate antioxidant balance, it may be impossible to achieve a protective concentration of antioxidants within an energy balanced diet. More research is needed.

PROLONGING LIFE

Caloric restriction is the only known method that increases the life span of rodents; studies currently underway suggest that this also applies to primates, and presumably to humans.[7] Energy restriction appears to increase the average life span by 15–20%. Caloric restriction exerts its aging retardation effect through at least two distinct mechanisms. One appears to be a metabolic shift, the other is through dietary antioxidants.[17] More specifically, caloric restriction boosts the antioxidant defence system, lowers production of free radicals, and reduces the age-related accumulation of advanced glycosylation end products (AGEs).[6] AGEs are formed by the nonenzymatic and irreversible reactions of proteins with glucose. AGEs have been linked with many indices of aging including the cross-linkage of molecules such as DNA, haemoglobin, collagen and elastin. Oxygen and free radical reactions significantly accelerate the formation of AGEs. Normal physiological functioning ranging from the transmission of axonal information, regulation of membrane-bound enzymes, control of ionic channels and various receptors are all highly dependent on membrane fluidity. Caloric restriction reduces the cell membrane rigidity associated with aging.[18]

Caloric restriction has been shown to decrease mitochondrial ROS production and oxidative damage to mitochondrial DNA (mtDNA).[11] Certainly, compared to short-lived animals, long-lived animals have lower rates of mitochondrial oxygen radical generation.[5] A low rate of mitochondrial ROS generation is postulated to extend life span both in long-lived and in caloric-restricted animals by determining the rate of oxidative attack and accumulation of somatic mutations in mitochondrial DNA.[11] A slow rate of ROS generation may be a primary cause of a slow aging rate.

Caloric restriction specifically decreases ROS production at complex I in mitochondria, i.e. it decreases free radical generation from the substrates pyruvate and malate. As oxygen consumption remains unchanged, caloric restriction achieves this end by decreasing the free radical leak, i.e. fewer electrons are diverted to free radical generation. Calorie restriction enables mitochondria to avoid generation of free radicals more efficiently. MtDNA is situated very close to the site of mitochondrial ROS production. Mutations in mtDNA, both deletions and point mutations, reach high levels in older individuals. Direct evidence that increases in mtDNA mutations increase the rate of aging has recently been obtained in mice.[11]

It would appear that caloric restriction retards the aging process through various metabolic alterations, only one of which involves modulation of antioxidant balance.[17] Nevertheless, if caloric restriction reduces ROS generation and prolongs life, can boosting antioxidants have a similar outcome? The concentration of endogenous antioxidants is negatively correlated with maximum longevity. Furthermore, antioxidants do help to control oxidative stress in cells in general. However, antioxidants do not appear to decrease the rate of aging. In fact, the concentration of anti-oxidants is lower in long-lived than in short-lived animals.[5] Furthermore, experimentally increasing antioxidant levels, whether by dietary supple-mentation, pharmacological induction or transgenic techniques, fails to affect the maximum longevity of vertebrates.[11] The general lack of effect of antioxidants on maximum longevity indicates that they fail to slow down the endogenous aging process. Nonetheless, a review of the maximum longevity of different animal species that compared the relationship between endogenous antioxidant and prooxidant factors suggested anti-oxidant supplementation could increase mean survival.[5]

PREVENTING DISEASE

Boosting antioxidants may not extend the maximum life span of a species; however, increased antioxidant levels may improve the longevity and quality of life of an individual. Animal studies have shown that both alpha-lipoic acid and coenzyme Q_{10} suppress specific pathways responsive to oxidative stress.[17] Experimentally deleting genes encoding particular antioxidants, although not affecting the rate of aging, did influence the development of different pathologies. Mean life span is increased in antioxidant-treated or antioxidant-induced animals. These findings suggest antioxidants can non-specifically protect against many causes of early death. Part of this benefit is related to the capacity of antioxidants to react induc-tively and then protect against increases in oxidative stress of exogenous origin. Furthermore, experiments showed antioxidant protection was most effective when animals were exposed to sub-optimum conditions. This would support arguments for boosting antioxidant intake given the oxida-tive stresses of modern life. Although antioxidants are unable to control the rate of aging, they do provide a measure of protection against various age-related diseases.[11] Individuals treated with antioxidants may live out their natural life span enjoying better health!

The dietary intake of antioxidants has been shown to be inversely related to the risk of premature death.[19] Immune function in the elderly improves on vitamin E 800 IU/day,[20] and vitamin E in doses exceeding 100 IU/day has been angiographically demonstrated to reduce the progression of coronary artery lesions.[21] Two prospective cohort studies suggested persons taking 100–250 IU of vitamin E a day were least likely to have a major coronary event and a randomized trial found patients with atherosclerosis on 400–800 IU of vitamin E daily were least likely to have a clinical cardiac event.[22]

Despite encouraging outcomes, overall results from such studies are inconsistent. One explanation for this inconsistency may be biological individuality. A randomized double-blind, placebo-controlled, primary-prevention trial over 7.5 years testing the efficacy of daily supplementation with low dosage antioxidant vitamins and minerals found total cancer incidence and all-cause mortality were lowered in men but not in women.[23] Supplementation at dosages 1–3 times the daily recommended dietary allowances provided these subjects with: vitamin C, 120 mg; vitamin E, 30 mg; beta-carotene, 6 mg; selenium, 100 μg; and zinc, 20 mg. In this study, men had a lower baseline status of some antioxidants, particularly beta-carotene.

Although the clinical impact of boosting antioxidants may be contro-versial, there is strong evidence that increasing antioxidant supplementation reduces the prevalence of suboptimal serum concentrations. A randomized placebo-controlled, double-blind trial found supplementation of healthy women aged 60 years and older with physiological dosages of antioxidant vitamins improved the blood concentration of these nutrients, even in relatively well-nourished elderly women.[24] The women were supplemented with 36 mg vitamin E, 150 mg vitamin C, and 9 mg beta-carotene over a 6-month period. It has also been found that 20 mg/day beta-carotene over 4 weeks reduces red cell susceptibility to peroxidation, 280 mg alpha-tocopherol acetate over 10 weeks reduces the concentration of exhaled per-oxidation end products in smokers, flavonoid rich vegetable juice extracts reduce plasma peroxidation, and 600 mg/day garlic over 2 weeks reduces susceptibility of apolipoprotein B lipoproteins to oxidation.[25]

The ability of antioxidant supplementation to change biochemical parameters is established; however, the pathophysiological benefit of such supplementation remains unproven. Even more questionable is the physio-logical benefit of antioxidant supplementation to athletes. Exercise appears to increase production of reactive oxygen species and many athletes take antioxidant supplements to counteract the oxidative stress of exercise. It remains unclear, however, whether strenuous exercise does indeed increase the need for additional antioxidants in the diet.[26] While some studies report that supplementation with vitamins C, E and/or other antioxidants reduces symptoms or indicators of oxidative stress resulting from exercise, these supplements fail to enhance performance.[27] Furthermore, exercise training seems to reduce the oxidative stress of exercise. Trained athletes show less evidence of lipid peroxidation for a given bout of exercise, and an enhanced defence system, compared to untrained subjects.[27] It appears the body may adapt to environmental demands.

The protective mechanism whereby the body adapts to free radical production during exercise appears to involve modulation of inflammatory biomediators. A cross-sectional study reported an inverse association between the level of recreational activity and the inflammatory markers interleukin-6 and C-reactive protein in older persons.[28] Other studies have found that inflammation, as measured by high levels of interleukins and C-reactive proteins, is significantly associated with poor physical performance and muscle strength in older persons.[29,30] Certainly, exposure to severe mental or physical stressors results in excess cytokine production and age-related increases of interleukin-6 appear to be associated with osteoporosis, sarcopenia, disability, and mortality in older adults.[31] There is increasing evidence to suggest that excessive activation of the cytokine network, with its pro-inflammatory biomediators, has a detrimental effect on the neuro-endocrine system, skeletal muscle, bone, the central nervous system and the vascular tree, perhaps via increased production of oxygen free radicals that produce oxidative tissue damage leading to subsequent organ damage and systemic functional decline.

While it has been established that boosting antioxidant intake favourably modifies biochemical parameters, the biological benefit of such modulation remains uncertain. Nonetheless, given current knowledge, it would seem prudent to maximize antioxidant resources.

HEALTHY EATING

Eating a 'living' food diet provides a health advantage

A 'living food' diet is rich in germinated seeds, cereals, sprouts, berries, nuts, fruits and vegetables. It is antioxidant rich. The 'living food' diet is relatively rich in fibre substrates for lignan production and polyphenolic compounds such as quercetin, myricetin and kaempherol. It provides significantly more dietary antioxidants than a cooked omnivorous diet. Subjects eating a 'living food' diet demonstrate substantially increased serum levels of beta- and alpha-carotenes, lycopene and lutein, and vitamins C and E.[32] An uncooked vegan diet epitomizes the 'living food' diet. The calculated dietary antioxidant intakes by vegans, expressed as percentages of the US recommended dietary allowances, were as follows: 305% of vitamin C, 247% of vitamin A, 313% of vitamin E, 92% of zinc, 120% of copper and 49% of selenium.[33]

Eating whole foods enhances health

Persons who eat more whole grains, fruit and vegetables enjoy a health benefit.[34,35] Due to chemical and physical interactions, the effects of individual nutrients may differ when eaten as whole foods.[35,36] Whole foods have a lower glycaemic index than refined/processed foods. Eating whole grains avoids loss of food structure, fibre, nutrients and phytochemicals.[37] Both nutrients and phytochemicals are concentrated in the outer portion of grains. Wheat, initially processed to form bran and endosperm, is milled to form flour with 77% less thiamine, 67% less riboflavin, 72% less niacin, 86% less vitamin B6, 68% less folic acid and 83% less biotin than the whole grain.[38] Vitamin E, removed during the refining process, would normally protect polyunsaturated fatty acids in cell membranes from oxidative damage, inhibit nitrosamine formation and keep selenium in a reduced state. Whole grains deliver as many, possibly more, phytochemicals and antioxidants as do fruits and vegetables.[39]

Eating at least three servings of fruit and vegetables daily is beneficial;[34] consuming two servings of fruit and five of vegetables provides an even greater advantage.[40] The health gain is enhanced if fruits and vegetables with diverse colours are selected.[41] Red-purple foods such as grapes and berries contain anthocyanins, which are powerful antioxidants; orange foods such as carrots and canteloupe contain beta-carotene; orange-yellow foods, e.g. oranges and lemons, contain citrus flavonoids; green foods, e.g. broccoli and cabbage, contain glucosinolates; while white-green foods, e.g. onion and garlic, contain allyl sulfides.[42]

Different antioxidants have varying degrees of potency against particular free radicals. Although all berries (blackberries, blueberries, cranberries, raspberries and strawberries) have antioxidant activities against superoxide radicals (O_2^{*-}), hydrogen peroxide (H_2O_2), hydroxyl radicals (OH*), and singlet oxygen ($'O_2$), there are differences among the different antioxidants in their abilities to scavenge dissimilar reactive oxygen species.[42] Beta-carotene has by far the highest scavenging activity against $'O_2$ but absolutely no effect on H_2O_2. Ascorbic acid is unsurpassed at inhibiting H_2O_2 free radical activity. The scavenging capacities of OH* range from a high of 15.3% with alpha-tocopherol to a low of 0.88% with ascorbic acid. Glutathione has higher O_2^{*-} scavenging capacity compared to the other antioxidants. Quercetin is an effective protector against lipid oxidation in the cell membrane.[43] All substances containing the B-ring catechol group and the 2,3-double bond have a higher redox potential than ascorbate and are consequently able to oxidize it to the ascorbyl radical. Only the flavanone dihydro-quercetin was found capable of reducing the ascorbyl radical, thus fulfilling the so-called ascorbate-protective function.[44] While flavonoids are effective radical scavengers, the rather high redox potentials for most flavonols may explain their occasional prooxidative behaviour.

Food processing may deplete antioxidants

In general the vitamin content of most foods is most dramatically decreased by canning, with blanching and freezing causing smaller losses. Losses between 26% and 90% have been documented, depending on the vitamin and vegetable or fruit canned.[45] Up to one third of bioavailable beta-carotene can be lost on heating; frying for 15 minutes causes a 70% loss, boiling for 60 minutes a 40% loss; freezing, canning and controlled drying a 20% loss. Losses of up to 90% of vitamin C have been reported with cooking and canning. The vitamin C content of fresh vegetables is reduced by air exposure, drying, salting, cooking or slicing. Freezing usually has little effect. The antioxidant activity of green beans is reduced 20% by processing. Although the vitamin C and dietary folate content of green beans remains constant, a 32% reduction in phenolic compounds occurs under conditions of typical commercial processing.[46]

Food processing may enhance antioxidant activity

Processed beets have a 5% increase in their phenolic content. However, this increase is offset by a loss of vitamin C antioxidant activity so the overall antioxidant activity remains unchanged after processing.[46] Thermal processing at 115°C for 25 minutes elevates the total antioxidant activity of sweetcorn by 44%. The 25% loss of vitamin C is offset by increased phytochemicals e.g. ferulic acid increases by 550% and total phenolics by 54%.[47] Likewise, although the vitamin C content of tomato products decreases during thermal processing, the total concentration of phenolics and water soluble antioxidant capacity increases.[48] Another study reported that thermal processing enhanced the nutritional value of tomatoes by increasing the bioaccessible lycopene content and total antioxidant activity.[49]

Increasing antioxidant intake is not the only dietary measure that may delay the effects of free radicals on cellular aging. The other dietary option is to enrich mitochondrial, and other, membranes with monounsaturated fatty acids. Long-lived animals have a low level of fatty acid unsaturation in their cellular membranes.[11] Unsaturated fatty acids, owing to the presence of highly unstable electrons near their double bonds, are sensitive to free radical damage. Sensitivity to lipid peroxidation increases as a function of the number of double bonds per molecule. Membranes with a low level of unsaturated fatty acid are less susceptible to oxidative stress. Many studies have shown that the degree of fatty acid unsaturation of mammalian tissues is negatively correlated with maximum longevity.[50] Fatty acid analyses of heart phospholipids in eight mammals with a life span ranging from 3.5 to 46 years showed the total number of double bonds was negatively correlated with maximum life span. The low double bond content of long living mammals was not due to a low polyunsaturated fatty acid content but rather to a redistribution between types of polyunsaturated fatty acids from the highly unsaturated docosahexaenoic acid (22:6n-3) to the lesser unsaturated linoleic acid (18:2n-6). However, the low degree of fatty acid unsaturation of long-lived animals, rather than being determined by diet, appears to be largely attributable to low tissue delta-5 and delta-6 desaturase activities. These enzymes are limiting for the biosynthesis of highly unsaturated long chain n-6 and n-3 fatty acids. While diet may not be the major determinant of cell membrane composition, dietary fat intake nonetheless influences cell membrane composition and modulation of dietary fat does have physiological repercussions in both animals and man.[51,52] Dietary choices conducive to maintaining a low level of unsaturated cell lipids may, in theory, limit oxidative damage to lipids, proteins and mtDNA. Dietary supplementation with omega-9 cis-monounsaturated fats and an appropriate ratio of omega-3 to omega-6 fatty acids may be conducive to health, if not longevity. Certainly, the Mediterranean diet which is rich in antioxidants and monounsaturated fats has been associated with increased survival among older people.[53] Similarly, the vegetarian diet also offers a distinct health advantage.[54,55]

KEEPING PERSPECTIVE

The free radical theory is only one possible explanation for aging. Evidence for the free radical hypothesis of aging is strong but inconclusive. Although intraspecies studies show a lifetime of increased antioxidant protection is able to slow down physiological deterioration and aging at the individual level, not all longer-life species have more effective antioxidant defences than shorter-life species.[6] Nonetheless, many structural changes that develop with aging, such as lipid peroxidation of membranes, formation of age pigments, cross-linkage of proteins, DNA damage and decline of mitochondrial function, can be mediated by oxidative stress. Realistically, aging is more likely to be a multifactorial process than one reducible to a single cause. Certainly the possible role of the immune system, neuro-endocrine control, somatic mutation and error catastrophe in controlling aging should not be ignored.

However, even when contemplating an alternative hypothesis, free radical interaction may be implicated. For example, altered signalling in a growth regulating pathway has been found to confer both longevity and increased resistance to oxidative stress. A regulatory growth factor pathway, involving decreased levels of growth hormone–insulin-like growth factor–insulin family (GH–insulin–IGF–I), has been linked to an increased life span in various species.[56] Mice engineered to express fewer receptors for IGF-I live longer. These GH–insulin–IGF-I longevity mutants also have the ability to counter oxidants more effectively. As the key factor in common in the longevity mutants is hormonal regulation of metabolic pathways, it is possible that regulation of glucose metabolism, especially in mammals, is the secret to slowing aging processes. The ability of caloric restriction to extend maximum life span certainly envisages a fundamental change to metabolic processes not achieved by antioxidant boosting alone.[17]

Another cautionary note needs to be sounded regarding the potential of antioxidants to reduce the risk of disease. There is a discrepancy between the health-promoting and protective effects of fruit and vegetables and those achieved using antioxidant supplements. A large prospective cohort study of postmenopausal women identified an inverse association between death from stroke and intake of vitamin E rich foods e.g. mayonnaise, nuts and margarine; but this relationship was not apparent in women taking vitamin E, total vitamin A and carotenoid supplements.[57] The failure of individual nutrients to decrease oxidative DNA damage may be loss of the additive effect achieved by antioxidants' interactions in foods or may result from the chemical structure of the supplement. Natural vitamin E (RRR-alpha-tocopherol) is distinct from the chemically synthesized supplement. Synthetic vitamin E (dl-alpha-tocopherol or all-rac-alpha-tocopherol) is a mixture of stereoisomers of which d-alpha-tocopherol makes up 12.5%. The potency of the mixture is lower, with 1 mg of synthetic vitamin E being equivalent to 1.10 IU and 1 mg of natural vitamin E being equivalent to 1.49 IU. While dose requirements are changed by the stereo chemistry of the nutrient mixture, efficacy may depend on the presence of the appropriate i.e. functional, nutrient compound. Similarly, carotenes constitute a group of distinct compounds. A case-control study found significant inverse associations between prostate cancer and plasma concentrations of lycopene and zeaxanthin, borderline associations for lutein and beta-cryptoxanthin, and no obvious associations for alpha- and beta-carotenes.[58] Consumption of carotenoid-rich vegetable products (carrot juice, spinach powder and tomato juice) enhances lipoprotein carotenoid concentrations, but only tomato juice (330 ml/day) reduces low density lipoprotein (LDL) oxidation. The antioxidant potency of carotenes is known to vary, being greatest for lycopene followed by alpha-carotene, beta-carotene and lutein. Lycopene appears useful for cardiovascular health;[59] but may not be as effective as alpha-carotene against lung cancer or beta-carotene against stroke.[60] Nutrients grouped as a single category may have some but not all of their actions in common.

The dilemma that arises is that while antioxidant combinations in food appear more effective than supplementation, the effective dose of anti-oxidants may not be achievable in foods, particularly given the desirability of limiting energy intake. Supplementing with mixtures of biologically active antioxidants capable of metabolic interaction to achieve synergy at the cellular level may somewhat resolve this conundrum.[61] For example, with respect to cardiovascular disease, vitamin E acts as a first risk dis-criminator, and vitamin C as a second, whereas optimal health requires synchronous interaction of vitamins C, E, A, carotenoids and vegetable conutrients. Plasma values deemed desirable for primary prevention are equal to or greater than: 30 µmol/L lipid-standardized vitamin E with an alpha-tocopherol/cholesterol ratio of 5.0 µmol/mmol; 50 µmol/L vitamin C aiming at a vitamin C/vitamin E ratio of 1.3–1.5; 0.4 µmol/L of beta- or 0.5 µmol/L of alpha+ beta-carotene.[22] This translates roughly into: 1 mg vitamin A; 2–3.5 mg beta-carotene in non-smokers and 7–12 mg in smokers; 70–145 mg vitamin C in non-smokers and 130–175 mg in smokers; and at least 67 mg vitamin E daily. Furthermore desirable ratios of these nutrients may be: vitamin C/E > 1.3, carotene/vitamin E > 0.02 and vitamin C/carotene > 100 or vitamin C/beta-carotene > 125. The risk of cancer and cardiovascular disease is postulated to double if values of these antioxidants drop 20–50% below these target thresholds.[19]

Unbridled used of supplements is also inadvisable given the risk of toxicity. Beta-carotene, an antioxidant in non-smokers, assumes the role of a prooxidant in the lungs of smokers. On the other hand, beta-carotene is water soluble and may safely be consumed in megadoses by non-smokers. In the presence of vitamin E, *beta*-carotene can be converted to vitamin A, a fat soluble vitamin with a relatively narrow therapeutic window. However, vitamin A toxicity is not a concern when supplementing *beta*-carotene as there is a threshold beyond which *beta*-carotene is not converted to vitamin A. Flavonoids are useful antioxidants. Conversely, at higher doses flavonoids may act as mutagens, prooxidants generating free radicals, and inhibiting key enzymes involved in hormone metabolism. Caution should be exercised if ingesting flavonoids at levels above that which would be obtained from a typical vegetarian diet.[62]

GETTING IT RIGHT

Aging is an extremely complex multifactorial process regulated by a multi-plicity of mechanisms, with explanatory theories of aging ranging from evolutionary and gene regulatory postulates to cellular senescence, free radical, and neuro-endocrine-immunological hypotheses.[63] Age may manifest as frailty, functional dependence, chronic disability, memory disorders and/or sarcopenia. Sarcopenia, a constant of aging, may reflect a combination of: reduced digestion of proteins and absorption of amino acids, decreased number of hepatocytes and thus protein synthesis, an increased concentration of circulating catabolic cytokines, reduced production of anabolic hormones, restricted exercise due to osteoarthritis and respiratory insufficiency – all of which may be exaggerated by the effects of polypharmacy.[64] The ultimate clinical presentation, which is unique in any particular individual, is the outcome of multiple causes and interacting processes.

Notwithstanding the failure to fully comprehend the aging process, there is no doubt that people are living longer and it is possible this trend will continue. Society is already faced with the dilemma of caring for an aging population; increasing longevity without enhancing health may exacerbate this predicament. Despite good intentions, enhancing longevity without simultaneously improving health could create significant problems for society. Various strategies can be attempted to minimize the social burden of an incapacitated elderly population.

Specifically addressing particular risk factors offers one option. A 15-year-long observational study of the aging process in a group of healthier 70-year-old 'survivors' found that the average reductions in survival time in men and women respectively associated with smoking were 22 and 15 months; with diabetes, 18 and 18 months; with very high blood pressure, 16 and 9 months; with impaired peak expiratory flow, 14 and 17 months; with physical disability, 16 and 12 months; and with zero alcohol intake, 9 and 5 months.[65] Combinations of selected risk factors multiplied the risk; likewise, combined interventions lowered risk. Persons between 68 and 95 years old who do not smoke, maintain a desirable body weight and walk daily accrue the lowest total healthcare costs.[66] Population studies suggest that an overall healthy lifestyle could postpone disability by up to 5 years and disability-free years can even be increased by people merely remaining active.[67] There is good evidence that regular moderate activity protects against the development of diabetes in populations independent of body weight, reduces colon cancer risk, may reduce the risk of ischaemic stroke in the elderly, has a role in reducing breast cancer incidence in postmenopausal women, improves mental health and enhances the quality and duration of sleep.[67]

Another approach is to review explanatory theories of aging and target fundamental processes believed to generate pathophysiological changes characteristic of senescence. Based upon the free radical hypothesis, boosting antioxidant levels would seem a logical approach to minimize the risk of many disorders prevalent in old age. Selecting nutrient dense, energy poor foods enhances the potential to live a long healthy life. Enhancing antioxidant levels by thoughtfully supplementing with antioxidant combinations may further contribute to this end. In the interim, although there appears to be no reason to discourage older people from taking vitamin E and C supplementation, the best advice may be to reduce their intake of xenobiotics, to drink tea instead of coffee, and to eat liberal amounts of fruit, vegetables, nuts, soybeans and lentils.[68]

The need for active intervention to address lifestyle choices of the whole population should not be underestimated. Analysis of birth cohorts using the National Health and Nutrition Examination Survey (1971–2002) showed obesity rates increased markedly, beginning earlier in life with each successive birth cohort.[69] Obesity is associated with a plethora of health problems, amongst which is arthritis. As the age of the US population has increased, so has the prevalence of arthritis. By the year 2020, it is predicted 59.4 million persons in the US will be affected by arthritis and the financial costs of this chronic disability will increase by more than 25%.[70] Increasing longevity without simultaneously ensuring a health status that provides an enhanced quality of life is a dubious endeavour.

CLINICAL CHALLENGE

The wife of a 65-year-old man presents asking for advice on how to prolong her husband's life. She says her husband is fat and refuses to discuss his health. He adamantly refuses to go near any health professionals. She feels her only option is to try surreptitiously to improve his lifestyle choices. You manage to establish his BMI is 33. He has never had his blood pressure, blood sugar or cholesterol levels recorded.

Given that case work-up is unacceptable, what advice would you give?

Questions arising

- Is it possible for a wife/mother to benefit her family's health without their consent?
- What changes are necessary to improve this patient's health?

Major clinical considerations

1. Weight reduction
2. Healthy eating

The wife may help her husband lose weight by:

- purchasing low-energy, nutrient-dense foods
- storing food out of sight—in the refrigerator or in opaque containers in the kitchen
- preparing low-energy meals in precise quantities to avoid leftovers
- using small plates and cups; servings appear larger
- lengthening the time between courses—preparing fewer courses
- celebrating with non-food rewards for goal attainment
- encouraging increased physical activity—find an exercise related hobby

Refer to Patient Handout 1.1 Prolonging Life.
  She may encourage healthy eating by providing a plant-based diet, rich in whole fresh foods.
Refer to Patient Handout 1.2 Preventing Disease.

PRACTICE GEMS

- ◆ Genetic composition determines the potential for health and disease but lifestyle choices influence genetic expression.
- ◆ Caloric restriction increases longevity.
- ◆ Boosting antioxidant intake reduces the risk of chronic diseases associated with aging—aim to die healthy!

- ◆ Maintaining a desirable body weight, eating a plant-based diet, limiting alcohol, not smoking and walking daily is good advice to give all elderly people.
- ◆ An overall healthy lifestyle could postpone disability by up to 5 years.
- ◆ It is never too late to adopt a healthy lifestyle.

References

1. Harman D. The free radical theory of aging. Antioxid Redox Signal 2003; 5(5):557–561.
2. Harman D. Aging: overview. Ann N Y Acad Sci 2001;928:1–21.
3. McCay C, Crowell M, Maynard L. The effect of retarded growth upon the length of life and upon ultimate size. J. Nutr 1989; 5:155–171.
4. Weindruch R. Caloric restriction: life span extension and retardation of brain aging. Clin Neurosci Res 2003; 2: 279–284.
5. Barja G. Rate of generation of oxidative stress-related damage and animal longevity. Free Radic Biol Med 2002; 33(9):1167–1172.
6. Wickens AP. Ageing and the free radical theory. Respir Physiol. 2001; 128(3):379–391.
7. Knight JA. The biochemistry of aging. Adv Clin Chem 2000; 35:1–62.
8. Stadtman ER. Protein oxidation in aging and age-related diseases. Ann N Y Acad Sci 2001; 928:22–38.
9. Yu BP, Lim BO, Sugano M. Dietary restriction downregulates free radical and lipid peroxide production: plausible mechanism for elongation of life span. J Nutr Sci Vitaminol (Tokyo) 2002; 48(4):257–264.
10. Ames BN, Shigenaga MK, Hagen TM. Oxidants, antioxidants, and the degenerative diseases of aging. Proc Natl Acad Sci USA 1993; 90:7915–7922.
11. Barja G. Aging in vertebrates, and the effect of caloric restriction: a mitochondrial free radical production-DNA damage mechanism? Biol Rev Camb Philos Soc 2004; 79(2):235–251.
12. Huang J, May JM. Ascorbic acid spares alpha-tocopherol and prevents lipid peroxidation in cultured H4IIE liver cells. Mol Cell Biochem. 2003; 247(1–2):171–176.
13. Steiner M. Vitamin E, a modifier of platelet function: rationale and use in cardiovascular and cerebrovascular disease. Nutr Rev 1999; 57:306–309.
14. Gey KF, Stahelin HB, Eichholzer M. Poor plasma status of carotene and vitamin C is associated with higher mortality from ischemic heart disease and stroke: Basel Prospective Study. Clin-Investig 1993; 71(1):3–6.
15. Halliwell B. Why and how should we measure oxidative DNA damage in nutritional studies? How far have we come? Am J Clin Nutr 2000; 72(5):1082–1087.
16. Eastwood MA. Interaction of dietary antioxidants in vivo: how fruit and vegetables prevent disease? QJM 1999; 92(9):527–530.
17. Lee CK, Pugh TD, Klopp RG, et al. The impact of alpha-lipoic acid, coenzyme Q10 and caloric restriction on life span and gene expression patterns in mice. Free Radic Biol Med 2004; 36(8):1043–1057.
18. Yehuda S, Rabinovitz S, et al. The role of polyunsaturated fatty acids in restoring the aging neuronal membrane. Neurobiol Aging 2002; 23(5):843–853.
19. Gey KF. Vitamins E plus C and interacting conutrients required for optimal health. A critical and constructive review of epidemiology and supplementation data regarding cardiovascular disease and cancer. Biofactors 1998; 7(1–2):113–174.
20. Meydani M, Meisler J. A closer look at vitamin E: can this antioxidant prevent chronic disease. Postgraduate Medicine 1997; 102:199–207.
21. Hodis HN, Mack WJ, et al. Serial coronary angiographic evidence that antioxidant vitamin intake reduces progression of coronary artery atherosclerosis. JAMA 1995; 273:1849–1854.
22. Haskell WL, Luskin FM, Marvasti FF. Complementary/alternative therapies in general medicine: cardiovascular disease. In: Spencer JW, Jacobs JJ, eds. Complementary alternative therapy: an evidence-based approach. Mosby: St Louis; 1998: 90–106.
23. Hercberg S, Galan P, et al. The SU.VI.MAX study: a randomized, placebo-controlled trial of the health effects of antioxidant vitamins and minerals. Arch Intern Med 2004; 164(21):2335–2342.
24. Wolters M, Hermann S, Hahn A. Effects of 6-month multivitamin supplementation on serum concentrations of alpha-tocopherol, beta-carotene, and vitamin C in healthy elderly women. Int J Vitam Nutr Res 2004; 74(2):161–168.
25. Lampe JA. Health effects of vegetables and fruit: assessing mechanisms of action in human experimental studies. Am J Clin Nutr 1999; 70(suppl):475S–490S.
26. Urso ML, Clarkson PM. Oxidative stress, exercise, and antioxidant supplementation. Toxicology. 2003; 189(1–2):41–54.
27. Clarkson PM, Thompson HS. Antioxidants: what role do they play in physical activity and health? Am J Clin Nutr. 2000; 72(2 Suppl):637S–46S.
28. Reuben DB, Judd-Hamilton L, et al. MacArthur studies of successful aging. The associations between physical activity and inflammatory markers in high-functioning older persons: MacArthur studies of successful aging. J Am Geriatr Soc 2003; 51(8):1125–1130.

29. Cesari M, Penninx BW, et al. Inflammatory markers and physical performance in older persons: the InCHIANTI study. J Gerontol A Biol Sci Med Sci 2004; 59(3):242–248.

30. Cohen HJ, Harris T, Pieper CF. Coagulation and activation of inflammatory pathways in the development of functional decline and mortality in the elderly. Am J Med 2003; 114(3):180–187.

31. Penninx BW, Kritchevsky SB, et al. Inflammatory markers and depressed mood in older persons: results from the Health, Aging and Body Composition study. Biol Psychiatry 2003; 54(5):566–572.

32. Hanninen O, Rauma AL, et al. Vegan diet in physiological health promotion. Acta Physiol Hung 1999; 86(3–4):171–180.

33. Rauma AL, Torronen R, et al. Antioxidant status in long-term adherents to a strict uncooked vegan diet. Am J Clin Nutr 1995; 62(6):1221–1227.

34. Huang HY, Helzlsouer KJ, Appel LJ. The effects of vitamin C and vitamin E on oxidative DNA damage: results from a randomized controlled trial. Cancer Epidemiol Biomarkers Prev 2000; 9(7):647–652.

35. Anderson JW. Whole grains protect against atherosclerotic cardiovascular disease. Proc Nutr Soc 2003; 62(1):135–142.

36. Liu S, Lee IM, et al. Intake of vegetables rich in carotenoids and risk of coronary heart disease in men: the physicians' health study. Int J Epidemiol 2001; 30(1):130–135.

37. Slavin JL, Martini MC, et al. Plausible mechanisms for the protectiveness of whole grains. Am J Clin Nutr 1999; 70:495S–463S.

38. Prochaska LJ, Nguyen XT, et al. Effects of food processing on the thermodynamic and nutritive value of foods: literature and database survey. Med Hypotheses 2000; 54(2):254–262.

39. Jones JM, Reicks M, et al. Becoming proactive with the whole-grains message. Nutr Today 2004; 39(1):10–17.

40. Miller MR, Pollard CM, Coli T. Western Australian Health Department recommendations for fruit and vegetable consumption—how much is enough? Aust N Z J Public Health 1997; 21(6):638–642

41. Heber D, Bowerman S. Applying science to changing dietary patterns. J Nutr 2001; 131(11 Suppl):3078S–3081S.

42. Wang SY, Jiao H. Scavenging capacity of berry crops on superoxide radicals, hydrogen peroxide, hydroxyl radicals, and singlet oxygen. J Agric Food Chem 2000; 48(11):5677–5684.

43. Chen ZY, Chan PT, et al. Antioxidant activity of natural flavonoids is governed by number and location of their aromatic hydroxyl groups. Chem Phys Lipids 1996; 79(2):157–163.

44. Bors W, Michel C, Schikora S. Interaction of flavonoids with ascorbate and determination of their univalent redox potentials: a pulse radiolysis study. Free Radic Biol Med 1995; 19(1):45–52.

45. Prochaska LJ, Nguyen XT, et al. Effects of food processing on the thermodynamic and nutritive value of foods: literature and database survey. Med Hypotheses 2000; 54(2):254–262.

46. Jiratanan T, Liu RH. Antioxidant activity of processed table beets (Beta vulgaris var, conditiva) and green beans (Phaseolus vulgaris L.). J Agric Food Chem 2004; 52(9):2659–2670.

47. Dewanto V, Wu X, Liu RH. Processed sweet corn has higher antioxidant activity. J Agric Food Chem. 2002; 50(17):4959–4964.

48. Gahler S, Otto K, Bohm V. Alterations of vitamin C, total phenolics, and antioxidant capacity as affected by processing tomatoes to different products. J Agric Food Chem 2003;51(27):7962–7968.

49. Dewanto V, Wu X, et al. Thermal processing enhances the nutritional value of tomatoes by increasing total antioxidant activity. J Agric Food Chem 2002; 50(10):3010–3014.

50. Pamplona R, Portero-Otin M, et al. Double bond content of phospholipids and lipid peroxidation negatively correlate with maximum longevity in the heart of mammals. Mech Ageing Dev 2000 Jan 10; 112(3):169–183.

51. Ghafoorunissa R, Ibrahim A, Natarajan S. Substituting dietary linoleic acid with alpha-linolenic acid improves insulin sensitivity in sucrose fed rats. Biochim Biophys Acta 2005; 1733(1):67–75.

52. Saldeen P, Saldeen T. Women and omega-3 fatty acids. Obstet Gynecol Surv 2004; 59(10):722–730; quiz 745–746.

53. Trichopoulou A, Orfanos P, et al. Modified Mediterranean diet and survival: EPIC-elderly prospective cohort study. BMJ 2005 Apr 30; 330(7498):991.

54. American Dietetic Association; Dietitians of Canada. Position of the American Dietetic Association and Dietitians of Canada: Vegetarian diets. J Am Diet Assoc 2003; 103(6):748–765.

55. Leitzmann C. Vegetarian diets: what are the advantages? Forum Nutr 2005; (57):147–156.

56. Brown-Borg HM. Hormonal regulation of aging and life span. Trends Endocrinol Metab 2003; 14(4):151–153.

57. Yochum LA, Folsom AR, Kushi LH. Intake of antioxidant vitamins and risk of death from stroke in postmenopausal women. Am J Clin Nutr 2000; 72:476–483.

58. Lu QY, Hung JC, Heber D, et al. Inverse associations between plasma lycopene and other carotenoids and prostate cancer. Cancer Epidemiol Biomarkers Prev 2001; 10(7):749–756.

59. Arab L, Steck S. Lycopene and cardiovascular disease. Am J Clin Nutr 2000; 71:1691S–1695S.

60. Ascherio A. Antioxidants and stroke. Am J Clin Nutr 2000; 72:337–338.

61. Pryor WA. Vitamin E and heart disease: basic science to clinical intervention trials. Free Radic Biol Med 2000; 28(1):141–164.

62. Skibola CF, Smith MT. Potential health impacts of excessive flavonoid intake. Free Radic Biol Med 2000; 29(3-4):375–383.

63. Weinert BT, Timiras PS. Invited review: theories of aging. J Appl Physiol 2003; 95(4):1706–1716.

64. Carreca I, Balducci L, Extermann M. Cancer in the older person. Cancer Treat Rev 2005; 31(5):380–402.

65. Simons LA, Simons J, et al. Impact of smoking, diabetes and hypertension on survival time in the elderly: the Dubbo study. Med J Aust 2005; 182(5):219–222.

66. Leigh JP, Hubert HB, Romano PS. Lifestyle risk factors predict healthcare costs in an aging cohort. Am J Prev Med 2005; 29(5):379–387.

67. Bauman AE, Smith BJ. Healthy ageing: what role can physical activity play? MJA 2000; 173:88–90.

68. Ward JA. Should antioxidant vitamins be routinely recommended for older people? Drugs Aging 1998;12(3):169–175.

69. Leveille SG, Wee CC, Iezzoni LI. Trends in obesity and arthritis among baby boomers and their predecessors, 1971–2002. Am J Public Health 2005; 95(9):1607–1613.

70. Elders MJ. The increasing impact of arthritis on public health. J Rheumatol Suppl 2000; 60:6–8.

PATIENT HANDOUT 1.1 – PROLONGING LIFE

Caloric restriction prolongs life—severe caloric restriction may increase average longevity by several years. Wise individuals limit their energy consumption.

Persons with a body mass index in excess of 25 are less likely to reach the age of 85 years than those with a body mass index of 20.

Calculate your body mass index(BMI) to determine your chances of living longer:

BMI = weight(kg)/height(m^2)

Increase your chance of a long life span by having a lower energy intake.

The energy concentration of various foods varies depending on their concentration of macronutrients:

- 1 g fat = 37 kJ (9 C)
- 1 g alcohol = 29 kJ (7 C)
- 1 g protein = 17 kJ (>4 C)
- 1 g carbohydrate = 16 kJ (4 C)

Strategies for decreasing energy intake revolve around choosing foods rich in nutrients and low in energy:

1. Avoid/limit your intake of energy dense foods (see table 1.1).
2. Eat generously from nutrient dense foods (see Table 1.2).
3. Limit your intake of foods with low nutrient density.

Other tips:
- Eating whole foods decreases your energy intake while increasing your nutrient and fibre intake.
- Calorie counters and booklets listing the energy value of various foods can be purchased—eat foods with fewer calories.
- Beware hidden fats—fats are energy dense and are plentiful in sausages, creamy sauces and many baked goods. Even health foods such as nuts are rich in fat.
- Avoid visible fat—cut visible fat off meat, spread bread with avocado, honey or jam rather than butter, margarine or lard.
- Always select low fat options. Reduced fat margarine contains 60% fat, reduced fat cheeses may contain 7–25% fat. Choose low fat dairy products and avoid cream.
- Although exercise increases free radical production, the body adapts and regular exercise promotes health.

Table 1.1 Energy density of foods

Energy Density	Food Sources
Very high (>2000 kJ/100 g or 100 mL)	Cream-filled biscuits, butter, cooking oil, margarine, nuts
High (1000–1999 kJ/100 g or 100 mL)	Plain biscuits and cakes, cheese, grilled sausages, fatty lamb or steak, honey, sugar, spirits, confections
Medium (400–999 kJ/100 g or 100 mL)	Boiled egg, bread, fried fish, grilled lean lamb or steak, canned salmon, spaghetti, boiled rice
Low (200–399 kJ/100 g or 100 mL)	Apple, fruit salad, avocado, creamed soup, milk, jelly, potato, steamed fish
Very low (<200 kJ/100 g or 100 mL)	French beans, broccoli, carrot, marrow pumpkin, skimmed milk, clear soup, beer

Table 1.2 Nutrient density of foods

Nutrient Density	Food Sources
Very high	Eggs, green leafy and yellow vegetables, liver, milk, oysters
High	Beans, cheese, oranges, pork, nuts
Medium	Bread, chicken, fish, steak
Low	Apples, beer, margarine
Very low	Butter, polished rice, soft drinks, spirits, sugar, wine

PATIENT HANDOUT 1.2 – PREVENTING DISEASE

THE AIM

To reduce oxidative stress.

THE OBJECTIVES

1. Decrease free radical formation
   a. eat fewer calories
   b. avoid lifestyle choices that increase free radical production
2. Increase free radical neutralization by boosting antioxidant levels
   a. eat a diet rich in fruit and vegetables
   b. consider antioxidant supplementation

GENERAL GUIDELINES

Make prudent lifestyle choices:

- Favour nutrient dense, low energy foods—refer to Patient Handout 1.1; Prolonging Life.
- Exercise moderately—exercise increases the demand for energy and coincidently increases free radical production.
- Avoid tissue damage—inflammation involves production of free radicals.
- Choose a diet rich in fruit, vegetables and whole grains.
- Consider supplementing with antioxidants to protect against specific diseases.

GENERAL GOOD DIETARY CHOICES:

Include foods from all food groups but be selective. It is a good idea to:

- Eat a fresh plant-based diet with at least:
  - 2 fruits
  - 5 vegetables
  - 5 different coloured items
- Have fish on alternate days
- Eat only low fat dairy food
- Limit your intake of
  - fat especially that from animal products
  - processed foods
  - alcohol
- Choose monounsaturated rich spreads in preference to butter or margarine. Use
  - olive oil
  - avocado pear
  - peanut butter
- Boost antioxidants.

The following contain equivalent amounts of antioxidant activity:[2]

- 1 glass (150 ml) red wine
- 12 glasses white wine
- 2 cups of tea
- 4 apples
- 5 portions of onion
- 5.5 portions egg plant (aubergine)
- 3.5 glasses of blackcurrant juice
- 3.5 (500 mL) glasses of beer
- 7 glasses of orange juice
- 20 glasses of apple juice (long life).

A HEALTHY LIFESTYLE PLAN

The guidelines above in Boxes 1.1–1.3 can be used to make healthy dietary choices.[1]

Box 1.1   Macrobiotic diet

Major inclusions
- Legumes
- Wholegrain cereals
- Vegetables

Lesser inclusions
- Fruit
- Nuts
- Seeds

Box 1.2   Mediterranean diet

High intake
- Vegetables
- Legumes
- Fruit
- Cereals—largely unrefined
- Unsaturated lipids, e.g. olive oil

Moderate to high intake
- Fish

Low to moderate intake
- Dairy products—milk, yoghurt

Low intake
- Saturated fat—meat

Box 1.3   Lacto–ovo vegetarian diet[a]

Dietary inclusion	Dietary exclusion
■ Grains	■ Meat
■ Vegetables	■ Fish
■ Fruit	■ Fowl
■ Legumes	
■ Seeds	
■ Nuts	
■ Dairy products	
■ Eggs	

[a]Lacto-vegetarians exclude eggs but combine legumes with cereals to ensure a protein intake of high biological value. Options include:

■ Corn and green peas or lima beans (succotash)
■ Peas with wheat
■ Peanuts, rice and dried beans
■ Rice and soybeans, dried beans or green peas
■ Lentils with wheat or rice
■ Seeds and green peas or soybeans
■ Dried beans and corn or barley or bulgur (wheat)
■ Yeast with peanuts
■ Sunflower seeds with wholegrains

References

1. Willett WC, Sacks F, et al. Mediterranean diet pyramid: a cultural model for healthy eating. Am J Clin Nutr 1995; 61(suppl 6):S1402–1406.
2. Paganga G, Miller N, Rice-Evans CA. The polyphenolic content of fruit and vegetables and their antioxidant activities. What does a serving constitute? Free Radic Res 1999; 30(2):153–162.

PATIENT HANDOUT 1.3 – A BRAIN TEASER

A couple with three identical triplets had an acrimonious divorce a year after the boys were born. The mother got custody of Peter and John, the father of Paul. When the siblings met for the first time after the divorce some 40 years later, Peter was horrified to see that Paul was emaciated. He was slight compared to John and a mere shadow compared to his rather robust self. While getting reacquainted over a meal Peter was amazed at how little his brother ate. He was bemused to find Paul was a vegetarian. As Peter tucked into his large steak, fries and vegetables he was pleased that he and John had similar tastes—although John was always on a diet. As the brothers ate, Peter couldn't help wondering if the weight problem, which he had put down to his father's genes, may not have something to do with his hearty appetite and sweet tooth.

A challenge: Who is likely to die first and who last?

Post script

Peter died of a heart attack at the age of 60.
John lived for 79 years.
Paul recently celebrated his 85th birthday.

Points to ponder

- Lifestyle choices affect genetic expression.
- A health promoting lifestyle increases the chances of a healthy old age.
- The vegetarian diet offers distinct health advantages – it is rich in antioxidants.
- Limiting energy intake may increase longevity.

Internet Resources:

http://www.niapublications.org/
publications on aging from the US National Institutes of Health

http://www.niapublications.org/engagepages/supplements.asp
Dietary supplements: more is not always better

http://www.niapublications.org/engagepages/lifeext.asp
Life extension: science fact or science fiction?

http://www.niapublications.org/engagepages/pills.asp
Pills, patches and shots: can hormones prevent aging?

http://www.nia.nih.gov/HealthInformation/ResourceDirectory.htm
Resource directory for older people

http://www.agingwell.state.ny.us/eatwell/index.htm
Dietary advice for elderly people

http://www.agingwell.state.ny.us/selfcare/articles/links.htm
Self-care links

Chapter **2**

Managing stress: A longevity strategy?

A 64-year-old man was within weeks of retiring when his wife of 40 years died unexpectedly.

- Do these lifestyle changes potentially increase the man's health risk?
- What pathophysiological processes have been proposed to explain how psychosocial stressors influence biology?
- Can good stress management reduce disease risk and increase longevity?

INTRODUCTION

The prevalence of older adults in the United States and other developed countries is growing at a substantial rate. By 2030, nearly one-fifth of Americans will be in their sixties or older.[1] In 1990 the over-65 age group represented only 4% of the US population; by 1998 it accounted for 12.4% and in 2030 it is projected to account for 22%.[2] Furthermore, the per capita cost of seniors (aged ≥65 years) in the US is three to five times greater than that of younger persons, and costs are anticipated to escalate as the proportion of frail elderly increases.[3]

The frail elderly are particularly susceptible to disability, becoming increasingly dependent on others for the activities of daily living.[4] Exposure of frail persons to minor stresses may cause severe and lasting functional compromise. A Frailty Index, based on the accumulation of deficits categorized as signs, symptoms and disease classifications, has determined that length of life correlates more closely with degree of frailty than with chronological age.[5] Box 2.1 provides some insight into the variables that are considered when attempting to measure frailty objectively. Frailty has been defined as a state of reduced physiological reserve.[4]

Box 2.1 Dimensions of frailty

Biological challenges associated with increasing age
Deteriorating organ system function contributes to:

- allergies
- cancer
- musculoskeletal problems: arthritis, rheumatism, backache
- respiratory disorders: chronic bronchitis, sinusitis
- cardiovascular diseases: heart disease, hypertension, migraine
- gastrointestinal problems: ulcers, bowel disorder
- endocrine disorders: diabetes, thyroid condition
- CNS dysfunction: Alzheimer's disease, other forms of dementia, epilepsy
- ocular problems: cataracts, glaucoma.

Lifestyle challenges associated with increasing age
Impaired quality of life due to functional difficulties can be attributable to:

- a stroke
- vision impairment
- hearing loss
- speech deficits
- impaired mobility
- loss of dexterity
- cognitive dysfunction
- emotional problems
- severe pain to persistent discomfort.

Loss of independence may result in help being required to:

- prepare meals
- shop
- do housework
- carry out heavy household chores
- move about at home.

ALLOSTASIS

Adaptive or allostatic responses of the body maintain 'homeostasis' by reacting to stressors to achieve stability through change. Whereas homeostasis posits an ideal set state of conditions for maintenance of the internal environment, allostasis recognizes that there is no single ideal set of steady-state conditions. Allostasis differs from homeostasis in that it recognizes that set points change with aging, e.g. blood pressure increases with age. Allostasis allows for continued function despite reduced physiological reserves due to aging.

Mediators of allostasis are produced by the hypothalamo–pituitary–adrenal (HPA) axis and the immune and autonomic nervous systems.[6] Primary mediators of allostasis include thyroid hormones, insulin, pituitary hormones, glucocorticoids, catecholamines, cytokines, serotonin, neurotransmitters, e.g. gamma aminobutyric acid (GABA), and neuropeptides, e.g. endorphins. While these mediators are adaptive in the short term, they can cause damage if persistent.[7]

Both repeated challenges and/or persistent activity of allostatic systems, in the absence of stimulation, can produce wear and tear. In fact, 'Taking into account the metabolic consequences of stressful environments, the free-radical theory of aging becomes a general stress theory of aging'.[8]

AGE AND THE ALLOSTATIC LOAD

The allostatic load tends to increase with aging. The term 'allostatic load' has been coined to refer to the consequences of sustained or repeated activation of the mediators of adaptation.[9] A study of older men and women found a higher allostatic load score was associated with and predictive of larger decrements in cognitive and physical functioning as well as an increased risk of cardiovascular disease.[10] These findings were independent of sociodemographic and health status risk factors. The allostatic load score included:[11]

- blood pressure as an index of cardiovascular activity
- the waist–hip ratio as an index of chronic levels of metabolism and adipose tissue deposition as influenced by increased glucocorticoid activity
- serum high density lipoprotein (HDL) and total cholesterol as an index of the propensity to develop atherosclerosis
- blood plasma levels of glycosylated haemoglobin as an integrated measure of glucose metabolism over several days
- serum dehydroepiandrosterone-sulfate, a measure of a functional HPA axis antagonist
- overnight urinary cortisol excretion, an integrated measure of 12-hour HPA axis activity
- overnight urinary norepinephrine and epinephrine excretion levels, an integrated index of 12-hour sympathetic nervous system activity.

THE STRESS HYPOTHESIS

Stress hormones appear to play a vital role in determining the rate of physical and mental aging. The stress response to psychological and physical challenges is similar, i.e. in both instances adenocorticotrophic hormone (ACTH) and cortisol secretion, heart rate, and blood pressure increase. Psychological stress, however, is different in that it is not tied to an increased metabolic demand, nor is there a clear initiation or termination of the psychosocial stressor. The 'glucocorticoid cascade hypothesis' of aging exemplifies how stresses can create an allostatic load that triggers a maladaptive feed forward mechanism. Under persistent psychosocial stress, gradual dysregulation of the HPA axis promotes pathophysiological changes in various tissues and organs throughout the body.[11] Frequent stress-related activation of the HPA axis with concomitant increase in cortisol has been linked to visceral obesity, hypertension, hyperlipidaemia, and insulin resistance. It has also been associated with an increased risk for chronic conditions including cardiovascular disease and diabetes—conditions more common in the aging population and listed in the Frailty Index. It is noteworthy that there is a higher prevalence of diseases associated with greater activation of the HPA axis in males, and elderly men respond to psychological stress with greater increases in cortisol than older women.[12] Furthermore, a recent study comparing young and older women reported aging was associated with greater HPA axis activation in response to a psychological challenge.[13]

Any patient management approach which incorporates consideration of the stress systems hypothesis of aging needs to bear discrepancies between psychosocial and physiochemical triggers in mind. While both psychological and physical stressors are equally efficient triggers of the stress mechanism, the biological changes induced produce maladaptive outcomes to psychosocial triggers.

MANAGING STRESS

While the impact of stress hormones can, in part, be determined by processes generating excess free radicals overwhelming natural protective mechanisms and agents such as oestrogens and flavonoids,[11] clinical management goes beyond antioxidant supplementation. It needs to address the whole stress phenomenon.

Holmes and Rahe developed a scale to measure stress-provoking events in terms of 'life change units'.[14] Using their scale, it was found that those who scored over 300 life change units have an 80% risk of minor illness in the near future, a score of less than 150 carrying a 30% risk. Illness was most likely to occur within 3 months of experiencing the life change, the probability and severity of illness correlating with the total score. The elderly are exposed to a number of high scoring life change events identified by Holmes and Rahe. Death of a partner was allocated a top rating of 100 life change units, the death of a close family member 63, retirement 45 and a change in responsibility at work 29. Loss of family, friends and professional identity along with decreasing physical mobility are inevitable age-related stresses faced by the elderly. Moreover, it is not only major stressors that pose a health risk; persistent minor stresses can have an equal or even greater impact on health. This scale, while useful and predictive of illness, focuses on events and failed to take individuals' reactions into consideration.

It is now recognized that an individual's response to stress is less influenced by the nature or intensity of an event than by their appraisal of the stimulus, their perceived ability to cope with the problem and their outcome expectations. The physical effects of stress are more closely linked to how individuals view the event than to the situation itself. While events perceived as stressful may induce chemical and histological changes in one individual, identical events perceived as non-threatening may produce little physiological change in another. The perception of psychosocial events influences the impact of the stimulus on the underlying 'tone' of nervous system arousal.

Modern stress management focuses on optimizing the individual's response to a stressor rather than on the nature of the stimulus itself. Good stress management can be enhanced by helping people to change their perception of self, specific stressors and their general life situation. Mind–body interventions ranging from relaxation, biofeedback and meditation to cognitive behavioural therapies and imagery have variously been found helpful in managing problems as diverse as insomnia and chronic pain.[15,16]

THE CONUNDRUM

Psychosocial stress has a biological impact. While life in modern society does contribute to the allostatic load, it has yet to be clearly demonstrated that improved management of psychosocial stressors prevents disease and increases longevity.

CLINICAL CHALLENGE

A 70-year-old man is the principal caregiver for his wife who has Alzheimer's disease. He comes to his doctor complaining of insomnia, fatigue and anxiety. His doctor finds his blood pressure has increased.

Questions arising

- Is the man showing evidence of carer fatigue?
- How can his load be lightened?

Clinical considerations

Somatic complaints can be a 'call for help'.

Options for decreasing the stress associated with caring for a demented spouse include:

- information on Alzheimer's Associations and support networks
- respite visits to allow the man to get out and regroup
- advice on personal stress management techniques.

Refer to Handouts for chapters 12 and 16 at www.jamisonhealth.com for information on:

- remaining calm, e.g. deep breathing, despite acutely stressful situations such as when his wife is being inappropriate in company
- relieving muscle tension, e.g. trigger point therapy to relieve stress-related headaches
- reducing background physiological arousal by relaxation, visualization or meditation
- how to enhance problem solving skills and get a balanced view of the situation.

PRACTICE GEMS

- Stressful social situations may carry a health risk.
  - The body does not discriminate between physical, chemical, psychological and social stressors.
- Stress mechanisms are primed to deal with physical stressors; the physiological response to social stressors may deplete physiological reserves and when persistent may lead to pathological changes.
- The nature of the stressor, the way individuals view a situation and their ability to cope with stressors all determine the physiological impact of the event.
- Persistent minor stresses may have even more serious health consequences than isolated major lifestyle challenges.
- When it is not possible to eliminate a social stressor, successful stress management can be achieved by changing the individual's response to the stressor.
- The biological response to a psychosocial stressor can be altered either by the individual changing their perception of a stressful situation or by modifying their physiological response.
- Muscle relaxation, breathing exercises, improved problem solving/coping skills and/or affirmative self-talk all have the ability to change the physiological response to social stressors.
- Stress is a vicious cycle – it exemplifies a positive feed back system.
- Frailty is not synonymous with aging – many aged persons are not frail.
- Moderate exercise regimens are anxiolytic, but vigorous activity may have less effect, or even be counterproductive, among older adults.

References

1. Centers for Disease Control and Prevention. Trends in aging: United States and worldwide. MMWR Morb Mortal Wkly Rep 2003, 52:101–104.
2. Elders MJ. The increasing impact of arthritis on public health. J Rheumatol Suppl 2000; 60:6–8.
3. Leigh JP, Hubert HB, Romano PS. Lifestyle risk factors predict healthcare costs in an aging cohort. Am J Prev Med. 2005; 29(5):379–387.
4. Chin MJ, Paw A, et al. How to select a frail elderly population? A comparison of three working definitions. J Clin Epidemiol 1999; 52:1015–1021.
5. Mitnitski AB, Mogilner AJ, et al. The accumulation of deficits with age and possible invariants of aging. The Scientific World Journal 2002; 2:1816–1822.
6. Tsigos C, Chrousos GP. Hypothalamic–pituitary–adrenal axis, neuroendocrine factors and stress. J Psychosom Res 2002; 53(4):865–871.
7. McEwen BS. Interacting mediators of allostasis and allostatic load: towards an understanding of resilience in aging. Metabolism 2003; 52(10 Suppl 2):10–16.
8. Parsons PA. From the stress theory of aging to energetic and evolutionary expectations for longevity. Biogerontology 2003; 4(2):63–73.
9. Goldstein DS, McEwen B. Allostasis, homeostats, and the nature of stress. Stress 2002; 5(1):55–58.
10. Seeman TE, Singer BH, et al. Price of adaptation— allostatic load and its health consequences. MacArthur studies of successful aging. Arch Intern Med. 1997; 157(19):2259–2268.
11. McEwen BS. Sex, stress and the hippocampus: allostasis, allostatic load and the aging process. Neurobiol Aging 2002; 23(5):921–939.
12. Traustadottir T, Bosch PR, Matt KS. Gender differences in cardiovascular and hypothalamic–pituitary–adrenal axis responses to psychological stress in healthy older adult men and women. Stress 2003; 6(2):133-140.
13. Traustadottir T, Bosch PR, Matt KS. The HPA axis response to stress in women: effects of aging and fitness. Psychoneuroendocrinology 2005; 30(4):392–402.
14. Holmes TH, Rahe RH. The social adjustment rating scale. J Psychosom Res 1967; 11:2133–2138.
15. NIH Consensus Statement: Integration of behavioral and relaxation approaches into the treatment of chronic pain and insomnia. http://odp.od.nih.gov/consensus/ta/017/017_sta tement.htm http://odp.od.nih.gov/consensus/ta/017/017_statement.htm
16. Astin JA, Shapiro SL, et al. Mind–body medicine: state of the science, implications for practice. J Am Board Fam Pract 2003; 16(2):131–147.

PATIENT HANDOUT 2.1 – PSYCHOSOCIAL STRESS: A HEALTH RISK

Social stress is a health risk!

Aging is associated with many social changes likely to cause psychological stress. Unfortunately, the body is primed to cope with physical rather than psychosocial stressors. Stress management systems have adapted poorly to life in the twenty-first century. Concern about the effect of situational stress on health has resulted in the development of a new area of medicine. Psychoneuroimmunology provides evidence about ways in which stressful social situations can be translated into physical changes.[1]

Prolonged and persistent exposure to psychosocial stress is thought to deplete physiological reserves and increase the risk of disease. It is possible to predict the likelihood of future illness based on analysis of recent stressful experiences. Elderly persons are exposed to many high rating stressful experiences, e.g. death of a partner or family member. Retirement or any change in work circumstances also causes substantial stress. Even going on vacation, one of the perks of leaving the workforce, is stressful. Furthermore, it is not only major life events that may increase the risk of stress-related illness; chronic minor stressors may be even more harmful.

Stress may unbalance the immune system. Negative emotions can trigger immune dysregulation.[2] Stress induced immune dysregulation is one explanation for a spectrum of conditions associated with aging, including heart attacks, osteoporosis, arthritis, type 2 diabetes, certain cancers, frailty and functional decline.[3] Psychoimmune imbalance appears a particularly important health risk— even in otherwise healthy aged people.[4]

Good stress management can reduce the physiological impact of stress. Mind–body interventions such as relaxation, cognitive behavioural therapies, meditation, imagery, biofeedback and hypnosis have all been found helpful in managing problems as diverse as insomnia and arthritis, coronary artery disease and chronic low back pain.

We all need to develop good stress management strategies!

References

1. Glaser R, Kiecolt-Glaser JK. Stress-induced immune dysfunction: implications for health. Nat Rev Immunol 2005 Mar; 5(3):243–251.
2. Kiecolt-Glaser JK, McGuire L, et al. Psychoneuroimmunology: psychological influences on immune function and health. J Consult Clin Psychol 2002 Jun; 70(3):537–547.
3. Guidi L, Tricerri A, et al. Psychoneuroimmunology and aging. Gerontology 1998; 44(5):247–261.
4. Astin JA, Shapiro SL, et al. Mind–body medicine: state of the science, implications for practice. J Am Board Fam Pract 2003 Mar–Apr; 16(2):131–147.

PATIENT HANDOUT 2.2 – COPING WITH STRESS

Become aware!

Step I: Are you overlooking the warning signs of stress?

Check whether you have any warning signs suggesting that stress is negatively impacting on you:

- physically. See *www.jamisonhealth.com* Handout 16.3
- emotionally. See *www.jamisonhealth.com* Handout 16.4
- cognitively. See *www.jamisonhealth.com* Handouts 16.3 and 16.5.

If you are at risk do something about it!

You can selectively improve your coping skills. Go to *www.jamisonhealth.com* and target your intervention to improve:

- physical coping by implementing the suggestions in Handouts 12.8 and 16.13
- emotional coping by implementing the suggestions in Handouts 12.7 and 16.12
- cognitive coping by implementing the suggestions in Handouts 12.6 and 16.12.

Step II: Are you having an acute stress reaction?

Check *www.jamisonhealth.com* Handout 16.2 to see if you need help coping with acute stress.

There are strategies you can use to help you cope!

You can choose from a number of options.

For strategies to help you become calm see *www.jamisonhealth.com*:

- Handout 16.7 provides tips on assuming a calm posture
- Handout 16.8 shows how breathing can be used to induce tranquility.

You can use these strategies when alone or in company—you can use them whenever you need to.

Step III: Are you chronically stressed?

Check to see if you have residual tension even when the stressful situations have passed. See *www.jamisonhealth.com* Handouts 12.9 and 16.6.

Stress creates a vicious cycle. Muscle tension tells your brain you are anxious, your brain registers stress and increases muscle tension. Respond by using the relaxation intercept: muscle relaxation tells your mind you are not stressed, the brain receives less somatic arousal and overall stress levels decrease.

There are many ways of reducing muscle tension. See *www.jamisonhealth.com*:

- If you have a particularly tight group of muscle try Handout 16.11
- If you want to loosen whole groups of muscles try Handout 16.9
- You also have the option of combining breathing and gentle exercises to enhance serenity (see Handouts 16.10 and 16.13).

Step IV: People with a positive outlook on life have a health advantage

Improve your mental health by:

- Becoming more optimistic: see *www.jamisonhealth.com* Handout 12.5
- Improving your self-concept: see *www.jamisonhealth.com* Handout 12.4
- Increasing your capacity to problem solve: see *www.jamisonhealth.com* Handout 12.3
- Reviewing tips for coping: see *www.jamisonhealth.com* Handout 12.2.

Other useful handouts are:

- Hot tips about psychosocial stress. see *www.jamisonhealth.com* Handout16.1
- Handout 16.14 at *www.jamisonhealth.com* provides a guide to developing a personal stress management program. Select the stress management options most suited to you!

A lifetime of stress exposure depletes physiological reserves. Stress management strategies can help to reduce your biological response to psychosocial stimuli and may diminish your health risk.

Chapter 3

Medication: A two-edged sword

Tom, a 77-year-old man, presents a little confused, even disorientated, and admits having lost his appetite and having had diarrhoea and weakness for the last 10 days.

You check his file and find he has been treated for hypertension and cardiac failure for some 3 years. His heart failure has been well controlled by digoxin and a diuretic since initial diagnosis. Some 4 weeks ago he developed atrial fibrillation with a heart rate of 95 beats per minute. His digoxin dose was increased.

- Is this patient's alteration of mental status due to disease or medication?
- Could this man's current problem be drug-related?

INTRODUCTION

Polypharmacy, defined as a daily intake of more than two drugs, is an increasingly prevalent practice amongst the elderly.[1,2] More than 90% of people over 65 years of age use at least one medication each week; up to 40% of elderly people use five or more drugs per week.

DRUGS: A CAUSE OF IATROGENIC DISORDERS

Errors in prescription or administration can have untoward effects. Fortunately, the majority of these medication errors do not cause injury; however, extensive drug use by the elderly is potentially dangerous. In the USA the overall rate of adverse drug events was approximately 50 cases per 1000 patients over 1 year; 27% were considered preventable.[3] Of the adverse drug events, 38.0% were categorized as serious, life-threatening or fatal and 42.2% of these more severe events were deemed preventable. Many persons over 70 years of age are prescribed drugs over prolonged periods for heart conditions, depression, anxiety and pain. Indeed, cardio-vascular medications (24.5%), followed by diuretics (22.1%), nonopioid analgesics (15.4%), hypoglycaemics (10.9%) and anticoagulants (10.2%) were found to be the most common medication categories associated with preventable adverse drug events.[3] Errors associated with preventable adverse drug events occurred most often at the stages of prescribing (58.4%) and/or monitoring (60.8%).

PRESCRIBING CONSIDERATIONS

Factors that need to be considered when prescribing include the disease state, the concentration of the drug at the receptor site and the influence of homeostatic regulation. Pharmacokinetic considerations that influence the concentration of drug at the receptor site include absorption, distribution, hepatic metabolism and renal elimination. Aging affects all these parameters to varying degrees. In general, elderly people require a smaller drug dose.

Drug absorption, diffusion, distribution and particularly elimination decline with age. Although gastric acidity is reduced and the surface area of the small bowel is diminished in the elderly, any resultant drug mal-absorption is usually not clinically relevant. It is those physiological changes associated with aging that increase the effective drug concentration that have a more substantial impact.

Drugs reach higher concentrations in the elderly due to a number of interacting factors. Reduced total body water and lean body mass, changes in protein binding, increased body fat prolonging the elimination half-life of fat soluble drugs and a decline in hepatic and renal function all play a role. In addition to reduced liver mass and perfusion, the primary biochemical pathway for hepatic drug metabolism declines with age. After the fifth decade of life progressive decline of the cytochrome P(450) system reduces the effective drug dose required. While elimination of drugs by the hepatic route declines even more in individuals over 70 years of age,[4] declining renal function poses an even greater problem. Reduced renal blood flow and glomerular filtration rate substantially retard elimination of drugs and their metabolites. Glomerular filtration rate declines by 50% between the ages of 20 and 90 years. Tubular secretion decreases 1% every year after the age of 40. Renal drug excretion is further compromised by renal disease, prostatic disorders, a febrile illness or dehydration in the elderly. Drug doses need to be adjusted for elderly people.

Drug–age interaction

The impact of age on different drugs varies, making generalization difficult. For example, aging enhances the clinical effect of:

- levodopa
- the psychomotor activity of triazolam
- the postural sway, psychomotor and sedative effect of temazepam
- the acute sedation of diazepam
- the acute antihypertensive effect of verapamil
- the analgesic effect of morphine, pentazocine
- the prothrombin time of warfarin.

In contrast, aging reduces the:

- onset and peak diuretic response of furosemide
- chronotropic effect of prazosin and isoproterenol
- acute sedative effect of haloperidol
- acute hypoglycaemic effect of tolbutamide.

On the other hand, the following drug actions are not altered by aging:

- gastroduodenal mucosal damage due to aspirin
- heparin's modification of the activated partial thromboplastin time
- bronchodilation with either albuterol or ipratropium
- minute ventilation and heart rate responses to adenosine
- acute venoconstriction and the acute hypertensive effect of phenylephrine
- chronotropic effect of timolol
- psychomotor effect of diphenhydramine.

Polypharmacy: drug–drug interaction

Drug interaction is an important consideration in caring for the elderly. It is emerging as a major concern in an age group in which persons on average take 4.5 prescription and 2 non prescription drugs on a regular basis. Drugs modify physiological parameters and drug interaction has important repercussions on drug selection and dosage. For example:

- Drugs vary in their binding power.
  —When a patient whose blood sugar has been stabilized on tolbutamide, a weak binder, is given salicylates, which are strong binders,

tolbutamide is displaced and blood sugar levels are affected. In the presence of an increased concentration of free tolbutamide, blood sugar levels fall and hypoglycaemia may be precipitated.

—Indometacin competes with warfarin for binding sites. Hence, if a patient whose coagulation has been stabilized on warfarin is given indometacin, bleeding may result.

- Hepatic drug activation and detoxification may be modified. Aspirin may inhibit tolbutamide metabolism. Patients on tolbutamide need to have their dose reduced if they are placed on salicylates for pain relief. Reduced hepatic mass may aggravate drug metabolism in the elderly both with respect to first pass metabolism and biotransformation. Stage 1 of hepatic drug metabolism involves reduction, oxidation or hydrolysis and is achieved by microsomal enzymes. Stage 2 involves conjugation of the metabolites produced in stage 1. Once the metabolite has been conjugated with glucuronic or sulphuric acid it usually assumes a more soluble form that is readily excreted.

In view of the polypharmacy practised in the elderly population some awareness of important drug interactions is necessary. For example:

- Antacids decrease the absorption of digoxin.
- Metoclopramide decreases the rate of gastric emptying, resulting in increased drug absorption.
- Aspirin and furosemide may displace warfarin bound to plasma proteins, resulting in increased anticoagulation and bleeding.
- Warfarin may predispose persons on aspirin to gastrointestinal bleeding.
- Barbiturates induce metabolism of warfarin and phenytoin resulting, respectively, in decreased anticoagulation and loss of seizure control.
- Smoking induces drug metabolism of theophylline, increasing dyspnoea.
- NSAIDs may interact with diuretics to reduce renal perfusion, resulting in impaired renal function.

Drug–disease interaction

The pathophysiology of diseases prevalent in the elderly can further enhance the risk of drugs and drug combinations. Older patients are at risk of digitalis toxicity due to heart disease, hypokalaemia and chronic obstructive airways disease. Patients with an underlying heart conduction disorder may have heart block precipitated by beta-blockers or tricyclic antidepressants. Patients with chronic obstructive airway disease may develop bronchoconstriction on beta-blockers or respiratory depression on opioids. NSAIDs may result in acute renal failure if given to patients with chronic renal impairment. Patients with dementia may become confused if given anticholinergics. Anticholinergics may also exacerbate glaucoma, or precipitate urinary retention in males with prostatism. Alcohol, corticosteroids, beta-blockers and/or benzodiazepine may precipitate or exacerbate depression, a common problem in the elderly. Corticosteroids may aggravate osteopenia and further predispose osteoporotic bones to fractures. Other disease interactions worthy of note include patients with:

- heart block responding adversely to drugs used to control cardiac conduction disorders, e.g. beta-blockers, tricyclic antidepressants, digoxin
- chronic obstructive airways responding adversely to beta-blockers with bronchoconstriction and to opioids with resultant respiratory depression
- dementia becoming more confused when medicated on antiepileptics, anticholinergics and levodopa
- diabetes having their blood sugar levels raised by diuretics or corticosteroids
- depression becoming more down when taking alcohol, benzodiazepines, beta-blockers, corticosteroids or centrally acting antihypertensive agents
- glaucoma being exacerbated by anticholinergic agents
- chronic renal failure developing acute failure on taking NSAIDs
- hypertension having further elevations in blood pressure by taking NSAIDs
- hypokalaemia developing cardiac toxicity on taking digoxin
- orthostatic hypotension becoming dizzy, falling or fainting when taking antihypertensives, diuretics, tricyclic antidepressants or L-dopa
- peptic ulcers having an upper gastrointestinal bleed after taking NSAIDs and/or anticoagulants
- peripheral vascular disease developing intermittent claudication on taking beta-blockers
- prostatism developing urinary retention if treated with anticholinergics or a-agonists.

Drug–alcohol interaction

In addition to medication, alcohol is a social drug that deserves mention. Older persons are more susceptible to alcohol-related problems[5] as:

- changes in body composition in the elderly, with the relative increase in fat, mean that one standard drink results in a higher blood alcohol level than in a younger person
- they are more likely to be on prescription drugs (especially psychoactive drugs—hypnotics, anxiolytics and narcotic analgesics) and drug–alcohol interactions are therefore more likely.

Drug–diet interaction

Food may interact with various medications. Warfarin prescribed to protect against thrombosis impairs the synthesis of vitamin K dependent clotting factors. Foods rich in vitamin K may impair the efficacy of warfarin. These include broccoli, cabbage, cauliflower, lettuce, kale, spinach, egg yolk, canola and soybean oil.[6] On the other hand, foods may enhance the effects of drugs. The dose of digoxin required to improve cardiac function may be decreased by green tea, and various fruit juices, including apple, orange and grapefruit, may increase the clinical effects of digoxin. Grapefruit juice has been found to affect the bioavailability, transport and metabolism of a number of medications. Grapefruit enhances the side effects of licorice, another problematic food.

Patients on digoxin, thiazide diuretics or antihypertensive agents require medical supervision if they eat licorice in amounts greater than 100 mg daily.[7] Licorice increases the risk of hypokalaemia with lasix and other loop diuretics and halves the bioavailability of nitrofurantoin, a urinary antiseptic. It is contraindicated in persons with cholestasis, cirrhosis, hypertension or hypokalaemia.

Drug–nutritional supplement interaction

When nutrients are taken in large doses they assume drug status. For example, taking 12 g fish oil daily increases the bleeding time in patients on anticoagulants.[6] It also increases the requirement for vitamin E. Furthermore, vitamin E at levels above 400 IU daily may increase clotting times. Vitamin E may enhance the anti-inflammatory effect of aspirin and decrease the dose of anticoagulant, insulin and digoxin required. Plasma levels of vitamin E may be reduced by anticonvulsants, oral contraceptives, sucralfate, colestyramine and/or liquid paraffin. In addition to nutrient–drug interactions, vitamin E has a number of nutrient–nutrient interactions.[7]

Vitamin E supplementation may impair the haematological response to iron, large doses of iron or copper may increase the requirement for vitamin E, while zinc deficiency reduces vitamin E plasma levels. Vitamin C has a sparing effect on vitamin E, and moderate doses of vitamin E have a sparing effect on vitamin A. On the other hand, large doses of vitamin E may deplete vitamin A and increase the requirement for vitamin K.

The elderly are prone to osteoporosis and self-medication with calcium and vitamin D is common. Persons with heart failure on this combination are at increased risk of arrhythmia due to hypercalcaemia if also treated with a thiazide diuretic and digoxin.[8]

Drug–herbal interaction

Many herbal remedies, readily available without prescription, interact with medications.[9] Although St John's wort (hypericum) is generally regarded as a safe herb, serious concerns exist about its interactions with several drugs frequently prescribed to elderly patients. Hypericum may lower the dose of digoxin required by up to 25%! Care should also be exercised when this drug is used in patients on theophylline and warfarin. Use of this herb should be avoided in patients on medications that affect neurotransmitters, such as tricyclic antidepressants or monoamine oxidase inhibitors. Patients should also be cautioned to avoid self-medicating with cough mixtures containing pseudoephedrine or ephedrine when taking hypericum.

Even some dietary choices require caution. Although safe in small amounts, ginger when taken as a supplement or in large quantities in the diet may have untoward effects. Drugs frequently prescribed for elderly patients that may interact with ginger include aspirin, NSAIDs, other antiplatelet agents and antiarrhythmic agents.[7] Ginger may also have a glycaemic effect and should be rationed in diabetics.

Drug compliance

However, pathophysiological changes in the elderly and their propensity to be on medication are not the only factors that complicate management of elderly patients. Behavioural variables also compromise therapy. In addition to being altered by the pharmacokinetics of the drug itself, drug concentration is determined by patient compliance. In fact, over 1 in 5 preventable adverse drug effects involve patient adherence. Compliance with treatment regimes, especially where polypharmacy is involved, may be problematic.

Factors that contribute to poor compliance include:

- sensory impairment such as failing vision and poor hearing
- cognitive impairment such as poor memory and dementia
- communication failure leading to misunderstanding of instructions and confusion with medication regimes
- unsuitable packaging. Childproof packaging is often aged person proof.

It is not uncommon to find cabinets full of outdated prescription drugs in the homes of elderly persons. Careful monitoring is required to detect any imbalances early. Particular care needs to be taken when diuretics and psychotropics such as antidepressants, tranquillizers and psycho-mimetics are prescribed. The most 'toxic' drugs taken by the elderly are the psychotropic drugs, and those used to treat Parkinson's disease and hypertension.

GETTING IT RIGHT

Prescribing for the elderly is challenging. The need for multiple medications, the underlying disease state and the physiological changes of aging all interact, making it particularly important to monitor carefully the responses of elderly persons to new treatments or any changes in their medication regime. It has also been suggested that the best way to reduce the prevalence of adverse drug reactions in the elderly is to limit drug prescription to essential medications, to explain clearly how prescribed agents should be taken, and to give drugs for as short a period as possible.[10]

A 75-year-old tourist develops chest tightness while travelling overseas. His discomfort is most pronounced after the evening meal. He explains he has difficulty swallowing.

On taking his history you find he has also recently experienced dizziness, slight blurring of vision and difficulty with urination. He has a long history of clinical depression that is controlled by imipramine.

Before coming on holiday he says his long-standing problem of abdominal pain and loose stools was troublesome. His local doctor prescribed mebeverine and his stool is now well formed. He has no history of blood in the stool.

Questions arising

- Is the patient's current problem attributable to an underlying medical problem or drug interaction?
- How may his medication be influencing his presentation?

Clinical considerations

Two medical conditions require investigation. Given his age, cardiac ischaemia is a likely explanation for his chest pain. In view of his dysphagia, blurred vision and dizziness, a possible cerebellar lesion also needs to be explored.

His drug therapy may, however, also be contributing to his presentation.

Points to note are:

- There has been a recent change in the patient's medication.
- Imipramine is an antidepressant; mebeverine is an anticholinergic.
- Anticholinergics and antidepressants interact and may be responsible for blurred vision, a dry mouth with resultant dysphagia, urinary retention and dizziness.

Further longer term considerations include:

- Screening for underlying benign prostatic hyperplasia
- Measuring intraocular pressure to exclude glaucoma.

A 55-year-old woman presents in your clinic with severe acute backache. You recommend ice and 5 g aspirin in divided doses for the next 24 hours and then return for reassessment. The patient has a history of diabetes but is well controlled on tolbutamide.

The patient returns the next day. Although her backache is much improved, she is confused, anxious and complains of palpitations and double vision. On examination you note she is sweating and has a tremor.

Questions arising

- Is the patient demonstrating drug toxicity?
- Can the clinical presentation be due to a drug overdose or drug interaction?

Clinical considerations

- Recommended drug dosage: the peak analgesic effect of aspirin is between 2.0 and 5.0 g per day. The analgesic effect lasts for about 4 hours and therefore about 1 g should be taken every 5 hours.
- Drug toxicity: a vast array of symptoms are potentially attributable to long term high dose salicylate use. However, in this case salicylates have only been taken for 24 hours at the maximum level permitted. While impaired renal function may have contributed to the present problem, the possibility of drug interaction needs to be explored. Salicylates bind to albumin, displacing tolbutamide. The patient's presentation is consistent with hypoglycaemia—evidence of acute 'salicylate toxicity' in this patient. Diabetics controlled on tolbutamide should not be given aspirin.

A 77-year-old patient appears a little confused, even disorientated. He has lost his appetite and had diarrhoea and weakness for the last 10 days. He is on diuretics and recently had his dose of digoxin increased.

Question arising

- Is this drug toxicity or a gastro-intestinal problem?

Clinical considerations

Digoxin toxicity must be ruled out. Digoxin toxicity is a possibility as

- His dose has been increased and digoxin has a very small therapeutic range.
- He is in the high risk age group. Digoxin toxicity is more than twice as likely in persons over 75 than those under 65 years of age.
- Diarrhoea and hypopotassaemia predispose to digoxin toxicity. His diuretic may further aggravate the situation.

The clinical presentation of acute digoxin toxicity includes:

- anorexia, nausea and vomiting
- confusion and disorientation in the elderly
- an arrhythmia e.g. premature ventricular beat, sinus arrhythmia, ventricular tachycardia, sino-atrial block.

Working Diagnosis: digoxin toxicity

PRACTICE GEMS

- ◆ Elderly people are more often than not on more than one prescribed or over-the-counter medication.
- ◆ The effects of aging on absorption, metabolism and excretion require that drug doses be adapted for elderly people.
- ◆ Older persons are prone to drug interactions due to declining function and polypharmacy.
- ◆ Always inquire about self-medication.
- ◆ Adverse medication effects and drug withdrawal, in addition to medical illness and depression, are frequently responsible for the appearance of anxiety in older women.

References

1. Linjakumpu T, Hartikainen S, et al. Use of medications and polypharmacy are increasing among the elderly. J Clin Epidemiol 2002; 55(8):809–817.
2. Jyrkka J, Vartiainen L, et al. Increasing use of medicines in elderly persons: a five-year follow-up of the Kuopio 75+ Study. Eur J Clin Pharmacol 2006; 12:1–8.
3. Gurwitz JH, Field TS, et al. Incidence and preventability of adverse drug events among older persons in the ambulatory setting. JAMA 2003; 289(9):1107–1116.
4. Anantharaju A, Feller A, et al. Aging liver. A review. Gerontology 2002; 48(6):343–353.
5. Reid MC, Anderson PA. Geriatric substance use disorders. Medical Clinics North America 1997; 81:999.
6. Braun L, Cohen M. Herbs and natural supplements: an evidence based guide. Marrickrille, NSW: Elsevier; 2005: 28–46.
7. Jamison JR. Clinical guide to nutrition and dietary supplements in disease management. Edinburgh: Churchill Livingstone; 2003: 587–589, 547–550, 733–742.
8. Mason P. Dietary supplements. London: Pharmaceutical Press; 2001: 234–239.
9. Philp R. Herbal remedies: the good, the bad and the ugly. J Comp Med & Integrated Med 2004; 1(1):4 http://www.bepress.com/jcim/vol1/iss1/4/
10. Merle L, Laroche ML, et al. Predicting and preventing adverse drug reactions in the very old. Drugs Aging 2005; 22(5):375–392.

Further reading

Hanlon JT, Shimp LA, Semla TP. Recent advances in geriatrics: drug-related problems in the elderly. Ann Pharmacother 2000; 34(3):360–365.

PATIENT HANDOUT 3.1 – TIPS FOR TAKING MEDICATION

WHAT TO DO

- Take medications as instructed—tablets are usually taken with a full glass of water.
- Always take the recommended dose of a medication—and take it for the time suggested.
- Read warning labels—ask the pharmacist if you are not sure what they mean.
- Always tell your doctor if you are taking over-the-counter medications, herbs or nutritional supplements.
- Flush medications that have expired down the toilet.

WHAT NOT TO DO

- Never mix medications with food or hot drinks or other drugs without first checking with your doctor or pharmacist.
- Never take medications left over from one illness to treat a different condition.
- Never take medication in the dark or without checking the label.

A CAUTION

- You often feel better before the medication has fully treated the underlying problem—always take the full course of treatment prescribed.
- Over-the-counter medications, including vitamins and other nutrients, can interact with prescribed medication—check with your pharmacist before self-medicating.
- Alcohol interacts with a number of medications—check with your doctor.

HELPFUL HINTS

- You can request your medications are provided in non-childproof containers.
- Develop a plan so that you remember to take your medication:
  —always take your pills at the same time
  —use a check-off calendar
  —buy a medication box with compartments to store your tablets for each day of the week.

Internet resources

See *http://www.niapublications.org/engagepages/medicine.asp*
for tips on the safe use of medications.

PATIENT HANDOUT 3.2 – DRUG INTERACTIONS: TIPS FOR REDUCING THE RISK

The required dose of prescribed medication may be increased or decreased by over-the-counter purchases or even by a substantial change in diet. The following is a list—by no means complete—to alert you to some of the hazards of self-medication.

'Pain relievers'

■ Paracetamol may cause liver damage—reduce the risk by taking garlic.
■ Aspirin interferes with vitamin C—increase the dose of vitamin C supplements when taking aspirin.

'Blood thinners'

Persons on warfarin or other anticoagulants risk bleeding and bruising if they self-medicate with any one of the following: celery, evening primrose oil, feverfew, fenugreek, fish oils, garlic, ginger, grape seed extract, licorice, turmeric, vitamin E, willowbark or aspirin. Exercise caution!

'Heart tablets'

■ The toxicity of digoxin is increased by aloe vera and/or licorice.
■ The dose of digoxin prescribed may need to be altered by taking herbs— hawthorn reduces the dose of digoxin required, St John's wort increases the dose required.

'Water tablets'

■ Thiazide diuretics increase the need for calcium, magnesium and zinc.
■ Beware of licorice when taking diuretics—it increases potassium excretion.

'Cholesterol lowering tablets'

■ Chromium, garlic, oats and vitamin B3 all reduce blood cholesterol.
■ Cholestyramine reduces absorption of all fat soluble vitamins (A, D, E, K), folate and iron.
■ The lipid lowering effect of pravastatin is increased by fish oils.
■ The dose of simvastatin needs to be increased if St John's wort is taken.

'Blood sugar lowering tablets'

■ The dose of hypoglycaemic agents, e.g. metformin, may need to be reduced if aloe vera, green tea, bilberry, chromium or alpha-lipoic acid is taken.
■ The dose of oral hypoglycaemic agents and insulin may need to be increased if glucosamine is taken.

Managing the 'blues'

■ The dose of prescribed antidepressants needs to be modified if taking L-tyrosine, St John's wort or S-adenosyl-methionine (SAMe).

'Sleeping/calming tablets'

- The sedative effect of barbiturates is increased by lemon balm, valerian, kava kava and passion flower.
- The effects of benzodiazepine withdrawal may be reduced by chamomile, kava kava or valerian.

'Heartburn'

- Antacids reduce absorption of folate and iron.

'Prostate problems'

- Difficulty passing urine due to benign prostatic hyperplasia may be eased by prescribed drugs, e.g. 5-alpha-reductase inhibitors (e.g. finasteride), and further eased by saw palmetto and nettle root.

'Anti-inflammatory drugs'

- The effective drug dosage of NSAIDs may be reduced if also taking chondroitin, glucosamine, ginger, fish oils, nettle, New Zealand green lipped mussel, SAMe, vitamin E or willowbark.

'Alcohol'

- The liver damage caused by alcohol may be reduced by Korean ginseng, SAMe, St Mary's thistle.

Before purchasing over-the-counter medications including herbs, nutrients and other dietary supplements ask your pharmacist to check if there are any possible adverse interactions with your current medication.

Chapter **4**

Functional decline: Triggering social isolation

Alistair was becoming increasingly concerned about his wife, aged 70. Jocelyn used to be the life and soul of a party but now resisted going out, and when friends came visiting she seemed withdrawn, saying very little. Even when one of their five children visited she seemed unusually quiet.

- Is social withdrawal a normal part of aging?
- What psychological and physical changes increase the risk of social withdrawal?
- What contributes to healthy aging?

INTRODUCTION

Industrialized countries are characterized by an aging population. In 1994, 13.6% of Americans were over 65 years of age; by 2030, 20% of the US population will be over 65 years.[1] This trend is not confined to the USA. The proportion of the population over 65 years is increasing, and the oldest old, i.e. those over 85 years, are increasing most rapidly.[2] An aging population is troubled by declining function and burdened by high disease prevalence. Some 70% of people over 80 years have at least one chronic condition while most have two—commonly arthritis and hypertension.[2]

In addition to an increased risk of disease in elderly persons, aging is associated with a marked functional decline.[3,4] While differences in lifestyle, psychological and social factors have long been recognized to explain socio-economic status differences in mortality, more recently biological dys-regulation has been acknowledged as a substantive consideration. The cumulative index of biological risk is thought to explain over 35% of the difference in mortality risk between those with higher versus lower socio-economic status as measured by level of education.[5] The cumulative measure of biological dysregulation or *allostatic load* reflects the function of multiple regulatory systems. The concept of allostatic load is based on the notion that healthy functioning requires on-going adjustments of the internal physiological milieu. With increasing age and depleted reserves physiological systems respond more slowly and adapt less readily to environmental demands. Functional impairments provide important explanatory information regarding differential mortality risks among older adults.

FUNCTIONAL IMPAIRMENT: A CONSEQUENCE OF AGING

Older adults' definition of successful aging is multidimensional, encompassing physical, psychological, social and functional health.[6] Remaining socially engaged has emerged as an important stimulus to wellness in the elderly. Functional impairments associated with the aging process can make continued social participation by elderly persons problematic.

Functional decline in various organ systems contributing to the cumulative allostatic load can be partially explained by the free radical theory.[3,4,7] Free radical damage to mitochondria can lead to numerous mitochondrial DNA mutations which result in a progressive reduction in energy output and various signs of aging, ranging from loss of memory, through impaired hearing and vision to declining stamina.[7] Maximal oxygen consumption decreases by 10% in men and 7.5% in women with each decade of adult life. Arterial walls thicken and blood pressure increases 20–25% between 20 and 75 years of age. The maximum ventilation capacity decreases 40% between the ages of 20 and 80. Strength also declines. Muscle strength declines 22% in women and 23% in men between 30 and 70 years of age. Hand grip strength declines 45% by age 75. Exercise can delay loss of muscle strength. Sedentary older adults are 1.5 times as likely to experience functional dependence as fit persons of similar age.[2] Declining vision also presents a problem in the elderly. Difficulty with focusing starts around the age of 40 years. Increased susceptibility to glare and difficulty seeing at low illumination levels becomes problematic after the age of 50. By 70 the ability to distinguish fine details may decline and memory and reaction time start to decrease. The Second Longitudinal Study of Aging showed that persons with lower levels of cognitive functioning were more likely to die or become disabled than those with higher levels of cognition.[8] Memory problems are an important cause of functional decline in an aging population. Dementia is considered in a separate chapter.

In addition to cognitive changes, two physiological changes associated with aging that strongly predispose to social withdrawal are incontinence and hearing loss. The decline in bladder capacity and increasing deafness are sources of embarrassment and social isolation. Keeping the elderly interested and involved is conducive to wellness; addressing incontinence and deafness in this age group warrants careful attention.

INCONTINENCE: A SOCIAL EMBARRASSMENT

Incontinence has a profound social and psychological impact resulting in significant changes in social activities outside the home, social isolation, depression, anxiety and enforced changes in sexual activity. A study of community dwelling adults aged 50 years and older found those with urinary incontinence were more likely to have psychological distress than were other older adults.[9] Another study reported that an overactive bladder, with and without incontinence, had a clinically significant impact on quality of life, quality of sleep and mental health.[10]

Worldwide, 1 in 5 elderly men and more than 1 in 3 elderly women suffer urinary leakage. Urinary incontinence is highly prevalent in women across their adult life span, and its severity increases linearly with age, from 8% in 30- to 39-year-old women to 33% in 80- to 90-year-olds.[11] Until the age of 60 years the incidence in women outnumbers men by 7:1. Incontinence is particularly common in the elderly living in institutions.

Bladder control

Continence is achieved by homeostatic mechanisms that adapt to filling and storage of urine and respond to voluntary expulsion of urine. A compliant bladder of sufficient capacity to accommodate increasing volumes of urine while maintaining bladder pressure below urethral pressure is a prerequisite for continence. To achieve this an intact system involving local and central neurological bladder control coordinating the detrusor muscle, the vesicourethral angle and the bladder sphincters is required. The storage phase entails both an intact sphincter mechanism and a stable detrusor muscle that inhibits contraction and permits bladder distension. A competent sphincter mechanism incorporates an internal and external sphincter. The external urethral sphincter can be voluntarily contracted to interrupt voiding and prevent leakage with sudden increases in intra-abdominal pressure. Spinal reflex contractions are continually generated between the spinal column and the expanding bladder. Inhibitory signals from the central nervous system continuously block the initiation of bladder voiding. Loss of central nervous system inhibition in the elderly can result in bladder contraction and leakage.

An unstable bladder may result when intravesical pressure rises and the spinal reflex stimuli are inadequately blocked. As urine accumulates in the bladder, no significant increase in intravesical pressure occurs due to stretching of the muscle and connective tissue of the bladder wall. When 150–250 mL of urine have accumulated in the bladder, mechanoreceptors in the bladder wall are stimulated and the desire to void is experienced. Bladder outlet resistance is increased by reflex stimulation of receptors in the smooth muscle of the bladder neck and urethra. As soon as intravesical pressure becomes greater than the resultant intraurethral pressure, urine is voided. Sacral reflexes contract the detrusor muscle and relax the external urethral sphincter. Bladder contraction should be powerful enough to completely empty the bladder leaving no residual urine.

Normal voiding is a voluntary act coordinated through interaction of the autonomic and voluntary nervous systems. It involves relaxation of the urethra, decreasing urethral pressure, and contraction of the bladder, increasing intravesical pressure. Voiding is terminated when the base of the empty bladder is elevated by the striated muscles of the urethra and pelvic floor, the intraurethral pressure is raised and detrusor contraction is inhibited. The vesicourethral angle resulting from elevation of the bladder helps to maintain the anatomical integrity of the bladder neck, helping to prevent leakage during physical activity, coughing or sneezing. Over-stretching of the pelvic muscles in childbirth and oestrogen deprivation resulting in relaxation of pelvic muscles after menopause may compromise the vesicourethral angle and contribute to the prevalence of incontinence in females.

The Aging Bladder

Aging tends to be associated with an increase in unstable bladder contractions, smaller bladder capacity, lower flow rates and increased residual volume. In general, incontinence may be attributable to factors that raise intravesical pressure and/or lower urethral resistance. Elderly persons are at increased risk of neurological lesion leading to:

- *An atonic bladder.* Diabetics are at risk due to autonomic neuropathy.
- *A reflex neurogenic bladder.* Disc lesions or osteophytes may result in disruption of innervation and a reflex bladder that fills and voids in the absence of sensory information.
- *A dystonic bladder.* Dementia, a cerebral tumour or infarct may produce an unstable bladder that empties recurrently due to bladder sensory impairment with loss of bladder inhibition.
- *Detrusor–sphincter dyssynergia.* Spinal cord lesions may trigger urethral sphincter inhibition of urine expulsion at the same time the bladder contracts.

In summary, factors predisposing to incontinence in the elderly include:

1. *Increased residual urine.* This predisposes to infection and incontinence. Faecal impaction and benign prostatic hyperplasia are important underlying causes in elderly patients. The prostate accounts for the marked increase in urinary incontinence in males over 60 years of age.
2. *Reduced bladder capacity.* Decreased compliance of the bladder wall may halve bladder capacity from 600 to 300 ml in elderly persons. Bladder lesions such as calculi, polyps or cancer may further aggravate the problem.
3. *Detrusor instability.* Age-related changes to the cerebral cortex and spinal arc predispose to uninhibited muscle contractions. Elderly persons have a short 'holding time'—the time lapse between the urge to void and urine loss is short. The overactive bladder associated with detrusor instability may be a primary problem or secondary to bladder inflammation, e.g. urinary tract infection, or outlet obstruction, e.g. benign prostatic hyperplasia. Uninhibited bladder contraction is a problem in a number of diseases encountered in elderly patients, including Parkinson's disease, cerebrovascular accidents, brain tumours and multiple sclerosis.
4. *Lowered urethral resistance.* Urethral resistance is lowered by oestrogen deficiency, straining at stool, disc lesion and cauda equina syndrome. Medications that block α-adrenergic receptors, e.g. phenoxybenzamine, prazosin, labetalol, all lower urethral resistance.
5. *Mobility problems.* Bladder sensitivity is decreased in the elderly and when the desire to void is experienced, the bladder may be near its functional capacity. The functional inability to reach the toilet rapidly may result in leakage. Impaired mobility, whether attributable to arthritis or neuropathy (cerebrovascular accident or Parkinson's disease), aggravates the problem.
6. *Nocturia.* Renal function diminishes with age and it is normal for the elderly to pass urine up to twice a night. Use of diuretics may aggravate the problem.
7. *Cognitive impairment.* Frail elderly, confused or demented persons are at increased risk. Disorientation may result from acute illness but may also be due to a change in location.
8. *Increased abdominal pressure.* Obesity and coughing associated with smoking further aggravate problems with urinary continence.

Incontinence

Urinary incontinence may be transient or persistent. Transient incontinence may result from confusional states, urinary infection, atrophic vaginitis/urethritis, drugs, restricted mobility or stool impaction. Alcohol may precipitate functional transient incontinence due to a combination of impaired mobility, sedation and diuresis.

Persistent urinary incontinence is clinically categorized as:

- *Stress incontinence.* Stress incontinence is associated with sphincter incompetence and/or urethral instability. It is the involuntary loss of urine associated with a rise in intra-abdominal pressure in the absence of detrusor activity. Stress incontinence is largely a daytime phenomenon and is encountered in women with genital prolapse and men with sphincter weakness following prostatectomy. Drugs that predispose to stress incontinence include: nicotine, alpha-sympathetic agonists and alpha- blockers which decrease bladder outlet and urethral resistance.

- *Urge incontinence.* Urge incontinence is associated with bladder instability or detrusor hyperactivity. It involves the involuntary loss of urine associated with a strong desire to void. Associated precipitancy is characterized by motor urgency, a fear of leakage and sensory urgency due to discomfort. Compared with stress incontinence, persons with urge and/ or mixed incontinence report significantly worse health-related quality of life.[12] Urinary frequency and nocturia may be due to local bladder problems, e.g. cancer, infection, interference with spinal inhibition, e.g. spondylosis, or central nervous system lesions, e.g. stroke, Alzheimer's disease or Parkinson's disease. Drugs that cause urge incontinence include: caffeine; diuretics which precipitate polyuria, frequency and urgency; sedatives/hypnotics/tranquillizers which may diminish awareness of bladder filling, and decrease outlet resistance and the ability to inhibit bladder contraction.
- *Overflow incontinence.* Overflow incontinence is due to outlet obstruction and/or underactive detrusor muscle activity. Patients experience hesitancy, straining to void and a weak, often interrupted, urinary stream. Prostatic hypertrophy or urethral stricture may cause obstruction to outflow or bladder contraction may be impaired by a herniated disc or diabetic neuropathy. Overflow incontinence may result from anticholinergic agents decreasing the strength of bladder contraction and the urge to void.
- *Functional incontinence.* Functional incontinence may be encountered in a normal urinary tract due to impaired mobility or long term cognitive problems. It may also aggravate any of the above.

Urinary Tract Infection—a treatable cause and consequence of incontinence

Urinary tract infection is an important cause of urge incontinence. Bacteriuria is present in up to 1 in 5 elderly women and 1 in 10 elderly men living in the community. The prevalence increases to 1 in every 2 or 3 hospitalized elderly patients. Factors predisposing the elderly to urinary tract infections include:

- incomplete bladder emptying
- decreased cell mediated immunity
- a decrease in bladder epithelium mucopolysaccharides resulting in less resistance to bacterial adherence to epithelial cells
- in males: loss of prostatic antibacterial secretions
- in females: raised vaginal pH and mucosal atrophy.

Due to their short urethra all women are at increased risk; after menopause this risk escalates. Oestrogen deprivation affects the tone of the pelvic floor, the condition of the mucosa and the flora of the vagina. The hormonal changes of menopause result in decreased glycogen storage in vaginal cells. In menstruating woman glycogen conversion to lactic acid by commensal lactobacilli creates a hostile environment to many genital and urinary pathogens.

Management

In the absence of surgical correction of disorders such as prostatic disease in males or genital prolapse in females, management of incontinence in the elderly relies largely on patient endeavour. The importance of actively attempting to help elderly patients cannot be underestimated as, compared to control patients, those with an overactive bladder are more prone to falls and fractures, 25.3% versus 16.1%; depression, 10.5% versus 4.9%; urinary tract infections, 28.0% versus 8.4%; skin infections, 3.9% versus 2.3%; vulvovaginitis, 4.7% versus 1.8%; any of these comorbidities, 52.1% versus 27.9%.[13] Bladder health in the elderly is enhanced by strengthening the pelvic floor.[14] Refer to Patient Handout 4.1.

Routinely taking precautions against urinary tract infections also deserves consideration. The risk of urinary tract infection can be reduced by a high fluid intake and dietary intervention. Frequent consumption of fresh juices, especially berry juices, is associated with a decreased risk of recurrent infection.[15] Daily ingestion of 300 ml of cranberry juice is acceptable to older people,[16] and its potential to prevent urinary infections is promising.[17,18] An open, randomized controlled trial over 1 year found 50 ml of cranberry-lingonberry juice concentrate daily for 6 months seemed to reduce the recurrence of urinary tract infection.[19] Drinking fermented milk products containing probiotic bacteria is less likely to be successful.[15,19]

HEARING IMPAIRMENT

Hearing impairment is a widespread problem in the elderly. At least 1 in 3 people over 65 years of age suffers from hearing loss with men experiencing hearing loss twice as rapidly as women between the ages of 30 and 80. A study of persons over 53 years of age found 28% had mild hearing loss and 24% had moderate to severe hearing loss.[20] Another study found most individuals (66%) perceived hearing loss as a severe handicap even though audiology revealed only mild to moderate impairment (pure tone average loss, 27–55 dB).[21] Certainly, depression is twice as prevalent in hearing impaired elderly persons and hearing impaired persons are at increased risk of sundowner syndrome, a behaviour pattern of confusion, anxiety and aggression, associated with reduced sensory stimulation. A study of elderly male veterans reported that hearing loss was associated with significant emotional, social and communication dysfunction.[21] Severity of hearing loss is associated with reduced quality of life in older adults.[20] In view of the prevalence and impact of hearing loss, older adults should be screened for hearing impairment by periodically questioning them about their hearing, and they should be made aware of the availability of hearing devices.[22]

Reversible hearing loss

Not all hearing loss is irreversible. Wax in the external auditory meatus is a reversible cause of conduction hearing loss at any age. Persons who complain of a 'fullness' in the ear or tinnitus may have wax impacted on the ear drum. Wax removal will improve hearing. However, before attempting to remove wax, after checking the eardrum is intact, soften wax using sodium bicarbonate, glycerine or mineral oil drops for several days prior to syringing. Olive oil drops may sooth dryness and itching of the ear canal. When inserting ear drops, flex the patient's head to one side so that the ear to receive the drops is facing upwards, insert the drops and compress the tragus for a few seconds. This encourages drainage of drops into the ear canal. When syringing the ear: cover the patient with a plastic sheet and have a container available to catch the water, use tepid water (at body temperature), pull the auricle upward, back and slightly outward and direct the stream superoposteriorly along the auditory canal. Do not insert the nozzle of the syringe too far into the external meatus. Dry the ear afterwards to ensure no residual water remains. Syringing is contraindicated in ears with perforated drums.

Wax in the external ear canal is not the only cause of deafness in the elderly.

Irreversible hearing loss

Age associated hearing loss

Presbycusis, the most common cause of deafness in the elderly, is a disorder of senescence. Presbycusis is permanent loss of the ability to detect high frequency sounds. Failure to detect high frequency tones may start at 20 years of age. Consonant sounds occur in the higher frequencies. Persons with presbycusis can hear vowel sounds but not consonants so words become unintelligible sounds. Hearing loss is progressive with age and ability to detect low frequency tones declines around 60 years of age. There appears to be a 10dB reduction per decade in hearing after the age of 60 years.

Presbycusis is a form of sensorineural deafness. Changes in the inner ear that may result in presbycusis include a loss of cochlear neurones (neural presbycusis), atrophy of the organ of Corti and related hair cells (sensory presbycusis), degeneration of a segment of the cochlear wall (mechanical presbycusis) and/or degeneration of the fibrous vascular lining of the cochlear duct that produces cochlear fluid (metabolic presbycusis).

Environmentally induced hearing loss

Noise induced hearing loss is the second most common cause of irreversible hearing impairment in the elderly. Noise induced hearing loss before old age reduces the effects of aging at noise-associated frequencies, but accelerates the deterioration of hearing in adjacent frequencies.[23] Both occupational and leisure exposure to noise in excess of 85 dB is detrimental to hearing. Individuals who engage in leisure activities with average sound levels greater than 90 dBA are significantly more likely to have a hearing loss than participants who don't.[24] The rate of hearing loss is influenced by noise intensity and the duration of noise exposure; more intense noise and longer exposure results in greater hearing loss. Noise induced hearing loss may be minimized by reducing the:

- intensity of sound, e.g. by wearing protective ear muffs
- duration of exposure—safe exposure time is largely determined by noise intensity.

In any 24-hour period limit exposure to:

- a power saw (110 decibels) to 1 minute
- a circular saw (100 decibels) to 15 minutes
- a power planer (97 decibels) to 30 minutes
- a jigsaw (94 decibels) to 60 minutes
- a disc sander (91 decibels) to 120 minutes
- a hand drill (88 decibels) to 4 hours
- a front-end loader (85 decibels) to 8 hours.

Early warning signs of potential noise induced hearing loss include headache, dizziness, tiredness, a sense of fullness in the ears, tinnitus and an altered sense of hearing. Hearing loss may also be exacerbated by other lifestyle choices. Smoking independently causes hearing deterioration at 4000 Hz, in males without noise exposure. The effect of smoking on hearing loss in middle-aged males was found to be dose-related and the combined effect of noise and smoking was additive.[25]

The need for a solution

Sensorineural damage resulting in irreversible hearing loss is the more prevalent problem in the elderly. In persons over the age of 85 years, 2 out of 3 report some hearing loss but fewer than 1 in 7 has a hearing aid and fewer than 1 in 12 actually uses a hearing aid! Hearing aids may make sounds louder but not necessarily clearer. It is more helpful to speak slowly and clearly than to shout when communicating with deaf people. Non-verbal communication is an important source of information for inter-action. Wearing spectacles may facilitate lip reading and therefore verbal communication.

SUMMARY

Vision, hearing and mood are significant predictors of overall self-reported health in persons over 65 years of age.[26] Depression, dementia, visual impairment and decreased mobility can also all predispose to social and functional impairment. Social isolation of the elderly would seem a particularly poignant problem. A cross-sectional study found that less than half of the elderly people over 80 years of age who were unable to open one or more of the containers received help with their medication.[27] Prevention strategies to help facilitate coping with the functional consequences of aging should always be actively pursued.[28]

CLINICAL CHALLENGE

A 70-year-old woman, a mother of five, self-consciously confides she is troubled by urinary incontinence. She has a long history of osteoarthritis and is finding it increasingly difficult to get around. She is afraid to go into hospital for a hip replacement in case she wets the bed. She has a 45 year history of smoking 10 cigarettes a day.

Questions arising

■ How may this patient's urinary incontinence be explained?
■ Which types of incontinence are most likely based on the above history?

Clinical considerations

Possible explanations for this patient's incontinence include:

■ Parity. A multiparous woman with several vaginal deliveries has had stretching and damage to the pelvic floor. This may predispose to incontinence due to loss of the vesicourethral angle.
■ Menopause. Atrophy of the genitalia and surrounding tissues in postmenopausal women as a result of oestrogen deprivation impairs the normal physiology of the area, resulting in pelvic and urethral muscle dysfunction. Mucosal changes predispose to bladder infection.
■ Age. Persons in this age group have a reduced bladder capacity.
■ Mobility. This patient has a mobility problem due to her osteoarthritis.
■ Smoking. Smoking may aggravate incontinence.

This patient may suffer from:

■ Stress incontinence due to loss of the vesicourethral angle and to coughing precipitating sudden increases in intra-abdominal pressure. The clinical presentation would be one of uncontrolled leakage of small volumes of urine from a full bladder precipitated by increases in intra-abdominal pressure, e.g. coughing or straining at stool.
■ Functional incontinence due to her impaired mobility.

A 70-year-old man complains of buzzing in the ears and loss of hearing. On examination you note his deafness is largely confined to his left ear. You placed a vibrating tuning fork in the centre of his forehead and find he now hears best in his 'deaf' ear.

Questions arising

■ How may this finding be explained?
■ What should you do next?

Clinical considerations

In conduction deafness sound lateralizes to the deaf ear. This can be confirmed by finding that bone conduction is better than air conduction on the left/deaf side.

The cause of the deafness should be sought—impacted wax abutting on the ear drum is a common and treatable cause.

PRACTICE GEMS

◆ Depression, incontinence and hearing impairment are all important treatable causes of social withdrawal.
◆ Urinary incontinence in the elderly is associated with small bladder capacity, increased residual urine and involuntary bladder contractions.
◆ Younger postmenopausal women have stress incontinence; older women are more likely to have urge incontinence.
◆ Urinary tract infection is a treatable and common cause of urge incontinence in elderly women.
◆ Medications may aggravate or precipitate incontinence.
◆ Always exclude and treat a reversible cause for hearing loss.
◆ Shouting does not help elderly people hear better; speaking clearly and slowly might.
◆ Counsel the elderly regarding the use of hearing aids.

References

1. US Bureau of the Census. Current population reports, special studies, P23–90, 65+ in the United States. Washington DC: US Government Printing Office; 1996.
2. Cobbs EL, Ralapati AN. Health of older women. Medical Clinics of North America 1998; 82:127–144.
3. US Department of Health and Human Services. With the passage of time: the Baltimore Longitudional Study of Aging. NIH Pub No 93–3685. Washington DC: Public Health Service; 1993:1–52.
4. US Department of Health and Human Services. In search of the secrets of aging. NIH Pub No 93–2756. Washington DC: Public Health Service; 1993:1–46.
5. Seeman TE, Crimmins E, et al. Cumulative biological risk and socio-economic differences in mortality: MacArthur studies of successful aging. Soc Sci Med 2004; 58(10):1985–1997.
6. Phelan EA, Anderson LA, et al. Older adults' views of "successful aging"—how do they compare with researchers' definitions? J Am Geriatr Soc 2004; 52(2):211–216.
7. Knight JA. The biochemistry of aging. Adv Clin Chem 2000; 35:1–62.
8. McGuire LC, Ford ES, Ajani UA. Cognitive functioning as a predictor of functional disability in later life. Am J Geriatr Psychiatry. 2006; 14(1):36–42.
9. Bogner HR, Gallo JJ, et al. Urinary incontinence and psychological distress in community-dwelling older adults. J Am Geriatr Soc 2002; 50(3):489–495.
10. Stewart WF, Van Rooyen JB, et al. Prevalence and burden of overactive bladder in the United States. World J Urol 2003; 20(6):327–336.
11. Melville JL, Katon W, et al. Urinary incontinence in US women: a population-based study. Arch Intern Med 2005; 165(5):537–542.
12. Coyne KS, Zhou Z, et al. The impact on health-related quality of life of stress, urge and mixed urinary incontinence. BJU Int 2003; 92(7):731–735.
13. Darkow T, Fontes CL, Williamson TE. Costs associated with the management of overactive bladder and related comorbidities. Pharmacotherapy 2005; 25(4):511–519.
14. Fonda D, Wellings C. Incontinence of urine. Australian Family Physician 1988; 17(8):657.
15. Kontiokari T, Laitinen J, et al. Dietary factors protecting women from urinary tract infection. Am J Clin Nutr 2003; 77(3):600–604.
16. McMurdo ME, Bissett LY, et al. Does ingestion of cranberry juice reduce symptomatic urinary tract infections in older people in hospital? A double-blind, placebo-controlled trial. Age Ageing 2005; 34(3):256–261.
17. Lynch DM. Cranberry for prevention of urinary tract infections. Am Fam Physician 2004; 70(11):2175–2177.
18. Jepson RG, Mihaljevic L, Craig J. Cranberries for preventing urinary tract infections. Cochrane Database Syst Rev 2004; (1):CD001321.
19. Kontiokari T, Sundqvist K, et al. Randomised trial of cranberry-lingonberry juice and Lactobacillus GG drink for the prevention of urinary tract infections in women. BMJ 2001; 322(7302):1571.
20. Dalton DS, Cruickshanks KJ, et al. The impact of hearing loss on quality of life in older adults. Gerontologist 2003; 43(5):661–668.
21. Mulrow CD, Aguilar C, et al. Association between hearing impairment and the quality of life of elderly individuals. J Am Geriatr Soc 1990; 38(1):45–50.
22. US Preventive Services Task Force. The periodic health examination: age-specific charts. Guide to clinical preventative services. 2nd edn. 1996. http://www.ahrq.gov/clinic/uspstf/uspshear.htm
23. Rosenhall U. The influence of ageing on noise-induced hearing loss. Noise Health. 2003; 5(20):47–53.
24. Dalton DS, Cruickshanks KJ, et al. Association of leisure-time noise exposure and hearing loss. Audiology 2001; 40(1):1–9.
25. Uchida Y, Nakashimat T, et al. Is there a relevant effect of noise and smoking on hearing? A population-based aging study. Int J Audiol 2005; 44(2):86–91.
26. Ostbye T, Krause KM, et al. Ten dimensions of health and their relationships with overall self-reported health and survival in a predominately religiously active elderly population: the cache county memory study. J Am Geriatr Soc 2006; 54(2):199–209.
27. Beckman A, Bernsten C, et al. The difficulty of opening medicine containers in old age: a population-based study. Pharm World Sci 2005; 27(5):393–398.
28. Giffords ED, Eggleton E. Practical considerations for maintaining independence among individuals with functional impairment. J Gerontol Soc Work 2005; 46(1):3–16.

PATIENT HANDOUT 4.1 – PROMOTING BLADDER HEALTH

TIPS FOR BLADDER WELLNESS

1. Have a good fluid intake. A rule of thumb is to drink 6–8 glasses or cups of liquid each day (Wt/2 = ounces of fluid required). A dilute urine is less likely to cause bladder irritation and become infected.
2. Avoid chemicals that may irritate the bladder, e.g. caffeine, carbonated drinks.
3. Promote regular bowel habits. A high fibre, high fluid diet and regular exercise promote bowel health.
4. Maintain a regular bladder schedule. Empty the bladder at 2–4 hourly intervals. Holding urine for more than 6 hours may predispose to infection. Voiding too often or too seldom can decondition the bladder.
5. Practice urge control. Urges are a reminder that the bladder is filling and do not signal the need to urinate. Standing or sitting still and breathing slowly to relax can help control urges. Pelvic muscles should be tightened 5–10 times while concentrating on controlling the urge. Distractions such as arithmetic may also help. Once the urge has subsided wait a few minutes before voiding.
6. Do pelvic exercises. Doing pelvic muscle exercises 30–80 times a day helps to maintain good muscle tone and control urges (see Box 4.1).
7. Consider drinking 300 ml of cranberry juice daily. Cranberry deodorizes urine and may be helpful for persons with an incontinence problem. It may also reduce the risk of urinary infection.
8. Get professional assessment at the first suggestion of:
   a. Urinary obstruction. Go to a doctor if when urinating you have:
      (i) hesitancy
      (ii) a poor stream
      (iii) a terminal dribble
      (iv) incomplete emptying
   b. Infection. Seek medical attention if you have:
      (i) burning or discomfort passing urine
      (ii) to pass urine more frequently
      (iii) sensory urgency
   c. Chronic retention. This could be due to anything from an abdominal mass such as a uterine or ovarian tumour to faecal impaction.

If incontinence remains a problem despite good bladder hygiene, put on an incontinence pad and go out and enjoy yourself!

A CAUTION

Never take sodium citrate to relieve burning unless you are on antibiotics/urinary antiseptic. Sodium citrate neutralizes an acid urine, relieves burning and masks the problem, encouraging multiplication of organisms.

Internet resources

See http://www.niapublications.org/engagepages/urinary.asp for more information on urinary incontinence.
See http://www.niapublications.org/engagepages/sexuality.asp to read about sexuality in later life.

Box 4.1   Pelvic muscle exercises

Stage 1: Identify the correct muscles to exercise

1. Identify the muscles around your back passage or rectum:
   a. sit or stand comfortably
   b. imagine that you are trying to control diarrhoea by consciously tightening the ring of muscles around the back passage
   c. hold this squeeze for 4 seconds each time.
2. Strengthen bladder support:
   a. go to the toilet and commence passing urine
   b. try to stop the flow of urine in midstream
   c. recommence voiding until the bladder has emptied

The muscles used to slow or stop the flow of urine are the front pelvic muscles which help support the bladder.

3. Check you are strengthening the correct muscles by inserting a finger into the vagina. Squeeze the finger by contracting the pelvic muscles. If the finger cannot be felt to be squeezed then either the wrong muscles are being exercised or the muscles are still very weak.

Don't:
- bear down as if trying to pass a bowel motion
- bear down as during childbirth.

This strengthens the wrong muscles and may make the incontinence worse.

Do:
- exercises to identify the correct pelvic muscles for at least 1 week.

Stage 2: Exercises to strengthen pelvic muscles

Slow and quick exercises are important to strengthen the pelvic muscles properly.

Slow exercises
- Sit or stand with thighs slightly apart.
- Contract the muscles around the back passage (rectum).
- Contract the front muscles around the vagina.
- Hold this contraction while counting to five slowly.
- Relax these muscles.
- Repeat this four times.

Try to be aware of the squeezing and lifting sensation in the pelvis that frequently occurs when these exercises are done correctly.

Quick exercises
- While sitting or standing, tighten the muscles around the front and back passage—together.
- Hold this contraction for 1 second and relax.
- Repeat this exercise five times in quick succession.

With practice the exercises should be quite easy to master. They can be carried out at any time.

Do:
- pelvic exercises every day while going about your daily chores
- ideally every hour but certainly no less than four times every day
- return to Stage 1 each 7–14 days to check that the correct muscles are being used.

Don't do these exercises while passing urine.

PATIENT HANDOUT 4.2 – DEALING WITH HEARING IMPAIRMENT

Hearing impairment increases with age. One in 3 people over 65 years of age has some degree of deafness; this increases to 2 in 3 for persons over 85 years of age.

Hearing loss may be due to:

- nerve damage (sensorineural deafness) or
- impaired transmission of sound (conduction deafness).

Ask your doctor to check for and remove wax from your ear if you have conduction deafness.

Suspect conduction deafness if:

- you hear speech better in a noisy environment
- talking loudly or shouting makes speech more intelligible.

Ask your doctor to send you for a hearing test and consider getting a hearing aid if you have sensorineural deafness.

Suspect sensorineural deafness if:

- people seem to be shouting—you are sensitive to small increases in sound
- you have difficulty understanding speech
- shouting makes speech less intelligible
- you have buzzing in the ears.

Noisy environments may damage hearing.

- The louder a noise the greater the risk of damage—avoid very loud noise and wear ear protection when in a noisy environment.
- The longer the exposure time the greater the risk of damage—spend as little time in a noisy environment as possible and interrupt noisy with quiet environments.

Chapter 5

Falls: Reducing the risk

Emily was a sprightly 78-year-old who enjoyed going out and visiting her friends. One day as she was rushing to answer her doorbell she slipped on the rug at her front door. She fell awkwardly but managed to crawl to a chair and get up with the help of her visitor. She was able to walk but had a lot of pain. An X-ray showed she had fractured her hip. She was hospitalized and scheduled for surgery.

Six weeks later she died of pneumonia.

- Was this fall preventable or an inevitable consequence of aging?
- How can the elderly reduce their risk of falling?
- How can the elderly reduce their risk of a fracture?

INTRODUCTION

With advancing age it becomes more difficult to perform many functional activities, even some basic activities of daily living become taxing. One

.contributing factor is the increased risk of falling. The annual incidence of falls is approximately 30% in persons over the age of 65 years and increases to around 50% in those over 80years of age.[1] In 1999 in the United Kingdom almost 1 in 3 persons over the age of 60 presenting at accident and emergency departments had a fall-related injury.[2] One third to one half of people over 65 years of age will have at least one fall annually.[3]

The health and financial repercussions of falls are substantial. In 1997, 9% of the non-institutionalized elderly population of the United States reported medical conditions related to falls; the estimated total direct medical cost of these conditions was $6.2 billion in 1997 and $7.8 billion in 2002.[4] The mean cost per person who had fallen was $2591 in 2002. The health ramifications of falls range from a fatal outcome through permanent incapacity to recovery with increased risk of a subsequent fall. The propensity to fall escalates with increasing age. Both the incidence of falls and the severity of fall-related complications rise steadily after age 60.[5]

THE ELDERLY AT RISK

Many elderly people appear unsteady. In general the risk of falling is increased by an unsafe environment and/or pathophysiological changes. Impaired sensory processes, musculoskeletal dysfunction and/or impaired central coordination directly increase the propensity to fall. Box 5.1 provides guidelines on how to assess those who are prone to falls.

Box 5.1   Falls: an approach to clinical assessment

Assessment of a patient who is prone to falls should include:

1. Sensory evaluation with respect to:
   a. vision
   b. proprioception
   c. vestibular function.
2. Central nervous system assessment incorporating evaluation of cerebral, cerebellar and basal ganglion function. Particularly useful information is obtained by assessing:
   a. gait
   b. muscle tone and reflexes
   c. any tremors that may be present.
3. Musculoskeletal system evaluation embracing consideration of :
   a muscle strength
   b joint mobility and stability
   c foot health
   d cervical range of motion and osteoarthritis.
4. Blood pressure fluctuations. Blackouts may result from:
   a. postural hypotension/syncope
   b. carotid sinus syncope
   c. exercise hypotension.

Sensory impairment

Sensory impairments are common among older adults. Among adults 70 years of age and over, 18.1% report vision impairment, 33.2% report hearing loss and 8.6% report both hearing and vision deficits.[6] Approximately 1 in 28 Americans over 40 years of age is affected by low vision or blindness.[7] Among community-dwelling adults, the prevalence of low vision and blindness increases dramatically with age, and between 2000 and 2020 the prevalence of blindness is expected to double.[7]

Physiological changes associated with the aging eye include: decreased tear viscosity, colour and light sensitivity, increased eyelid laxity and impaired lens accommodation. Problems with focusing start around the age of 40 years. More than 9 in 10 persons over the age of 65 years require glasses. Increased susceptibility to glare and greater difficulty in seeing at low illumination levels i.e. poor night vision, are noted after 50; by the age of 70 years the ability to distinguish fine details may decline.[8,9] By 85 years of age 1 in 4 persons is visually impaired and 1 in 9 is blind.

In addition to age-related changes, ocular diseases may further compromise vision. Particular problems encountered with aging are:

- Presbyopia. This is a degenerative condition. The relative inflexibility of the lens in this condition, first noted in late middle age, is associated with blurring of near vision. In elderly persons the ability of the lens to become sufficiently convex is impaired. Spectacles correct the problem.
- Senile cataracts. Cataracts cause a painless loss of visual acuity due to lens opacity. The condition is corrected by surgery. Persons with a history of prolonged unprotected exposure to sunlight/ultraviolet light are at increased risk of senile cataracts.
- Senile or age-related macular degeneration involves damage to the macular area. Age-related macular degeneration presents with loss of central vision. In senile macular degeneration peripheral vision is retained. Standing to the side rather than directly in front of a person with senile macular degeneration places you in their area of sight, i.e. in the peripheral visual field. Wet (neovascularization) macular degeneration is treatable with laser photocoagulation; dry (depigmentation) macular degeneration is progressive and does not respond to treatment.
- Glaucoma. Persons over 40 years of age should be screened for glaucoma. Glaucoma presents with loss of peripheral vision.
- Diabetic retinopathy. The risk of blindness due to diabetic retinopathy increases dramatically in persons who have had the disease for 15 or more years.

Although vision is the principal method used, vestibular function and proprioception also provide information about body position with increasing age. Vestibular input is essential to provide rapid accurate information for reflexively adapting to unexpected body displacements. The maculae provide information about the static position of the head relative to gravity and the semicircular canals provide input about acceleration. In addition to vestibular function deteriorating with age, the elderly are more prone to vestibular disorders such as acute labyrinthitis, Ménière's Disease and benign positional vertigo.

Proprioception may also be compromised in the elderly, particularly in those with diabetes, alcoholism, spondylosis and nutritional deficiencies whether due to dietary or absorption problems. Vitamin B12 deficiency in the elderly may result from, among other causes, dietary insufficiency and atrophic gastritis.

Musculoskeletal inadequacies

As sensory input is reduced in the elderly, postural tasks become more difficult and require greater attention than in younger people. The situation is further aggravated by normal aging which is associated with reduced muscle strength and tone.

An adequate motor response to sensory input requires both muscle strength and joint mobility. A small study concluded that the contribution of the support limb to prevent a fall after tripping was decreased in older adults and surmised that lower limb strength could be an underlying factor and strength training might help to reduce fall risk.[10] Muscle strength declines by 22% in women and 23% in men between 30 and 70 years of age.[8,9] While loss of muscle power may be minimized by exercise, disease processes such as arthritis and foot problems may make exercise and/or balance difficult.

The elderly are at increased risk of lower limb pathologies such as arthritis, peripheral vascular disease and foot pain especially due to calluses or corns. All these factors converge to increase the risk of falling. Tripping is a major cause for falls, especially in the elderly.

Coordination catastrophes

Along with insufficient quadriceps muscle strength and a history of falls, body balance deficits make up the three primary predictors of falls. Central processing of sensory data and mounting a coordinated response is the function of both the cerebrum and cerebellum. Speed, accuracy and coordination are essential to avoid imbalance. A common condition in the elderly which may impair this process at the cognitive level is dementia. Disorders of the central nervous system can have a substantial impact on gait and balance, e.g. Parkinson's disease with its disordered basal ganglion function, a cerebrovascular accident or cerebellar lesion.

Gait disorders predispose to falls. Parkinsonism, an imbalance between the concentration of dopamine and acetylcholine in the basal ganglion region of the brain, presents as a movement disorder. Bradykinesis, rigidity and a festinating gait combine to increase the risk of falls in elderly persons with this condition.

In addition to lower extremity weakness and gait disorders, the effects of medications on the nervous system are causally related to a substantial proportion of falls in the elderly.[1,11] Polymedication and abnormal mobility were associated with significant changes in gait[12] and gait changes in dual-task conditions have been associated with an increased risk of falling in older frail adults.

Elderly users of psychotropic drugs increased their risk of falling by almost 47%,[13] yet sedatives are available for over-the-counter purchase.[14] Using atypical antipsychotic drugs and benzodiazepine, regardless of the length of their half-life, increased risk.[13] Antihistamines, different classes of psychotropic medications, including antipsychotic agents, benzodiazepines and non-benzodiazepine sedative-hypnotics all increase the risk of falling.[13,14]

ENVIRONMENTAL RISKS

Environmental factors seem to be responsible for about half of the falls in the elderly. An Australian study found that 80% of homes in which persons over 70 years of age resided had at least one hazard and 39% had more than five hazards.[15] The bathroom was identified as the most hazardous room. Hazards related to floor surfaces and the absence of appropriate grab or handrails. Loose rugs, slippery floors, uneven door thresholds, poor lighting, unsafe stairs, the absence of handrails or handrails that are too high or too low, and chairs without arm supports all contribute to the environmental risk of falling in old age.

PREDICTING INDIVIDUAL RISK

A number of factors interact to increase the risk of falling. A study of community-dwelling elderly identified postural sway, number of falls in the previous year, hand grip strength and depression as four determinants of risk.[16] A study on hostel dwellers concluded that significant independent risk factors for falls in the elderly were poor balance, cognitive impairment, incontinence, higher illness severity rating and older age.[17] A study of nursing home residents reported depression, impaired cognitive function, poor balance and mobility independently and interactively increased risk.[18] And a hospital based study found older age, male gender, number of comorbidities, recent surgical procedure and longer duration of hospitalization were associated with an increased risk of falls.[19] Impaired integration of sensory inputs, increased response time to unexpected perturbation, visual impairment, reduced tactile sensitivity, lower limb proprioception and poor general health all contribute to postural unsteadiness and increase the propensity for elderly persons to fall.[20]

Assessment tools to identify frail elderly individuals at risk have been developed.[16,17] The Falls Risk Score based on Balance × Standardized Mini Mental Status Examination × Illness Severity × Age × Incontinence can be used to identify potential single, recurrent, or multiple fallers.[8] A person with a high score (≥7) would have almost a 2 in 3 chance of falling in the first 6 months, while someone with a low score (<3) would have only a 1 in 7 chance of falling.

FRACTURES: A POTENTIAL OUTCOME OF FALLING

Age is the most important independent indicator of the risk of fractures. The risk of a fracture is related both to the strength of the bone and the risk of falling. Advanced age is the best predictor of osteoporosis, but bone mineral density (BMD) is only one factor associated with risk of an osteoporotic fracture—only 44% of women with non-vertebral fractures were reported to have a T-score below −2.5 SD.[21] While the propensity to fall, visual impairment, and reduced mobility also all correlate with increasing age, patients with osteoporosis are at greatest risk. Hip and vertebral fractures are particularly important.

Factors predicting an increased risk of a hip fracture on falling due to underlying osteoporosis include: low BMD, a history of hip, radius or vertebral fracture in a first degree relative, a personal history of a fracture after the age of 40, current cigarette smoking, low body weight, certain medications/diseases, hip pain, the inability of the hip to bear weight and a shortened externally rotated leg. Studies[21] suggest:

- A predicted escalation from about 1.7 million new hip fractures worldwide in 1990 to 2.6 million in 2025.
- A 10% to 20% higher mortality than expected for their age in women who have sustained a hip fracture. Hip fractures among a relatively healthy group of women increased the relative risk of dying almost six-fold—some 24% of patients over the age of 50 years died in the year following the fracture!
- A three- to six-fold increase in the risk of a hip fracture from 50 to 80 years of age.
- Prolonged and severe disability with 25% of patients requiring long term care and only 15% of patients being able to walk across a room unaided 6 months after sustaining a hip fracture.

The statistics surrounding vertebral fractures are equally alarming and include:[21]

- 1 in 8 persons 50–79 years old with no history of fracture having evidence of vertebral deformity.
- A two- to three-fold increased risk of a subsequent fracture of a different type following a vertebral fracture. The relative risk of a fracture is 11.8 times greater if more than one vertebral fracture has been sustained.[22]
- Relatively healthy women with a vertebral fracture have a nine-fold increased risk of dying. Approximately half the deaths occur within a year of the fracture.
- Women with vertebral fractures may have decreased physical function, back pain, loss of height due to crush fractures of the spine, and impairment of social contact.

Factors predicating an increased risk of a spinal fracture due to the presence of osteoporosis include: backache lessened or intensified when not lying down, restricted spinal movement, flexion reduced more than extension, a pronounced kyphosis, loss of height, an arm span–height difference of over 3 cm (especially if over 70 years of age and less than 160 cm tall), decreased exercise tolerance due to postural changes, feeling bloated after small meals, a protruding abdomen and skin folds overlying the margin of the ribs/pelvis.

Compared with women who received normal medical care, screening and treatment over a 6-year period can reduce the incidence of hip fractures by 36%.[21] While the single strongest marker of a future fracture is a previous fracture, there are a number of modifiable factors that indicate an increased risk of an osteoporotic linked fracture. Tobacco use and a BMI of less than 23 individually increase the relative risk of a fracture by at least a factor of 5.[22] Smoking appears to accelerate bone loss from both the femoral neck and total body in the elderly.[23] Furthermore, quitting is associated with an increased body weight. Similarly, nutrition is important for bone structure. Elderly patients are prone to less efficient calcium absorption, particularly those with achlorhydria. Furthermore, the current recommended daily allowance of vitamin D and calcium for the elderly appears to be too low.[24] Elderly people and persons using heavy sun screens require a dietary intake of 400 to 800 IU of vitamin D per day.[25] Moreover, supplementing elderly persons with mild vitamin D deficiency not only has a positive effect on the functional health index but also appears to reduce the rate of falls.[26] Certainly, compared to those offered home safety inspection with dietary and health advice, females who took 1000 mg of elemental calcium as calcium carbonate and 400 IU vitamin D daily had a 12% risk reduction in severe falls.[27] Routine calcium and vitamin D supplementation of elderly persons deserves consideration.

REDUCING THE RISK OF FALLING

Given the plethora of risk factors, a multipronged approach to fall prevention is needed.[5,28] The risk of falling can be reduced by exercise programs aimed to increase muscle strength and improve balance. More recently it has been suggested that long term essential amino acid supplementation which includes excess leucine may further reduce falling by limiting sarcopenia.[29] Sarcopenia, calculated by dividing the appendicular skeletal muscle mass by height, is a relative skeletal muscle index below $5.45 \, \text{kg}/\text{m}^2$.[30] Age-related muscle mitochondrial dysfunction shown to be related to reduced mtDNA and adenosine triphosphate (ATP) production is believed to contribute to the functional muscular changes observed in the elderly.[31] Current research suggests progressive loss of muscle mass associated with aging may respond to amino acid supplementation.

The risk of falling can be reduced by minimizing environmental hazards, e.g. scatter rugs, by treating functional aberrations such as postural hypotension and extrapyramidal signs, and by avoiding unnecessary medications. Fall-prone persons are also most likely to stumble when attempting to perform attention-demanding tasks while walking.[32] In addition to reducing the risk of falling, the risk of fractures can be minimized by protecting bone mass and providing information on how to fall 'safely' (see Patient Handout 5.1). Devices such as hip protectors may offer a degree of protection by decreasing the skeletal impact of falling.

The best approach is to select a combination of the intervention strategies best suited to the needs of the individuals.

An 80-year-old woman presents for a check up. She says she has had a few nasty falls. She reports some dizzy spells recently. She has some neck stiffness and a slight headache, worst on waking. She does not report any vomiting. She is somewhat hearing impaired. She is on medication for her blood pressure and has placed herself on a 'salt-free' diet.

Questions arising

- Can the underlying problem causing this woman's falls be corrected?
- How may she reduce her risk of falling?
- What can be done to avoid sustaining a fracture should she fall?

Clinical considerations

The differential diagnosis includes:

- Cervical spondylosis
- Positional vertigo
- Postural hypotension
- Impacted ear wax
- Transient ischaemic attack (especially vertebral ischaemia)
- Anaemia.

Gather more information to reach a working diagnosis.

On further questioning you find that the patient's dizziness is transient and occurs on standing. Dizziness is not precipitated by wearing blouses with tight collars or by various head positions. You confirm she has limited neck mobility and cervical osteophytes are noted on X-ray. She has no neurological deficits. She has recently had her ears syringed.

Clinical considerations

The working diagnosis is postural hypotension precipitated by the changed drug therapy and her self-imposed low salt diet. Alpha-blockers, vasodilators and ACE inhibitors all predispose to postural hypotension.

Management considerations include:

- Modification of her medication
- Advice on falling safely (see Patient Handout 5.1).

- ◆ Falls contribute to morbidity and mortality statistics in old age.
- ◆ Age-related visual changes include intolerance of glare, impaired depth perception, reduced nocturnal acuity and diminished peripheral vision.
- ◆ Improving the intensity of lighting enhances visual acuity while increasing light–dark contrast enhances depth perception.
- ◆ Screening for diminished visual acuity with the Snellen chart is recommended for elderly persons.
- ◆ The risk of falls can be decreased by managing household hazards.
- ◆ Regular exercise protects bone, retards muscle weakening and improves coordination and balance.
- ◆ Falling 'carefully' can reduce the risk of injury.
- ◆ The risk of injury on falling can be minimized by good bone health.
- ◆ Elderly patients who are prone to falling are at increased risk when operating motor vehicles. Driving is an integrated activity involving cognition, a knowledge of road regulation and how to operate a motor vehicle, visual and auditory processes, and an intact musculoskeletal system capable of manual dexterity, coordination, strength and good reaction time.

References

1. Steinweg KK. The changing approach to falls in the elderly. Am Fam Physician 1977; 56(7):1815–1823.
2. Scuffham P, Chaplin S, Legood R. Incidence and costs of unintentional falls in older people in the United Kingdom. J Epidemiol Community Health 2003 Sept; 57(9):740–744.
3. Downton JH, Andrews K. Prevalence, characteristics and factors associated with falls among the elderly living at home. Aging (Milano) 1991; 3:219–228.
4. Carroll NV, Slattum PW, Cox FM. The cost of falls among the community-dwelling elderly. J Manag Care Pharm 2005;11(4):307–316.
5. American Geriatrics Society, British Geriatrics Society, American Academy of Orthopaedic Surgeons Panel on Falls Prevention. Guideline for the prevention of falls in older persons. J Am Geriatr Soc 2001; 49:664–672.
6. Campbell VA, Crews JE, et al. Surveillance for sensory impairment, activity limitation, and health-related quality of life among older adults—United States, 1993–1997. Mor Mortal Wkly Rep CDC Surveill Summ 1999 Dec 17; 48(8):131–156.
7. Gohdes DM, Balamurugan A, et al. Age-related eye diseases: an emerging challenge for public health professionals. Prev Chronic Dis 2005; 2(3):A17.
8. US Department of Health and Human Services. With the passage of time: the Baltimore Longitudinal Study of Aging. NIH Pub No 93–3685. Washington DC: Public Health Service; 1993:1–52.
9. US Department of Health and Human Services. In search of the secrets of aging. NIH Pub No 93–2756. Washington DC: Public Health Service; 1993:1–46.
10. Pijnappels M, Bobbert MF, van Dieen JH. Push-off reactions in recovery after tripping discriminate young subjects, older non-fallers and older fallers. Gait Posture 2005; 21(4):388–394.
11. Kane RL, Ouslander JG, Abrass IB. Essentials of clinical geriatrics. 3rd edn. New York: McGraw-Hill; 1994:200.
12. Beauchet O, Dubost V, et al. Relationship between dual-task related gait changes and intrinsic risk factors for falls among transitional frail older adults. Aging Clin Exp Res 2005; 17(4):270–275.
13. Landi F, Onder G, et al. Psychotropic medications and risk for falls among community-dwelling frail older people: an observational study. J Gerontol A Biol Sci Med Sci 2005; 60(5):622–626.
14. Francis SA, Barnett N, Denham M. Switching of prescription drugs to over-the-counter status : is it a good thing for the elderly? Drugs Aging 2005; 22(5):361–370.
15. Carter SE, Campbell EM, et al. Environmental hazards in the homes of older people. Age Ageing 1997; 26(3):195–202.
16. Stalenhoef PA, Diederiks JP, et al. A risk model for the prediction of recurrent falls in community-dwelling elderly: a prospective cohort study. J Clin Epidemiol 2002; 55:1088–1094.
17. Chen JS, March LM, et al. A multivariate regression model predicted falls in residents living in intermediate hostel care. J Clin Epidemiol 2005; 58(5):503–508.
18. Kose N, Cuvalci S, et al. The risk factors of fall and their correlation with balance, depression, cognitive impairment and mobility skills in elderly nursing home residents. Saudi Med J 2005; 26(6):978–981.
19. Halfon P, Eggli Y, et al. Risk of falls for hospitalized patients: a predictive model based on routinely available data. J Clin Epidemiol 2001; 54:1258–1266.
20. Kuczynski M, Ostrowska B. Understanding falls in osteoporosis: the viscoelastic modeling perspective. Gait Posture 2006; 23(1):51–58.
21. Reginster JY, Burlet N. Osteoporosis: a still increasing prevalence. Bone 2006; 38(2 Suppl 1): 4–9.
22. Ullom-Minnich P. Prevention of osteoporosis and fractures. Amer Family Phys 1999; 60: 194–202.
23. Krall EA, Dawson-Hughes B. Smoking increases bone loss and decreases intestinal calcium absorption. J Bone Miner Res 1999; 14(2):215–220.
24. Russell RM. New views on the RDAs for older adults. J Am Diet Assoc 1997; 97(5): 515–518.
25. Barrett-Connor E, Chang JC, Edelstein SL. Coffee-associated osteoporosis offset by daily milk consumption. The Rancho Bernardo Study. JAMA 1994; 271(4):280–283.
26. Nowson CA. The significance of vitamin D to health in Australia. Asia Pac J Clin Nutr 2005; 14 Suppl:S17.
27. Larsen ER, Mosekilde L, Foldspang A. Vitamin D and calcium supplementation prevents severe falls in elderly community-dwelling women: a pragmatic population-based 3-year intervention study. Aging Clin Exp Res 2005; 17(2):125–132.
28. Hogan D. Preventing falls in older adults. Canadian Medical Association leadership series: elder care 2005; 4:37–38.

29. Fujita S, Volpi E. Amino acids and muscle loss with aging. J Nutr 2006; 136(1):277S–280S.

30. Walsh MC, Hunter GR, Livingstone MB. Sarcopenia in premenopausal and postmenopausal women with osteopenia, osteoporosis and normal bone mineral density. Osteoporos Int 2006; 17(1):61–67.

31. Short KR, Bigelow ML, et al. Decline in skeletal muscle mitochondrial function with aging in humans. Proc Natl Acad Sci USA. 2005; 102(15):5618–5623.

32. Beauchet O, Dubost V, et al. Relationship between dual-task related gait changes and intrinsic risk factors for falls among transitional frail older adults. Aging Clin Exp Res 2005; 17(4):270–275.

PATIENT HANDOUT 5.1 – REDUCING THE RISK OF FALLS AND FRACTURES

Step I: Identify The Risk Of Falling

The more boxes you tick the greater the risk.

Unalterable risks

- ☐ Increasing age—especially after 60 years of age
- ☐ Female
- ☐ History of prior falls
- ☐ Dementia/Impaired cognition
- ☐ Dizziness due to inner ear disease
- ☐ Altered peripheral sensation

Potentially modifiable risks

- ☐ Stroke
- ☐ Lower extremity arthritis
- ☐ Impaired vision
- ☐ Weakness
- ☐ Lower extremity abnormality
- ☐ Impaired balance
- ☐ Abnormal gait
- ☐ Impaired ability to perform daily activities of living

Modifiable risks

- ☐ Taking four or more medications
- ☐ Taking psychotropic medication, e.g. benzodiazepine, hypnotic, antidepressant, antipsychotic
- ☐ Environmental risks, e.g. loose rugs, poor lighting

Step II: Tips for Preventing Falls

1. Have regular vision checks and replace spectacles as indicated.
2. Fit hand and grab rails.
3. Discard or replace loose or slippery floor coverings.
4. Ensure good lighting—consider using night lights.
5. Buy comfortable sensible foot wear.
6. Exercise regularly to increase muscle strength, flexibility, balance and endurance.
7. See if you can modify any of the risks in Step I you checked.

Step III: Reduce Injury From Falls

Fall 'safely'
When falling:

- ■ Fold your arms around your head.
- ■ Try to roll forward.
- ■ Relax your body.
- ■ Attempt to land on a well-padded area, e.g. buttocks, thigh, shoulder.

Strengthen bones

- ■ Take 1000 mg calcium and 400 IU vitamin D daily.
- ■ Exercise regularly—walk 30 minutes a day.
- ■ Consider resistance exercises to strengthen particular muscle groups.

Step IV: Use Internet Resources

Some advice about exercise:
http://www.niapublications.org/engagepages/exercise.asp—exercise for endurance, strength, balance and flexibility

http://www.niapublications.org/exercisebook/ExerciseGuideComplete.pdf—a complete exercise guide

http://www.agingwell.state.ny.us/fitness/index.htm—exercises to improve flexibility, strength and balance

Some facts about falls and hip fractures in older adults:
http://www.phppo.cdc.gov/cdcRecommends/showarticle.asp?a_artid=1111++++&TopNum=50&CallPg=Adv

Some tips for preventing falls:
http://www.phppo.cdc.gov/cdcRecommends/showarticle.asp?a_artid=P0000767&TopNum=50&CallPg=Adv

http://www.niapublications.org/engagepages/falls.asp

Chapter **6**

Menopause: Meeting the challenge

An obese 65-year-old woman presents complaining of fatigue. She says she is sleeping badly and feels generally anxious. She asks if she should be on hormone replacement therapy.

- Is this woman's presentation attributable to menopause?
- Would hormone replacement therapy (HRT) benefit this patient?
- Under what circumstances is HRT indicated and contraindicated?

INTRODUCTION

Menopause is that physiological stage of life during which women adjust to oestrogen deprivation. As the median age of menopause in women in developed countries is around 50 years of age, approximately 30 years of adult life are spent in an oestrogen deprived state. The nature and intensity of menopausal symptoms vary in different women and are related to oestrogen fluctuations. Hormone replacement therapy (HRT) is a therapeutic option. For maximum benefit it is necessary to start HRT shortly after the start of the menopause.[1]

THE MENOPAUSAL CHALLENGE

The biological impact of menopause is evident in both the short and long term. In the short term menopause presents with missed menstrual periods, vasomotor instability, urogenital atrophy and psychological changes. Vasomotor instability presents as hot flushes, night sweats, palpitations, insomnia and dizziness. Urogenital atrophy causes vaginal dryness, dyspareunia, vulvo-vaginal itching, dysuria, frequency, urgency and predisposes to incontinence. Symptoms that appear to be specifically related to hormonal changes of menopausal transition are vasomotor symptoms, vaginal dryness and breast tenderness.[2] Short term oestrogen replacement therapy benefits vasomotor and urogenital symptoms and may improve mood.

Prolonged withdrawal of oestrogen is associated with an increased health risk, particularly of developing osteoporosis and cardiovascular disease. In fact, after menopause the probability of developing various chronic diseases has been estimated to be around 46% for ischaemic heart disease, 20% for stroke, 15% for hip fracture, 10% for breast cancer and 2.6% for endometrial cancer.[3]

THE PARADOX

Hormone replacement therapy is readily available yet is not routinely recommended. In fact, the US Preventive Services Task Force (USPSTF) recommends against the routine use of combined oestrogen and progestin for the prevention of chronic conditions in postmenopausal women.[4] Despite there being good evidence that combined therapy reduces the risk of fractures and fair evidence it reduces the risk of colorectal cancer, the long term risk is deemed to outweigh any benefit. In addition to definitely posing an increased risk of breast cancer and venous thromboembolism, combined therapy may predispose to coronary heart disease. There is also fair evidence that combined therapy increases the risk of a stroke, cholecystitis and dementia and lowers global cognitive function.[4]

The USPSTF also recommends against the routine use of unopposed oestrogen for the prevention of chronic conditions in postmenopausal women even if they have had a hysterectomy.[4] While oestrogen alone may decrease a woman's risk for fractures, they feel there is insufficient evidence to determine its effects on colorectal cancer or all cause mortality. In fact, while both the combined and oestrogen only arms of the trial showed an increased rate of thromboembolic events and stroke and protection against fractures, only combined therapy appeared to protect against colon cancer and cause a non-statistically significant increased incidence of cardio-vascular events and breast cancer.[5]

Much of the concern surrounding use of hormone replacement therapy arose from the findings of the Woman's Health Initiative (WHI) randomized controlled trial which was conducted in 40 clinical centres and enrolled 10 739 postmenopausal woman aged 50–79 years.[6,7] Although well designed and executed, the relevance of the study's findings to standard hormone therapy for clinical practice is being questioned,[7,8] the major objection being that the target population used in the WHI trial was not representative of the target population for whom menopausal HRT is normally considered. It was also suggested, given the diverse pharmacokinetic properties of various hormone preparations, that benefits may be increased and risks reduced by careful drug selection e.g. *17beta*-estradiol at the lowest dosage level may provide safe and effective therapy for most indications. Other considerations include norethisterone acetate in preference to medroxyprogesterone acetate; or transdermal rather than oral hormone delivery.[9] There was consensus that HRT should be given to women with menopausal complaints to meet their individual needs, taking into account their individual risk profile and the overall therapeutic objectives. Timing with respect to initiating therapy and the duration of treatment was deemed critical.[7]

WEIGHING THE OPTIONS

Current thinking is that menopausal hormone replacement improves symptoms due to vasomotor imbalance and genital atrophy and prevents osteoporosis-related fracture but does increase the likelihood of venous thromboembolism.[10] There is irrefutable evidence that HRT increases the risk of thrombosis, both by early activation of coagulation and some reduction in circulating anticoagulants.[11] Nonetheless, it has been suggested that interpretation of the results of the WHI study should not put into question the validity of prescribing combined HRT in early menopause.[8] Furthermore, meta-analyses of numerous observational studies and the WHI trial, which confirmed an increased risk of ischaemic heart disease, stroke, thromboembolic events and breast cancer, found this risk occurred after 5 or more years of hormone replacement.[12] Short term therapy in appropriate circumstances appears a viable option, particularly in women who have no increased risk of breast cancer.

Breast cancer remains a concern. Analysis of the most current pivotal trials and observational studies suggests that the risk of breast cancer outweighs the benefits of osteoporosis prevention from HRT and confirms that any use of combined or oestrogen only replacement therapy should be limited to the shortest possible duration.[13] The increased risk of incident and fatal breast cancer appears to be substantially greater for oestrogen–progestogen combinations than for other types of HRT.[14]

Further controlled studies are required to determine the significance of any breast cancer risk and clarify the effects of hormone replacement on cardiovascular or central nervous system disease prevention.[10,15] Controversy continues and concern persists.

Alternatives to HRT for preventing postmenopausal osteoporosis have been advocated.[13] However, acceptance of herbs, botanicals and some foods for treatment of menopausal symptoms may be 'based on little more than advertising and consumers' desire to believe it'.[16]

PHYTO-OESTROGENS: A VIABLE ALTERNATIVE?

The chief problems with herbal and nutrient approaches have been lack of standards for sample selection, uncertainty about the concentration of active principles, and unclear or lax criteria for effectiveness.[16] Nonetheless, a review of randomized, controlled trials of complementary and alternative medicine (CAM) therapies for menopausal symptoms concluded black cohosh may be effective for menopausal symptoms, especially hot flushes, while soy might have modest benefit for hot flushes, although isoflavone preparations seemed less effective than soy foods.[17]

Phyto-oestrogens are a common denominator between soy and black cohosh. Phyto-oestrogens are a group of phytonutrients with oestrogen-like activity. With a high affinity for binding to the oestrogen receptor beta, these non-steroidal plant molecules show both agonist and antagonist activity. They are generally believed to be antagonistic in the oestrogen rich environment of the menstruating female but to act as stimulants in the oestrogen depleted environment of menopause. Various phytonutrients including isoflavones, indoles, coumestans, isothiocyanates and lignans have oestrogen-like activity. Although less potent than hormone replacement, phyto-oestrogens have greater tissue selectivity.[18] However, some studies suggest there is remarkably little evidence of benefit from phyto-oestrogen consumption.[19]

Twenty-four weeks of supplementation with soy (20 g/d, equivalent to 20 mg/d isoflavones) did not affect plasma levels of endogenous hormones (estradiol, follicle-stimulating hormone (FSH), luteinizing hormone (LH), prolactin, testosterone and dehydroepiandrosterone sulphate (DHEAS)) in a study of 16 postmenopausal women.[20] Similarly, a recent small study found that 50 g textured soy protein containing 60 mg total isoflavones daily for 10–14 days did not affect mean baseline or peak LH concentrations in pre- or postmenopausal women. While this suggested a lack of oestrogen-like effect at the level of the pituitary, mean LH secretion decreased after discontinuing soy in postmenopausal subjects.[21] A residual oestrogenic effect may explain this finding. Despite inconclusive scientific evidence and inadequate long term safety data, particularly on phyto-oestrogenic stimulation of the breast or endometrium, it may be premature to summarily dismiss the use of phyto-oestrogens for menopausal women.

DIETARY SOURCES OF PHYTO-OESTROGEN

Phyto-oestrogens are consumed in foods such as grains, beans, fruits and nuts. These foods contain varying quantities of isoflavones, lignans and other chemicals with recognized oestrogen-like activity. The main consumable plant sources of isoflavones are soybeans and chickpeas; of lignans, flaxseed; of indoles and isothiocyanates, cruciferous vegetables; while cereals, fruit and vegetables contain a variety of phenolic compounds. The North American Menopause Society commented that although the health effects in humans cannot be clearly attributed to isoflavones alone, foods or supplements that contain isoflavones do have some physiological effects.[22]

After 6 months on a diet rich in isoflavones, supplying an average daily dose of 50 mg genistein, the incidence of vasomotor episodes declines.[22,23] As little as 60–140 mg of soybeans daily may decrease hot flushes.[24] On the other hand, 3 months of soy supplements failed to provide symptomatic relief to older postmenopausal women with a high frequency of mild menopausal symptoms.[25] Nonetheless, within-group comparisons revealed that, unlike the placebo group, the active group reported a significant decrease in vaginal dryness. Furthermore, while some data would seem to support the efficacy of isoflavones in reducing the incidence and severity of hot flushes, the most convincing health effects are attributed to the actions of isoflavones on lipids and bone.[22,26]

An isoflavone-rich diet achieving a daily intake of 90 mg genistein reduces total cholesterol and low density lipoprotein (LDL) cholesterol and increases bone mineral density.[22,23] After 6 months on a soy rich diet, lipid profiles show a favourable outcome, similar to that observed in the hormone replacement group, even though compliance to the diet was low.[27] Consuming isoflavones (80.4 mg daily) in soy protein isolates appears to attenuate vertebral (lumbar) bone loss in perimenopausal women.[26]

A high intake of phyto-oestrogens may have untoward effects. Specific phyto-oestrogen compounds found in hop extracts exert oestrogen-like activities on bone metabolism; however, depending on their concentration, all compounds tested showed proliferative effects in MCF-7 breast cancer cells.[28] The biological impact of isoflavones is not limited to their oestrogenic and anti-oestrogenic effects. They can modify cell signalling conduction, and influence cell growth and death. Isoflavones have the potential to alter enzyme activities, inhibit protein tyrosine kinase, regulate gene transcription and modulate transcription factors.[29] Despite the potential for isoflavones to benefit cardiovascular and skeletal health, any recommendations suggesting long term high dose consumption of these phyto-oestrogens is premature.

HERBAL INTERVENTION

Dong quai, black cohosh, licorice root, red clover, evening primrose oil, St John's wort, Ginkgo biloba and ginseng are all popular menopausal remedies among peri- and menopausal women.[28,30,31] However, single clinical trials have questioned the efficacy of dong quai, evening primrose oil, a Chinese herb mixture, vitamin E, red clover and acupuncture.[17] Nonetheless, another study found women supplementing their diet with soy (29%), ginkgo biloba (16%), and black cohosh (10%) did perceive their quality of life to be improved, along with the overall control of menopausal symptoms, including vaginal dryness, libido and mood.[32] A word of caution. When dong quai, ginseng, black cohosh, and licorice root were tested in vitro it was found that dong quai and ginseng both significantly induced the growth of MCF-7 cells, a human breast cancer cell line.[30] Black cohosh and licorice root did not.

Black cohosh: herbal hope?

Black cohosh is a saponin containing herbs that may help adaptation to new hormonal levels.[33] A number of clinical studies using Remifemin, a standardized extract of black cohosh, have demonstrated its efficacy for the alleviation of menopausal complaints such as hot flushes, menopausal anxiety, sleep disturbances, mood swings and depression.[34] In fact, clinical trials suggest black cohosh extracts more effectively relieve menopausal symptoms than soy-rich diets.[35] Two recent studies found that black cohosh was effective against classic menopausal complaints, provided some osteoprotection and was deemed safe, even when the dosage was increased threefold.[35] Despite encouraging results,[36] some reservations persist. A randomized clinical trial among breast cancer patients concluded black cohosh was not significantly more efficacious than placebo against most menopausal symptoms—including the number and intensity of hot flushes.[37]

Targeting symptoms

Rather than attempting to modify menopausal symptoms globally, herbs may be selectively used to alleviate individual problems. St John's wort has been shown to substantially improve psychological and psychosomatic symptoms[38] and a randomized, multicentre, double-blind, parallel group study found ginseng reduced depression and enhanced wellbeing in postmenopausal women.[39] Kava, in conjunction with hormone replacement therapy, has been found to be effective against menopausal anxiety.[40] Its safety remains an issue.[41]

The ongoing dilemma

Safety and efficacy are problematic. While the evidence for black cohosh is promising, safety concerns for the use of other herbs may preclude their current use as a therapeutic option. Unlike pharmaceuticals, herbal products are not regulated for purity and potency and batch to batch variability is recognised to be associated with varying efficacy and side effects resulting from impurities.[42] Pharmacological differences have been reported within a single species of herb cultivated in two different locations.[43] The bioactive compounds present in different preparations of the same herb also vary depending on the plant species, the part of the plant used and the extraction method employed.[44] Plant identification, genetic variation, agronomic factors, the time and method of harvesting, post-harvest handling, manufacturing technique and stability all contribute to confusion regarding the clinical benefits of herbal therapy.[45]

Another problem encountered when considering the use of herbs for menopausal symptoms is whether an effect is clinically meaningful. A randomized, double-blind, placebo-controlled trial of menopausal women using isoflavones extracted from red clover detected a biological effect of Promensil but queried whether its effect on hot flushes or other symptoms of menopause was clinically important;[46] this despite other authors having suggested red clover may be useful for severe menopausal symptoms.[38] Until adequate standardization of preparations is achieved, the ongoing controversy and the absence of convincing evidence for alternative medicine options for menopause will persist.[38,47,48] Such reservations are not limited to herbal products but extend to include acupuncture.[17,49]

A HOLISTIC APPROACH

While it is premature to suggest that the use of alternative approaches provides satisfactory general management of menopausal symptoms, certain interventions may relieve particular symptoms in some patients. In the meantime using HRT for 5 or fewer years improves menopausal symptoms and does not adversely affect mortality.[50,51] A multidisciplinary approach that combines prevention, symptom management and health promotion may be most effective for women struggling to cope with the climacteric.[52,53]

Mrs Jones is a 49-year-old woman complaining of hot flushes and a disrupted menstrual cycle. She says she is sleeping badly, has night sweats and feels generally anxious. She asks if she should be on hormone replacement therapy.

Questions arising

- Are symptoms severe enough to warrant drug therapy?
- What is the benefit/risk ratio of HRT for this patient?
- Are there other options worth considering?
- Is the patient's major concern her current discomfort or the long term complications of oestrogen withdrawal?

Major clinical considerations

HRT is a personal choice. Counsel Mrs Jones and help her decide by asking her to complete Patient Handout 6.2.

In the event of Mrs Jones electing to take HRT to relieve her menopausal symptoms:

- monitor her progress
- screen for side effects
- advocate lifestyle measures to help her cope with symptoms
- encourage her to minimize the duration of HRT use.

Should she prefer not to take HRT, discuss the phyto-oestrogen option:

- a diet rich in soy products
- herbal supplementation with black cohosh.

Note that long term side effects of these interventions have not been clarified. While these oestrogen replacement options may alleviate most, if not all the symptoms of menopause, management of particular symptoms may also be considered.

Attacking individual problems

- Insomnia. Identify any factors, other than menopause, that may contribute to disturbed sleep. See www.jamisonhealth.com Handout 9.4.

  Provide her with tips for improving her sleep pattern. See www.jamisonhealth.com Handout 9.5. Other options are available—a warm glass of milk on retiring, taking tryptophan or a herbal remedy. Valerian and kava kava are both used to improve sleep and alleviate anxiety.
- Anxiety. In addition to chemical remedies, there are cognitive behavioural options for managing stress and reducing anxiety. See Handouts 16.7–16.14 at www.jamisonhealth.com.

  See Handout 16.14 to work out a comprehensive stress management program if necessary. Numerous options to decrease arousal are available. Select from Handouts 16.7–16.13.
- Long term consequences of hormone depletion. The side effects of HRT are most pronounced when it is taken over a number of years. Women concerned about the long term effects of oestrogen deprivation require long term management for osteoporosis prevention. In these instances careful consideration should be given to lifestyle and pharmaceutical interventions that minimize the risk of osteoporosis and other disorders prevalent in postmenopausal women, including coronary artery disease, stroke and cancer.

- For symptomatic relief of menopause, HRT should be curtailed within 5 years; for other benefits, therapy may be needed for 5–10 years.
- The risk/benefit ratio of HRT in women untroubled by climacteric symptoms is generally unfavourable.
- HRT in menopausal women reduces the osteoporotic fracture risk by 50–80% for as long as therapy is continued. For past users risk is reduced by 10–20%.
- Locally applied oestrogens are low risk and effective for relieving symptoms of urogenital aging.
- Women under 60 years of age benefit most from HRT for vasomotor and psychological symptoms of menopause.
- HRT does not provide contraceptive protection for perimenopausal women.
- Oestrogen relaxes the blood vessel wall and reduces anginal pain in women but not men.
- Lipoprotein (a) contains a protein that impedes the dissolution of blood clots. Lipoprotein a levels increase in menopause and HRT reduces these levels.
- The increased risk of venous thromboembolism, coronary heart disease and stroke arises within the first 1–2 years of combined HRT; other risks, e.g. breast cancer, only increase with longer term hormone replacement.
- Tobacco consumption may alter oestrogen metabolism and decrease responsiveness to oestrogen—smoking may diminish the benefits of oestrogen replacement.

- Boron deficiency may reduce the beneficial effects of hormone replacement therapy resulting in exacerbation of both osteoporosis and menopausal symptoms.
- Oestrogen may have a direct cardioprotective effect on endothelial cells which persists even when the lipid modulating benefit of oestrogen is counteracted by progestogens.
- Introduction of HRT should be considered in early menopause; it is probably no longer an option from 5 years from the onset of menopause.
- Phyto-oestrogens are routinely consumed in a diet containing plant foods—2 cups of soy milk or 200 g of tofu provides 50 mg of isoflavones.
- The physiological impact of dietary phyto-oestrogens is influenced by the hormonal status of the woman.
- Scientific evidence reporting the clinical impact of dietary phyto-oestrogens is contradictory.
- The potency of different phyto-oestrogens varies and genistein, found in soy products, promises to provide health benefits to oestrogen deprived women; however, potential adverse effects from ingestion of high doses of phyto-oestrogens have not been ruled out.
- Bio-identical hormone creams synthesized from wild yam or soya beans with 80% oestriol and 20% oestradiol are available—they appear to relieve hot flushes without side effects.

References

1. Shaywitz SE, Shaywitz BA, et al. Effect of estrogen on brain activation patterns in postmenopausal women during working memory tasks. JAMA 1999; 281:1197–1202.

2. Dennerstein L, Dudley EC, et al. A prospective population-based study of menopausal symptoms. Obstet Gynecol 2000; 96(3):351–358.

3. Grady D, Rubin SM, et al. Hormone therapy to prevent disease and prolong life in postmenopausal women. Ann Intern Med 1992; 117(12):1016-1037.

4. US Preventive Services Task Force (USPSTF). Hormone therapy for the prevention of chronic conditions in postmenopausal women. 2005. Online. Available: http://www.ahrq.gov/clinic/uspstf/uspspmho.htm

5. Harman SM, Brinton EA, et al. Is the WHI relevant to HRT started in the perimenopause? Endocrine 2004; 24(3):195–202.

6. Rossouw JE, Anderson GL, et al. Risks and benefits of estrogen plus progestin in healthy postmenopausal women: principal results from the Women's Health Initiative randomized controlled trial. JAMA 2002; 288(3):321–333.

7. Burger H. Hormone replacement therapy in the post-Women's Health Initiative era. Report of a meeting held in Funchal, Madeira, February 24–25, 2003. Climacteric 2003; (6 Suppl 1):11–36.

8. Lemay A. The relevance of the Women's Health Initiative results on combined hormone replacement therapy in clinical practice. J Obstet Gynaecol Can 2002; 24(9):711–715.

9. Modena MG, Sismondi P, et al. New evidence regarding hormone replacement therapies is urgently required. Transdermal postmenopausal hormone therapy differs from oral hormone therapy in risks and benefits. Maturitas 2005 Sept 16; 52(1):1–10.

10. Bhavnani BR, Strickler RC. Menopausal hormone therapy. J Obstet Gynaecol Can 2005; 27(2):137–162.

11. Hoibraaten E, Qvigstad E, et al. The effects of hormone replacement therapy (HRT) on hemostatic variables in women with previous venous thromboembolism—results from a randomized, double-blind, clinical trial. Thromb Haemost 2001; 85(5):775–781.

12. Nelson HD, Humphrey LL, et al. Postmenopausal hormone replacement therapy: scientific review. JAMA 2002; 288(7):872-881.

13. Deady J. Clinical monograph: hormone replacement therapy. J Manag Care Pharm 2004; 10(1):33–47.

14. Beral V, Million Women Study Collaborators. Breast cancer and hormone-replacement therapy in the Million Women Study. Lancet 2003; 362(9390):1160.

15. Craig MC, Maki PM, Murphy DG. The Women's Health Initiative memory study: findings and implications for treatment. Lancet Neurol 2005; 4(3):190–194.

16. Taylor M. Alternatives to HRT: an evidence-based review. Int J Fertil Womens Med 2003; 48(2):64–68.

17. Kronenberg F, Fugh-Berman A. Complementary and alternative medicine for menopausal symptoms: a review of randomized, controlled trials. Ann Intern Med 2002; 137(10):805–813.

18. Ariyo AA, Villablanca AC. Estrogens and lipids. Can HRT designer estrogens, and phytoestrogens reduce cardiovascular risk markers after menopause? Postgrad Med 2002; 111(1):23–30.

19. Pinn G. Herbs used in obstetrics and gynaecology. Aust Fam Physician 2001; 30(4):351–354, 356.

20. Foth D, Nawroth F. Effect of soy supplementation on endogenous hormones in postmenopausal women. Gynecol Obstet Invest 2003; 55(3):135–138.

21. Nicholls J, Lasley BL, et al. Effects of soy consumption on gonadotropin secretion and acute pituitary responses to gonadotropin-releasing hormone in women. J Nutr 2002; 132(4):708–714.

22. Consensus opinion. The role of isoflavones in menopausal health. The North American Menopause Society. Menopause 2000; 7(4):215–229.

23. Arena S, Rappa C, et al. A natural alternative to menopausal hormone replacement therapy. Phytoestrogens. Minerva Ginecol 2002; 54(1):53–57.

24. Glisson J, Crawford R, Street S. The clinical applications of Ginkgo biloba, St John's Wort, Saw Palmetto, and soy. Nurse Practitioner 1999; 24: 28–49.

25. Kotsopoulos D, Dalais FS, et al. The effects of soy protein containing phytoestrogens on menopausal symptoms in postmenopausal women. Climacteric 2000; 3(3):161–167.

26. Alekel DL, Germain AS, et al. Isoflavone-rich soy protein isolate attenuates bone loss in the lumbar spine of perimenopausal women. Am J Clin Nutr 2000; 72(3):844–852.

27. Chiechi LM, Secreto G, et al. The effects of a soy rich diet on serum lipids: the Menfis randomized trial. Maturitas 2002; 41(2):97–104.

28. Effenberger KE, Johnsen SA, et al. Regulation of osteoblastic phenotype and gene expression by hop-derived phytoestrogens. J Steroid Biochem Mol Biol 2005 Jul 11; [Epub ahead of print].

29. Ren MQ, Kuhn G, et al. Isoflavones, substances with multi-biological and clinical properties. Eur J Nutr 2001; 40(4):135–146.

30. Amato P, Christophe S, Mellon PL. Estrogenic activity of herbs commonly used as remedies for menopausal symptoms. Menopause 2002; 9(2):145–150.

31. Dailey RK, Neale AV, et al. Herbal product use and menopause symptom relief in primary care patients: a MetroNet study. J Womens Health (Larchmt) 2003; 12(7):633–641.

32. Kam IW, Dennehy CE, Tsourounis C. Dietary supplement use among menopausal women attending a San Francisco health conference. Menopause 2002; 9(1):72–78.

33. Mills S, Bone K. Principles and practice of Phytotherapy. Edinburgh: Churchill Livingstone; 2000:245.

34. McKenna DJ, Jones K, et al. Black cohosh: efficacy, safety, and use in clinical and preclinical applications. Altern Ther Health Med 2001; 7(3):93–100.

35. Viereck V, Emons G, Wuttke W. Black cohosh: just another phytoestrogen? Trends Endocrinol Metab 2005; 16(5):214–221.

36. Osmers R, Friede M, et al. Efficacy and safety of isopropanolic black cohosh extract for climacteric symptoms. Obstet Gynecol 2005; 105(5 Pt 1):1074–1083.

37. Jacobson JS, Troxel AB, et al. Randomized trial of black cohosh for the treatment of hot flashes among women with a history of breast cancer. J Clin Oncol 2001; 19(10):2739–2745.

38. Grube B, Walper A, Wheatley D. St. John's Wort extract: efficacy for menopausal symptoms of psychological origin. Adv Ther 1999; 16:177–186.

39. Wiklund IK, Mattsson LA, et al. Effects of a standardized ginseng extract on quality of life and physiological parameters in symptomatic postmenopausal women: a double-blind, placebo-controlled trial. Int J Clin Pharmacol Res 1999; 19:89–99.

40. De Leo V, la Marca A, et al. Evaluation of combining kava extract with hormone replacement therapy in the treatment of postmenopausal anxiety. Maturitas 2001; 39(2):185–188.

41. Huntley AL, Ernst E. A systematic review of herbal medicinal products for the treatment of menopausal symptoms. Menopause 2003; 10(5):465–476.

42. Cupp MJ. Herbal remedies: adverse effects and drug interactions. Am Fam Physician 1999; 59(5):1239–1245.

43. Yuan CS, Wu JA, et al. Gut and brain effects of American ginseng root on brainstem neuronal activities in rats. Am J Chin Med 1998; 26:47–55.

44. Linde K, ter Riet G, et al. Systematic reviews of complementary therapies—an annotated bibliography. Part 2: Herbal Medicine. BMC Comp & Alter Med 2001; 1:5.

45. Pinn G. Herbal medicine and overview. Aust Fam Phys 2000; 29(11):1059–1062.

46. Tice JA, Ettinger B, et al. Phytoestrogen supplements for the treatment of hot flashes: the Isoflavone Clover Extract (ICE) Study: a randomized controlled trial. JAMA 2003; 290(2):207–214.

47. Krebs EE, Ensrud KE, et al. Phytoestrogens for treatment of menopausal symptoms: a systematic review. Obstet Gynecol 2004; 104(4):824–836.

48. Barentsen R. Red clover isoflavones and menopausal health. J Br Menopause Soc 2004; 10 Suppl 1:4–7.

49. Wyon Y, Wijma K, et al. A comparison of acupuncture and oral estradiol treatment of vasomotor symptoms in postmenopausal women. Climacteric 2004; 7(2):153–164.

50. Pentti K, Honkanen R, et al. Hormone replacement therapy and mortality in 52- to 70-year-old women: the Kuopio Osteoporosis Risk Factor and Prevention Study. Eur J Endocrinol 2006; 154(1):101–107.

51. Barlow DH. Menopause and HRT—the state of the art in Europe. Maturitas 2005; 51(1):40–47.

52. Mitchell D. Menopause. J Comp Med 2006; 5(1):61–64.

53. O'Connell E. Mood, energy, cognition, and physical complaints: a mind/body approach to symptom management during the climacteric. J Obstet Gynecol Neonatal Nurs 2005; 34(2):274–279.

PATIENT HANDOUT 6.1 – MENOPAUSE: THE HRT OPTION

Menopause is a normal physiological event that occurs at an average age of 51 years. Most women will spend more than a third of their lives in a post-menopausal state. Hormone replacement therapy (HRT) is a popular option. It has been the accepted management for the symptoms and sequelae of menopause.

The advantages of HRT in postmenopausal women are that it modulates:

- vasomotor symptoms
- mood changes
- genito-urinary tissue atrophy
- osteoporosis and hip fractures
- heart disease
- colorectal cancer.

Other possible benefits of HRT are improved verbal memory and sleep.

Recently the benefits of HRT have been questioned.
Possible disadvantages include side effects and increased risk of disease:

- Side effects of oestrogen only replacement are:
  −breast discomfort
  −nausea
  −weight gain
  −temporary leg cramps.
- Additional side effects of combined HRT due to progesterone are:
  −pelvic bloating
  −irritability
  −depression.
- Women on combined HRT run an increased risk of:
  −a heart attack (29%). Reduce this risk by not smoking and by controlling blood cholesterol and blood pressure.
  −a stroke (41% increase). 8 more strokes in 10 000 women over 12 months. Reduce this risk by controlling hypertension.
  −venous thromboembolism (200% increase). Reduce this risk by having a diet rich in garlic and ginger or taking aspirin.
  −invasive breast cancer (26% increase – reports vary). Reduce this risk with regular screening: thermography/mammography.
  −endometrial cancer (200–300%) if unopposed oestrogen is used.

The decision to use hormone replacement therapy should be made by the informed patient.
The final decision to cease hormone replacement therapy rests with the patient.

Internet Resources

http://www.niapublications.org/engagepages/menopause.asp
menopause

http://www.niapublications.org/engagepages/hormonesafter.asp
hormones after menopause

PATIENT HANDOUT 6.2 – THE PATIENT'S CHOICE: WEIGHING THE EVIDENCE

(Adapted from Jamison JR. *Maintaining health in primary care*. Brochure 5.1. Edinburgh: Churchill Livingstone; 2001:92.)

The following quiz has been constructed to help you make an informed choice.

Determine your cost/benefit ratio in your decision whether or not to use hormone replacement therapy (HRT).

Women who benefit most from HRT are those:

- at high risk of osteoporosis
- at low risk of breast cancer
- severely troubled by the side effects of menopause
- who have no contraindications for oestrogen replacement.

Use these three steps to help you to weigh the evidence:

- Step 1: Identify the benefits of taking HRT
- Step 2: Identify the risks of taking HRT
- Step 3: Putting it together.

Step 1 Identify the benefits

a. Relief of menopausal symptoms

Ascertain how distressed you are by the major side effects of menopause which are:

Vasomotor instability leading to:

- hot flushes
- night sweats
- palpitations
- insomnia
- dizziness
- headaches/migraine.

Urogenital atrophy leading to:

- Painful intercourse (dyspareunia)
- vaginal dryness
- vulvo-vaginal itch
- difficulty or pain in passing urine (dysuria), frequency, urgency
- incontinence
- decreased libido.

Sleep disturbance leading to:

- insomnia
- fatigue.

Memory problems:

- forgetfulness
- difficulty concentrating.

Menopausal distress level HIGH MODERATE LOW

b. Personal risk of diseases that benefit from HRT

Osteoporosis:

- slender body build
- sedentary lifestyle
- low calcium, high salt and protein diet
- low bone mineral density.

(Every year for every 10 000 woman on HRT there are 5 fewer hip fractures.)

Bowel cancer:

- a first degree relative diagnosed with bowel cancer at age 50 years
- family history of familial polyposis coli
- a long history of inflammatory bowel disease
- a lifetime of constipation.

(Every year for every 10 000 woman on HRT there are 6 fewer colon cancers.)

Potential personal risk reduction by using HRT— HIGH   MODERATE   LOW

Step 2 Identify the risks

a. A perilous choice

Taking HRT is risky behaviour if you have:

- unexplained vaginal bleeding
- active liver disease
- chronic impaired liver function
- Recent vascular thrombosis
- Cancer of the breast
- Cancer of the uterus.

Do you have strong contraindications to HRT? YES   NO

b. A risky choice

Taking oestrogen may be risky if you have:

- seizure disorders
- hypertension

- uterine tumours (leiomyomas)
- familial hyperlipidaemia
- migraine headaches
- thrombophlebitis
- endometriosis
- gallbladder disease.

How do you rate the hazard to you of taking oestrogen replacement?
HIGH   LOW

c. Potential discomfort
Possible side effects from taking HRT:

- breast discomfort/tenderness
- endometrial bleeding
- nausea and headache.

How do you rate your level of disquiet about side effects?
MILD   MODERATE   SEVERE

d. Risking disease
Taking HRT increases the following risks:

- uterine cancer (2–3 fold if unopposed oestrogen is used)
- breast cancer (7 extra cases per 10 000 women each year)
- stroke (8 extra cases per 10 000 women each year)
- heart attack (8 extra cases per 10 000 women each year)
- blood clot (8 extra clots to the lung per 10 000 women each year).

How do you rate your unease about having an increased risk of disease?
MILD   MODERATE   SEVERE

e. Identifying personal risk
Pointers to increased risk of breast cancer:

- personal or family history of coronary heart disease
- first baby born after 30 years of age
- early menarche, before 12 years; and late menopause, after 50 years.

Pointers to increased risk of heart attack/coronary heart disease:

- family history
- high blood pressure
- a high waist–hip ratio
- cigarette smoker
- high LDL cholesterol, low HDL cholesterol.

Pointers towards stroke:

- high blood pressure
- 3 or more standard glasses of alcohol daily
- obesity.

Pointers towards clot (venous thromboembolism):

- personal history of pulmonary embolus
- first degree family history of venous thromboembolism.

How do you rate your personal risk of acquiring disease?
HIGH   MODERATE   LOW

Step 3 Putting it together
Summary of potential benefits of taking HRT
Menopausal distress level
HIGH   MODERATE   LOW

Potential personal risk reduction by taking HRT
HIGH   MODERATE   LOW

Summary of potential costs of taking HRT
Strong contraindications to taking HRT
YES   NO

Hazard taking oestrogen replacement
HIGH   LOW

Disquiet about side effects
MILD   MODERATE   SEVERE

Unease about disease risk
MILD   MODERATE   SEVERE

Personal risk of acquiring disease
HIGH   MODERATE   LOW

Use Step 3 to make a considered decision to either take or avoid HRT.

Patient's considered decision

Take HRT

- Menopausal with a uterus
  - Continuous oestrogen and cyclical progestogens. Treatment needs to be individualized to achieve cyclical withdrawal bleeding.
  - Continuous oestrogen and continuous progestogens. No withdrawal bleeding although spotting is common in the early phases.
- Menopausal without a uterus
  - Continuous oestrogen
  - Continuous oestrogen and progestogen for those with a history of endometriosis.
- Screening to reduce the risk of dying from cancer
  - Annual pelvic examination
  - Occasional endometrial sampling
  - Mammography.

Choose another option

- Relief of menopausal symptoms through diet
  Diets high in carrots, corn, apples, barley, soybean products and oats are rich in phyto-oestrogens. Types of phyto-oestrogens and their sources include
  - isoflavones: soy products, lentils and beans
  - lignans: linseed, whole grain cereals, (rye, wheat, barley and oats), carrot, corn, apples, pears, fennel
  - coumestans: soy bean sprouts, alfalfa.
  - Soy products contain diadzin, a particularly potent phyto-oestrogen
    - 45 g soy flour each day reduces hot flushes by 40%
    - 2–3 serves of soy products (30 g) per day can result in a decrease in total cholesterol, LDL cholesterol and triglycerides
    - soy products, especially those that are calcium enriched, can have a beneficial effect on osteoporosis.
  - Limit alcohol, caffeine, and spicy foods.
- Relief of symptoms through supplements
  - Black cohosh appears the most effective herbal option for relieving menopausal symptoms, particularly hot flushes.
- Relief of symptoms through exercise
  - Regular aerobic exercise benefits some symptoms and may attenuate the risk of certain diseases associated with menopause.
- Reduce the risk of particular conditions.

(Refer to the chapters on osteoporosis, cancer, coronary artery disease, depression.)

Chapter 7

Insomnia: Reality or perception?

Mrs Walker, a 70-year-old woman, presents complaining of insomnia. She says it takes her almost half an hour to fall asleep and then she only sleeps for a maximum of 6 hours. She says she seldom has a deep sleep and wakes early in the morning. She complains of tiredness mid-afternoon and often finds she naps in front of the television in the evening. On further consultation she is found to be cheerful and in good physical condition.

- Does this woman have primary insomnia?
- Should she be managed with long acting benzodiazepines to counteract her early waking?
- Will a tot of alcohol last thing at night help her fall asleep and stay asleep?

INTRODUCTION

Insomnia is a worldwide challenge.[1–9] More than 1 in 20 persons experience chronic and/or severe insomnia during their lifetime and around 1 in 3 adults has difficulty sleeping in any one year.[1] Common complaints are difficulty getting to sleep, staying asleep and non-restorative sleep. A survey of the general population in Finland found 37.6% of people surveyed experienced insomnia symptoms at least three nights each week. This study found 11.9% of the sample had difficulty initiating sleep, 31.6% had difficulty maintaining sleep, 11% complained of early morning waking and 7.9% woke feeling unrested.[4] A Canadian study found daytime fatigue (48%), psychological distress (40%), and physical discomfort (22%) were the main determinants prompting individuals with insomnia to seek treatment.[5]

Insomnia is a particularly prevalent complaint amongst the elderly.[6–9] A prospective cohort study of Canadians age 65 and older found almost 1 in 5 experienced early morning waking and/or had difficulty falling asleep, while almost 1 in 3 suffered daytime sleepiness.[6] Females are particularly prone to insomnia and this trend is consistent and progressive across age, being more significant in the elderly.[7] Various studies confirm that insomnia is more prevalent and more severe in older persons.[8] The prevalence of insomnia increases dramatically after the age of 70 years.[9]

INSOMNIA DEFINED

Insomnia may be defined as evidence of difficulty in sleeping, relative to age-appropriate norms, plus a subjective insomnia complaint and at least one type of perceived daytime impairment. Perceived daytime impairment may manifest as daytime fatigue, negative affect, cognitive inefficiency, impaired performance, reduced energy, social discomfort, non-specific physical symptoms (e.g. tension, headaches), unrefreshing sleep, daytime sleepiness, proneness to errors/accidents while driving, or excessive concern about sleep.[8] Insomnia may be transient or chronic. Chronic insomnia is diagnosed when the following three criteria are present:[10]

- sleep onset latency (taking more than 30 minutes to fall asleep) or wake time after sleep onset of more than 30 minutes
- occurring on 3 or more nights a week
- for 6 or more months.

CHANGING SLEEP PATTERNS WITH AGE

Insomnia in the elderly should not be confused with sleep pattern changes associated with aging.[8,9] The duration, overall quality and efficiency of sleep decreases with normal aging. Efficiency is determined by the total sleep time divided by the time spent in bed. Normal sleep efficiency is about 90–95%; in the elderly this decreases as they wake more often and have longer wakeful periods. Total sleep time decreases from around 18 hours in neonates to 11 hours in young children, 9 hours in adolescents, to 7.5 hours in adulthood. From mid-life until 80 years of age sleep time decreases a further 27 minutes per decade –more so for males than females. There is also a change in the quality of sleep.

Various stages of sleep have been defined on the basis of characteristic patterns of brain wave activity, eye movement and muscular activity. Adult sleep is divided into two broad categories. These are random eye movement (REM) and non-random eye movement (NREM) sleep. The former is associated with dreaming and memory.[11] The amount of REM sleep decreases with age. The latter is further divided into four stages according to the depth of sleep, ranging from stage 1 (the lightest and easiest to arouse) to stage 4 (the heaviest and most difficult to arouse). In the elderly there is increased light sleep (stages 1 and 2 NREM) The amount of light sleep doubles after middle age and may reach 13%. Shifts between sleep stages occur more often. Sleep is lighter and arousals more frequent. Arousals are brief periods, up to 15 seconds, of increased nervous system activation during sleep. The restorative benefits of sleep decrease as the frequency of arousals increases. In the elderly there is decreased deep sleep (stages 3 and 4 NREM), decreasing from 19% in middle age to 3.4% of total sleep time in the elderly. Slow wave sleep of stages 3 and 4 determines sleep intensity. Elderly people wake more often and remain awake longer. On average, elderly people have eight awakenings during the night, four times that of middle-aged persons. Awakenings are periods of wakefulness that interrupt sleep and last for several minutes. Patients report lighter and more fragmented sleep.

In addition to older adults experiencing aging-related changes in their sleep pattern they are prone to psychophysiological reactivity factors such as sub-clinical anxiety, over-arousal and negative conditioning.[8] Negative conditioning results from frequent nights with excessive amounts of time spent lying awake. It is sometimes compounded by poor sleep hygiene such as daytime napping, staying in bed late in the morning, irregular bedtimes, and trying too hard to sleep. Napping may cause homeostatic dysregulation. Daytime naps decrease the depth of subsequent major sleep episodes and increase latency to sleep onset. Excessive time in bed and irregular hours may disrupt the circadian rhythm, while conditioned arousal, i.e. doing mentally demanding work prior to retiring, may inhibit sleep due to excess mental arousal. Nightcaps can also have an adverse effect – as little as one cup of coffee or two cans of caffeinated soda (10 mg caffeine) slightly increases sleep latency while alcohol increases sleep fragmentation.[12] Although inadequate sleep hygiene is not considered a primary cause of insomnia, it is recognized to contribute to insomnia.

In addition to psychophysiological dysfunctions, the elderly are more prone to certain sleep disorders, e.g. sleep apnoea, gastro-oesophageal reflux, various diseases and medications that may disrupt sleep.[8]

SLEEP ASSESSMENT

In view of the pathophysiological changes associated with aging it is particularly important to do a comprehensive patient assessment. In view of the changing sleep pattern of the elderly, taking a thorough sleep history is indispensable in order to recognize normal for age sleep behaviour and to identify any factors that cause or contribute to the persistence of insomnia. Particular attention should be given to conditions that disrupt sleep such as pain and urinary frequency. In addition to the self-assessment sheet Handout 9.2, available at *www.jamisonhealth.com*, suggest the patient keep a sleep diary, available to download and personalize from *www.jamisonhealth.com* (Handout 9.3). It may also be helpful for the patient to become aware of the various lifestyle choices that may contribute to their problem (see *www.jamisonhealth.com* Handout 9.4).

SLEEP MANAGEMENT

Good sleep hygiene should feature in the management of any patient troubled by insomnia. Tips for good sleep hygiene are available at *www.jamisonhealth.com*, Handout 9.5.

In addition to good sleep hygiene, other self-help measures are available. Progressive relaxation, sleep restriction and stimulus control therapy may be combined with sleep hygiene. See *www.jamisonhealth.com* Handout 16.9, and Patient Handout 7.1. Reading and listening to music are other popular choices.[5] General routines may need to be modified in the elderly. To avoid muscle spasms or arthritic pain during progressive relaxation, elderly insomniacs may eliminate muscle tensing and focus on releasing tension passively. Older people who have difficulty walking may choose not to leave the bedroom when trying a stimulus control therapy. Napping may be used as an important adjunct in sleep restriction schedules. Cognitive behavioural therapy is the 'treatment' of choice for primary insomnia.[13] However, consensus has yet to be achieved on how best to identify appropriate candidates for this intervention.[14]

When self-help measures fail or as an interim adjunct to cognitive-behavioural options, drugs may be used. While behavioural therapies produce long-lasting and reliable changes among people with chronic insomnia, pharmacological therapies improve sleep maintenance, reducing the number of night-time awakenings as well as the wake time after an awakening,[15] both of which pose substantial problems for elderly insomniacs. To limit unwanted effects, pharmacotherapeutic treatment is best used for no more than 2–3 weeks.[16] However, about one-third of older adult hypnotic users will continue taking sleeping tablets for at least 5 years.

Older adults are more vulnerable to the hazards associated with hypnotics than are younger adults.[8] Age-related changes in drug absorption and elimination in later life can extend drug half life in the body and promote excess drug accumulation, can heighten the risk of residual day-time cognitive and motor impairment, and can exacerbate sleep-related breathing disorders. Drugs with a short half life of less than 6 hours are preferred.[16] Hypnotic agents, including benzodiazepines with longer pharmacological half lives, have been associated with side effects, including residual sedation, memory impairment and insomnia rebound, and have even been shown to increase the risk of falls, hip fractures and motor vehicle accidents in the elderly. Higher doses of benzodiazepines can similarly impair functioning.

Zaleplon, a new non-benzodiazepine hypnotic, has a short half life and does not appear to cause rebound insomnia or residual sedation, or adversely affect psychomotor function.[17] It can be taken within 2 hours of waking without 'hangover' effects. It does not, however, help with sleep maintenance. Another non-benzodiazepine agent, eszopiclone, which may specifically address sleep maintenance problems in elderly patients, has now been approved by the Food and Drug Administration (FDA).[18] Ultra short-acting drugs are useful when initiating sleep is the main problem, but short- and intermediate-acting substances are required for maintaining sleep. Although sedative hypnotics do improve sleep, the magnitude of effect is small and the increased risk of adverse events in people over 60 years old is statistically and clinically significant.[19] The use of these drugs in elderly patients with additional risk factors for cognitive or psychomotor adverse events is questionable.

Herbal preparations provide another alternative. A Canadian study found that 15% of subjects had used herbal/dietary products to facilitate sleep at least once in the year preceding the survey.[5] Valerian (Valeriana officinalis) has consistently been shown to have sleep-inducing, anxiolytic, and tranquillizing effects in both animal and human studies.[20] Clinical trials report 400–900 mg of valerian extract at bedtime improves sleep quality, decreases sleep latency, and reduces the number of night awakenings.[20,21] A randomized, controlled, double-blind trial concluded that neither single nor repeated evening administrations of 600 mg of native valerian root extract had any substantive adverse effect on reaction time, alertness and concentration the morning after.[22] Valerian tends to normalize the sleep profile, reducing periods of wakefulness and enhancing the efficacy of sleep periods.

L-tryptophan also tends to normalize the sleep profile of insomniacs.[23] Tryptophan-assisted sleep increases the third and fourth stage of NREM sleep and, unlike other hypnotics, appears to reduce wakefulness without decreasing the periods of REM sleep. Tryptophan is the amino acid precursor of serotonin, the neurotransmitter thought to induce sleep. A dose of 1–2 g of L-tryptophan has been reported to halve sleep latency and decrease waking time. Up to 5 g may be taken. Tryptophan is currently available by prescription. When taken with vitamin B6 (50 mg) and niaci-namide (500 mg), the conversion of tryptophan to serotonin is encouraged. Milk is rich in tryptophan –so perhaps a warm glass of milk before going to bed is not a bad idea.

Exogenous melatonin has been shown to decreases sleep onset latency and increase sleep efficiency and total sleep duration. Melatonin, a hormone produced by the pineal, influences the sleep–wake cycle. In humans, plasma melatonin level begins to increase steadily around 1900-2300 hours to attain peak values at around 0200–0400 hours. Plasma melatonin levels consistently decrease as aging progresses and the day/night rhythm alters with phase advance in the elderly. A meta-analysis found that exogenous melatonin treatment significantly reduced sleep onset latency by some 4 minutes, increased sleep efficiency by 2–3% and total sleep duration by around 13 minutes.[24] A 3% increase in sleep efficiency usually implies fewer awakenings, shortened periods of wakefulness and/or reduced sleep latency. Furthermore, unlike benzodiazepines, melatonin appears neither to affect stages 2 and 3–4 sleep, nor to produce a 'hangover' effect. Exogenous melatonin may improve the overall quality of sleep for elderly insomniacs.

SECONDARY INSOMNIA

Secondary insomnia is present when there is a persistent causal relationship between insomnia and another condition. The relationship between insomnia and various conditions is often difficult to establish. Epidemiological studies show that depression is one of the strongest risk factors for current insomnia, but recent evidence indicates that this relationship is bidirectional: current insomnia is a risk factor for future depression.[25] Valerian remains a safe, useful herbal option and in combination with St John's wort is particularly useful for insomniacs with depression or anxiety.[22,26]

There is a similar reciprocal relationship between sleep quality and pain. Sleep disorders are furthermore commonly encountered in persons complaining of pain,[27] and insomnia is in turn associated with increased pain and distress.[28] Although the poor sleep quality experienced by patients with chronic pain may sometimes be more an expression of depression or anxiety[29] than pain intensity or duration, this is not always the case and intervention to relieve pain should always be part of any management schema.

While attention to the underlying condition may alleviate insomnia in patients where insomnia is secondary to psychiatric problems, a medical condition or medication, simultaneous use of cognitive-behavioural intervention often appears to achieve the best results.[30]

IN PERSPECTIVE

Insomnia is a common complaint in elderly persons. Awareness of the changing sleep pattern associated with aging may increase acceptance of the 'problem'; however, a number of people will require more active intervention. Behavioural interventions should be part of any management regime; however, in view of older people's frequent waking and difficulty in getting back to sleep, drug therapy is often required. Attention should be paid to the dose and duration of any pharmaceuticals prescribed.

A plump 63-year-old woman presents, complaining of insomnia. On taking her sleep history you find she has difficulty falling asleep, wakes unrefreshed and has interrupted sleep on most nights. She says she is tired and irritable. She finds she nods off when trying to read. She says she has had trouble sleeping ever since she retired 11 months ago. She admits that for the first 6 months after her retirement she was worried about her finances but has now found she can cope. Prior to retirement she had no history of sleeping difficulties or taking hypnotics.

Questions arising

- How do you take a good sleep history?
- What sort of insomnia does she have?
- Based on her type of insomnia, how should she be managed?

Clinical considerations

A good sleep history includes checking if sleep is disturbed due to:

- arousals resulting from nocturia, pain, orthopnoea or restless legs or from environmental factors—noise, temperature, suitability of bed and pillow
- daytime naps
- a stress-related problem that may be responsible for acute insomnia
- underlying depression.

The differential diagnosis includes:

- primary insomnia
- secondary insomnia
- rebound insomnia
- chronic insomnia
- she doesn't have insomnia.

Based on a working diagnosis of chronic insomnia, possibly secondary to financial stress following retirement, a two-step management program includes:

1. Step I—describing the problem and trying to correct it by behavioural measures:
   a. Produce a sleep diary to determine the extent of the problem and provide a baseline for monitoring progress.
   b. Screen the patient to establish sleep routines and identify errors in sleep hygiene.
   c. Educate the patient to create sleep expectations consistent with her age, advise her on good sleep hygiene and consider trying relaxation therapy, stimulus control therapy or sleep restriction according to her preference.
2. Step II—resorting to short term drug intervention to break the insomnia cycle:
   d. If behavioural measures are unsuccessful, try to break her sleep habits first by adding valerian to her behavioural regime and, if necessary, try pharmaceuticals but for no more than 14 days. Melatonin may be a worthy choice.
   e. Persist with the behavioural regime.

- 1 in 5 people over the age of 65 years report a sleeping problem.
  - Chronic insomnia is linked to accidents, decreased quality of life, diminished productivity and an increased long term risk for medical diseases, e.g. diabetes, and psychiatric disorders, e.g. depression.
- Elderly people are generally more dissatisfied with their sleep performance than younger persons.
- Sleep patterns change with age—elderly persons who believe they have insomnia may need to be made aware of these changes:
  - Sleep latency is longer in elderly persons. One study of elderly females found the time lapse between deciding to sleep and falling asleep was 40 minutes.
  - The number and duration of awakenings after sleep onset increase with age.
- A sleep diary and good sleep history are required in the diagnosis and treatment of insomnia.
- Patient education and an attempt to improve sleep hygiene should be included in any insomnia management regime.
- Sleep maintenance, rather than sleep initiation, is the most common sleep problem reported by elderly people.
- Insomnia correlates with an increased risk of falling.
- There is a strong correlation between depression and insomnia in the elderly.

- Patients with medical or psychiatric conditions associated with insomnia should have their underlying problem plus their insomnia managed.
- Cognitive-behavioural therapy offers effective interventions for late-life insomnia, whether it be primary, secondary or rebound insomnia from hypnotic usage.
- Elderly insomniacs usually respond to about half the standard dose of hypnotic generally recommended.
- Ultra-short acting hypnotics are helpful for treating sleep latency; short to medium acting hypnotics may be needed to improve sleep maintenance.
- Avoid using hypnotics on a regular basis for more than 14–21 days.
- Gradually tapering the dose of hypnotics over 8–12 weeks may reduce withdrawal symptoms in patients with rebound insomnia.
- Overall there are fewer and less severe negative outcomes associated with non-benzodiazepine hypnotics than with the benzodiazepines.
- The ideal hypnotic is one that has a rapid onset, lasts through the night but has no residual daytime effects, and no adverse side effects.
- Unlike benzodiazepines, tryptophan and melatonin tend to leave the physiological sleep pattern unaltered.

References

1. Ohayon MM. Epidemiology of insomnia: what we know and what we still need to learn. Sleep Med Rev 2002; 6(2):97–111.
2. Olson LG. A community survey of insomnia in Newcastle. Aust N Z J Public Health 1996; 20(6):655–657.
3. Martikainen K, Partinen M, et al. The impact of somatic health problems on insomnia in middle age. Sleep Med 2003; 4(3):201–206.
4. Ohayon MM, Partinen M. Insomnia and global sleep dissatisfaction in Finland. J Sleep Res 2002; 11(4):339–346.
5. Morin CM, Leblanc M, et al. Epidemiology of insomnia: prevalence, self-help treatments, consultations, and determinants of help-seeking behaviors. Sleep Med 2006 Feb 1; [Epub ahead of print].
6. Rockwood K, Davis HS, et al. Sleep disturbances and mortality: results from the Canadian Study of Health and Aging. J Am Geriatr Soc 2001; 49(5):639–641.
7. Zhang B, Wing YK. Sex differences in insomnia: a meta-analysis. Sleep 2006; 29(1):85–93.
8. Nau SD, McCrae CS, et al. Treatment of insomnia

in older adults. Clin Psychol Rev 2005; 25(5):645–672.

9. Petit L, Azad N, et al. Non-pharmacological management of primary and secondary insomnia among older people: review of assessment tools and treatments. Age Ageing 2003; 32(1):19–25.

10. Lichstein KL, Durrence HH, et al. Quantitative criteria for insomnia. Behav Res Ther 2003; 41(4):427–445.

11. Lee Kavanau J. Evolutionary approaches to understanding sleep. Sleep Med Rev 2005; 9(2):141–152.

12. Stepanski EJ, Wyatt JK. Use of sleep hygiene in the treatment of insomnia. Sleep Med Rev 2003; 7(3):215---225.

13. Edinger JD, Means MK. Cognitive-behavioral therapy for primary insomnia. Clin Psychol Rev 2005; 25(5):539–558.

14. Smith MT, Perlis ML. Who is a candidate for cognitive-behavioral therapy for insomnia? Health Psychol 2006; 25(1):15–19.

15. Benca RM. Diagnosis and treatment of chronic insomnia: a review. Psychiatr Serv 2005; 56(3):332–343.

16. Norup PW. Sleeping disturbances and pharmacological/nonpharmacological interventions in old people. Ann Univ Mariae Curie Sklodowska [Med] 2002; 57(1):530–534.

17. Weitzel KW, Wickman JM, et al. Zaleplon: a pyrazolopyrimidine sedative-hypnotic agent for the treatment of insomnia. Clin Ther 2000; 22(11):1254–1267.

18. McCall WV. Diagnosis and management of insomnia in older people. J Am Geriatr Soc 2005; 53(7 Suppl):S272–S277.

19. Glass J, Lanctot KL, et al. Sedative hypnotics in older people with insomnia: meta-analysis of risks and benefits. BMJ 2005; 331(7526):1169.

20. Attele AS, Jing-Tian Xie, Chun-Su Yuan. Treatment of insomnia: an alternative approach. Altern Med Rev 2000; 5(3):249–259.

21. Donath F, Quispe S, et al. Roots I. Critical evaluation of the effect of valerian extract on sleep structure and sleep quality. Pharmacopsychiatry 2000; 33(2):47-53.

22. Kuhlmann J, Berger W, et al. The influence of valerian treatment on 'reaction time, alertness and concentration' in volunteers. Pharmacopsychiatry 1999; 32(6):235–241.

23. Jamison JR. Clinical guide to nutrition and dietary supplements in disease management. Edinburgh; Churchill Livingstone; 2003:339–344.

24. Brzezinski A, Vangel MG, et al. Effects of exogenous melatonin on sleep: a meta-analysis. Sleep Med Rev 2005; 9(1):41–50.

25. Buysse DJ. Insomnia, depression and aging. Assessing sleep and mood interactions in older adults. Geriatrics 2004; 59(2):47–51; quiz 52.

26. Wheatley D. Medicinal plants for insomnia: a review of their pharmacology, efficacy and tolerability. J Psychopharmacol 2005; 19(4):414–421.

27. Lobbezoo F, Visscher CM, Naeije M. Impaired health status, sleep disorders, and pain in the craniomandibular and cervical spinal regions. Eur J Pain 2004; 8(1):23–30.

28. Wilson KG, Eriksson MY, et al. Major depression and insomnia in chronic pain. Clin J Pain. 2002; 18(2):77–83.

29. Sayar K, Arikan M, Yontem T. Sleep quality in chronic pain patients. Can J Psychiatry 2002; 47(9):844–848.

30. Smith MT, Huang MI, Manber R. Cognitive behavior therapy for chronic insomnia occurring within the context of medical and psychiatric disorders. Clin Psychol Rev 2005; 25(5):559–592.

PATIENT HANDOUT 7.1 – MANAGING INSOMNIA: A SELF-CARE GUIDE[1,2]

Step 1: What is my sleep pattern?
Construct a sleep diary. Refer to
www.jamisonhealth.com Handout 9.3.

Step 2: Do I have a sleep problem?
Sleep patterns change with aging. Acceptable
sleep behaviours for older people are:

- sleep latency time, i.e. time to fall asleep, up to 30 minutes
- 5–10 hours sleep nightly, average 6 hours
- sleep efficiency, i.e. total sleep time/bed time, of 80–85%
- no daytime impairment because of sleepiness
- earlier to bed and earlier to wake –shift in circadian rhythm
- tiredness mid-afternoon and before bed at night.

If your sleep pattern conforms to the above you
do not have a sleep problem.

If you remain concerned about your sleep
pattern try to describe your sleeping problem. Do
you find you:

- [ ] can't stay awake during the day
- [ ] are irritable and/or anxious
- [ ] can't concentrate or remember
- [ ] are listless
- [ ] are prone to making errors/having accidents
- [ ] wake unrefreshed
- [ ] take longer than 30 minutes to fall asleep
- [ ] wake frequently (8 or more times)
- [ ] stay awake for 30 or more minutes after an awakening?

If you ticked a number of boxes go to Step 3 and
try some of the strategies outlined to help you
sleep better.

Step 3: Strategies for managing insomnia
Behavioural options
Avoid risky sleep behaviours:

1. Don't indulge in daytime napping—don't sleep for more than an hour or after 3.00 pm if you do nap.
2. Don't have variable bedtimes and waking up times.
3. Don't have an extended time in bed.
4. Don't try to sleep in an uncomfortable environment—check bed and bedding, light, temperature, noise, ventilation.
5. Don't have caffeine, nicotine or other chemical stimulants within 4 hours of retiring.
6. Don't exercise vigorously within 2 hours of going to bed—avoid being physically aroused.
7. Don't go to bed upset—being emotionally provoked isn't conducive to sleep.
8. Don't concentrate hard before going to bed—avoid being too mentally stimulated.
9. Don't review problems or plan strategies in bed.
10. Don't use the bed for non-sleep related activities—studying, watching television, arguing.

Cognitive therapy: sleep hygiene
The aim is to identify and change dysfunctional
beliefs and attitudes towards sleep.
  The procedure:

1. Limit the time spent in bed. Spending too long in bed encourages broken and shallow sleep.
2. Raise core body temperature by taking a hot bath before retiring or regular daily exercise in the late afternoon or early evening.
3. Establish a pattern of going to bed and getting up at the same time each day. This strengthens the circadian rhythm.
4. Avoid stimulation at bedtime—don't argue, drink alcohol or coffee or smoke (nicotine) or do vigorous exercise in the evening.
5. Eat a light bedtime snack. Cheese prevents night time hunger and may encourage sleep. Avoid heavy meals 2 hours before retiring. Avoid fluids after supper to prevent frequent night-time urination.
6. Prepare an environment conducive to sleep— have a comfortable mattress, a quiet room,

good ventilation and suitable bedclothes—neither too hot nor too cold.

7. Don't struggle to fall asleep. Relax, think pleasant thoughts and if still wakeful get up and do something relaxing.

8. Get rid of the bedroom clock. Checking the time increases mental arousal!

9. Avoid any stimulating activities or environments after 5.00 pm—go to bed mentally and physically relaxed. Set aside time to relax before going to bed.

10. Beware of regularly taking hypnotics—reserve sleeping tablets for special occasions.

Stimulus control therapy

The aim is to associate the bed/bedroom with falling asleep rapidly.

The procedure:

1. Go to bed when you feel tired—not before!
2. Limit using the bed to sleep (and sex).
3. If you don't fall asleep within 35 minutes—get up. If ambulatory go to another room. Do this until you do fall asleep within half an hour.
4. Always get up the same time in the morning—regardless of when you went to sleep the night before.
5. Avoid napping.

Sleep restriction therapy

The aim is to increase the efficiency of sleep, i.e. reduce the time spent in bed relative to the time spent sleeping.

The procedure:

1. Determine the average estimated sleep time—keep a sleep diary for 14 days.
2. Restrict the time in bed to average estimated sleep time.
3. Each week calculate sleep efficiency. (Sleep efficiency = total hours of sleep/time in bed × 100)
4. When sleep efficiency ≥89%, increase the total time in bed by 15–20 minutes. When sleep efficiency ≤75% decrease the total time in bed by 15–20 minutes.
5. Adjust total time in bed to achieve a sleep efficiency of 75–90%.
6. Do not reduce time in bed to less than 5 hours.
7. Daytime naps are permissible and may be desirable for the elderly.

Drug options

Caution: avoid risky drug use.

1. Prolonged use—don't take hypnotics regularly for more than 2–3 weeks.
2. Take less than the dose recommended for younger adults.
3. Don't rely on drugs to improve sleep—always try behavioural measures.

Benzodiazepine hypnotics

Effective but may cause:

- rebound insomnia on drug withdrawal
- increased risk of falling and hip fracture
- drowsiness
- dizziness
- cognitive impairment
- motor vehicle accidents.

Non-benzodiazepine hypnotics

Newer drugs have fewer adverse effects but may not be as effective for sleep maintenance. Melatonin has been approved for therapeutic use.

Herbs

Valerian is regarded as a safe option.

References

1. Zhang B, Wing YK. Sex differences in insomnia: a meta-analysis. Sleep 2006; 29(1):85-93.
2. Lichstein KL, Durrence HH, et al. Quantitative criteria for insomnia. Behav Res Ther 2003; 41(4):427-445.

Chapter **8**

Osteoporosis: Skeletal failure

An 85-year-old man presents, complaining of the sudden onset of back pain. He explains he has had vague backache for a number of years. Rest relieves the pain. His current problem started when he leant over backwards in his chair to retrieve a cushion. He has no history of trauma. The pain is aggravated by straining and standing and relieved by rest. On examination there is marked restriction of movement, muscle spasm and deformity. He reports he is in good health. He is eating and sleeping well. His blood pressure is well controlled, his weight unchanged.

- Can this be an osteoporotic fracture? Are elderly men at risk?
- What clinical findings would suggest osteoporosis? What would you look for?
- If this is osteoporosis, what intervention options are available?
- What special investigations are available to make a definitive diagnosis of osteoporosis and monitor progress?
- Is the patient at risk of a second osteoporotic fracture?

INTRODUCTION

In 2003, osteoporosis affected up to 1 in 3 women and 1 in 12 men. In 1990 there were 1.6 million hip fractures per annum worldwide; this is expected to have reached 6 million by 2050.[1] Hip fractures are associated with 20% mortality and 50% permanent loss in function.[2] A UK study reported 12.8%, 46.8% and 63.0% of women were osteoporotic in the under 65 year, 65–75 year and over 75 year age groups, respectively.[3] Another study reported that, compared to 50–54 year old women, the odds of osteoporosis were 5.9 times greater in 65–69 year olds and 14.3 times higher in 75–79 year olds.[4] At any given bone mineral density, both the absolute and relative excess fracture risk increases with advancing age.[5] The prevalence of osteoporosis and the absolute risk of a fracture for all fracture sites increases with age.

THE PROBLEM: PROGRESSIVE AGE-RELATED BONE LOSS

Although remodelling of bone takes place throughout adult life, bone depletion starts during the third or fourth decade of adulthood. Osteoclasts resorb old bone and osteoblasts create new bone with 3% of cortical and 25% of trabecular bone being remodelled annually. Osteoporosis results when bone resorption outstrips bone formation. A peak period of accelerated bone loss occurs during the first 5–10 years following menopause with 1–6% of bone tissue lost annually. Persons with a high peak bone mass have the reserves to tolerate more bone loss before reaching the fracture threshold.

OSTEOPOROTIC FRACTURES

Peak bone mass is achieved in adolescence and early adulthood. It is determined by genetic and environmental factors. Although up to 75% of the predisposition to osteoporosis may be genetically determined, genetic predisposition becomes less important with increasing age. Furthermore, while genotype may be an important determinant,[6] it is not the only factor influencing the risk of an osteoporotic fracture. Although it is too late to intervene to achieve a high peak bone mass in this age group, intervention focusing on reducing bone resorption and decreasing the risk of falling can reduce the risk of fractures. Indeed falling, not osteoporosis, is the strongest single risk factor for a fracture.[7] In addition to these immediate risk factors for fractures in the elderly, more distant risk factors include aging, a previous vertebral fracture, disease, medication, functional impairment, disabilities, inactivity, poor nutrition, use of alcohol and smoking.[1,7] While Handouts 21.1–21.5 at *www.jamisonhealth.com* may be used to screen lifestyle choices that impinge on skeletal health, in elderly patients a more definitive evaluation of bone status is desirable.

PREDICTING PERSONAL RISK

Persons with a previous vertebral fracture and/or a body mass index (BMI) of under 23 are at increased risk of an osteoporotic fracture.[1] Vertebral deformity is a strong predictor of subsequent fracture risk.[8] A random sample of individuals 60 years and over found the prevalence of asymptomatic vertebral deformity was 31% in men and 17% in women. While changes detected clinically are helpful, radiological assessment can provide information before clinical indicators are apparent.

Osteopenia and osteoporosis can be determined using dual-energy X-ray absorptiometry, quantitative ultrasonography, radiographic absorptiometry, single energy X-ray absorptiometry, peripheral dual-energy X-ray absorptiometry, and peripheral quantitative computed tomography. Osteoporosis is defined as a bone mineral density (BMD) of more than 2.5 standard deviations below the mean for a young healthy adult woman (t > –2.5), osteopenia as a BMD between 1 and 2.5 standard deviations below the mean (t = –1.0 to –2.5) (see Box 8.1). The risk of a fracture increases steadily as bone

---

Box 8.1   Diagnostic screening for osteopenia[a]

RECOGNIZING RISK

Recognizing genetic predisposition
Predisposition to osteoporosis is 75% genetically determined.
Screen variations in gene receptors for vitamin D. Blood tests can determine if an individual has a gene variant.

Recognizing age-related muscle wasting
- Relative skeletal muscle index = appendicular skeletal muscle (kg)/height (m[2])
- Sarcopenia = relative skeletal muscle index = <5.45 kg/m[2].

Recognizing lifestyle risk
Refer to *www.jamisonhealth.com.au* handout 21.1

DIAGNOSING CURRENT STATUS

Biochemical measures
Markers of bone formation:

- alkaline phosphatase
- serum osteocalcin.

Markers of bone resorption:

- N-telopeptides
- hydroxyproline
- urinary calcium.

Biochemical markers guiding therapy:

- High bone turnover—treat with hormone replacement therapy or calcitonin
- Low bone turnover—treat with fluoride.

Bone mass measurement (BMD)

- Single-photon adsorptiometry of the distal forearm
- Dual-photon absorptiometry
- Computed tomography.

COMBINATION OF ABOVE MARKERS
- predict bone mass 15 years later
- predict risk of vertebral fracture
- BMD osteopenia BMD t = –1.0 to –2.5; osteoporosis t > –2.5
- risk of osteoporosis/fracture in next 10 years: 10% if t < –1.4; 56% if t > –1.4

[a]serum calcium and phosphate are usually within normal limits.

density declines, with no threshold. However, in any individual, a baseline BMD t-score less negative than –1.4 at both femoral neck and lumbar spine sites has been shown to be associated with a 10-year risk of less than 10% of developing an osteoporotic BMD or fracture.[9] In contrast, participants with t-scores more negative than –1.4 had a 56% risk. A BMD measurement performed in the first 2 years following menopause is a strong long term predictor of bone mineral density in healthy women.

While detecting structural change may be useful in identifying current bone status, biochemical measures may be more useful in monitoring bone changes. Use of bone turnover markers to complement BMD measurement is advocated in the management of osteoporosis. Biochemical markers of bone formation include procollagen type I, carboxy amino terminal peptides and serum bone-specific alkaline phosphatase, while markers of bone resorption include urinary hydroxyproline, urinary pyridinoline, urinary deoxypyridinoline, urinary amino terminal crosslinked telopeptide, and urinary and serum carboxy terminal crosslinked telopeptide. Although elevated marker levels have been shown to be associated with an increased risk of fracture in elderly women, their utility in predicting fracture has yet to be established.[10] Nonetheless, several clinical trials have established the potential utility of markers to identify patients with rapid bone loss, aid in therapeutic decision-making, and monitor therapeutic efficacy of various treatments.[10]

MANAGEMENT

Osteoporosis is an important underlying factor in hip fractures in the elderly, but falling is the immediate cause of fractures. Management in this age group targets both bone density and mobility. It includes consideration of diet, supplements, drug therapy and exercise.

Calcium intake

The dominant mineral in bone is calcium, and calcium supplementation has a significant effect on a number of biomarkers of bone remodelling, an effect that is, in turn, correlated with decreased fracture risk.[11] It is therefore possible cause for concern that a review of past and current data concluded that the current recommended daily allowance for the elderly is too low for vitamin D and calcium.[12] However, not everybody agrees.

It has been postulated that osteoporotic fractures result from age-related exhaustion of osteoblasts' replicative capacity.[13] This hypothesis proposes that calcium restriction may preserve bone health by retarding the decrease in the age-related osteoblast capacity to form new bone. The argument is that a high calcium intake leads to an increased activity of osteoblasts. Increased osteoblast activity and cell differentiation coincide with increased osteoblast apoptosis rate. The proposal is to prevent osteoporosis by reducing mean calcium intake to 300–500 mg/day, the approximate calcium consumption level of countries where the incidence of osteoporotic fractures is lowest.[13] Another study suggests an appropriate recommended daily allowance (RDA) for elderly persons is around 18.1–18.5 mg/kg body weight.[14] This would suggest 1000 mg daily may be more appropriate. Dietary calcium is not the only determinant.

One study of early postmenopausal woman found calcium supplementation and alcohol use were significantly associated with reduced levels of markers for bone resorption, and a lower mean serum osteocalcin, a marker of bone formation.[15] Calcium and alcohol would appear to dampen remodelling. Other lifestyle choices may also affect calcium metabolism. A 3-year placebo-controlled study concluded that smoking accelerated bone loss from the femoral neck and total body in the elderly.[16] Less efficient calcium absorption was postulated to be one contributing factor.

Vitamin D

Vitamin D enhances calcium absorption. About 50% of the population has the heterozygous vitamin D receptor gene which, on calcium supplementation, slows the rate of bone density loss. The situation is further aggravated by many of those aged 65 years and over having a vitamin D deficiency.[17] The elderly are at high risk of developing vitamin D deficiency, especially those with malabsorption. Mild vitamin D deficiency, serum 25 hydroxyvitamin D (OHD) levels 30–50 nmol/L, are associated with increased parathyroid hormone secretion, and levels between 12.5 and 25 nmol/L are associated with reduced bone density, high bone turnover and increased risk of hip fracture in the elderly. Vitamin D supplementation (10 000 IU weekly or 1000 IU daily) together with calcium (600 mg daily) has been found to reduce the incidence of falls and may aid fracture prevention in persons with serum 25 OHD levels below 50 nmol/L.[18] Daily supplementation with calcium-vitamin D fortified milk (1000 mg calcium and 800 IU of vitamin D3) over 2 years is effective in suppressing parathyroid hormone (PTH) and slowing bone loss. In contrast to elderly institutionalized individuals, in community-dwelling older people vitamin D, either alone or in combination with calcium supplementation, is ineffective in the primary or secondary prevention of fractures.[19] Institutionalized elderly people commonly have vitamin D deficiency and secondary hyperparathyroidism.

A systematic review of oral vitamin D supplementation concluded 700–800, but not 400, IU vitamin D daily reduced the risk of hip and other non-vertebral fractures in ambulatory elderly persons.[20] However, 800 IU daily oral vitamin D3, either alone or combined with 1000 mg calcium, did not appear to prevent low trauma fractures in elderly people who had had a previous fracture.[21] Nonetheless, 2 years of treatment with calcium (500 mg/day) and vitamin D3 (400-600 IU/day) improved bone mineralization in postmenopausal women—with or without additional supplementation with an oestrogen receptor agonist.[22] Another year long study of supplementation with calcium citrate (800 mg/day) plus exercise (aerobic, weight-bearing and weight-lifting exercise three times per week) confirmed an increase in trochanteric bone mineral density among women who did not use hormone replacement therapy (HRT).[23] This randomized, multi-arm study of non-smoking postmenopausal women did, however, find that only those on HRT who exercised and took calcium also increased their femoral neck and lumbar spine bone mineral density. A prospective, randomized 2-year trial with postmenopausal women over 60 years of age with low lumbar bone mineral density confirmed HRT as a low dose of conjugated oestrogen (0.31 mg/day) with or without medroxyprogesterone acetate (2.5 mg/day) plus alfacalcidol (1.0 microg/day) was more effective than HRT alone.[24]

Phyto-oestrogens

The most important single non-genetic factor determining the risk of osteoporosis in postmenopausal women is oestrogen deficiency,[25] and when initiated at menopause, HRT undoubtedly reduces the risk of osteoporotic fractures.[26] Continued use of HRT is, however, associated with adverse effects. Phyto-oestrogens provide an alternative to oestrogen.

Laboratory studies of postmenopausal osteoporosis suggest the soy isoflavones genistein and daidzein have a significant bone-sparing effect, but human studies, although promising, have had variable results.[27] Studies suggest genistein may prevent bone loss through upregulating production of osteoprotegerin by human osteoblasts.[28] Certainly, bone mineral densities, adjusted to weight and years since menopause, are significantly different in persons with high and low intakes of soy isoflavones.[29] In early, but not late postmenopause, significant differences were also found with respect to backache between the high and low intake categories. Taking 40 g soy protein daily, with isoflavone content of 2.25 mg or more per gram of protein, appears to protect against spinal bone loss.[28] A cup of firm tofu contains around 13 g of soy protein, 6 g is found in a soy 'sausage', 10–12 g in a soy 'burger', 14 g in a soy protein bar, 19 g in a quarter cup of roasted soy nuts and 10 g in an 8-ounce glass of plain soymilk. Other good sources of isoflavones are chickpeas, kidney beans, lentils and red clover.

Other dietary considerations

In addition to calcium, vitamin D and soy products, other nutritional factors worthy of mention include protein and various micronutrients. A higher protein intake (72 g/day) was associated with greater bone mineral density among women with calcium intake exceeding 408 mg/day in a study of postmenopausal women aged 65–77 years.[30] High protein diets do, however, increase urinary calcium excretion. The calciuria induced by high dietary protein may be minimized by consumption of protein-rich foods that are also rich in phosphorus, such as meat and dairy products.

The other micronutrient needs for optimizing bone health may be met by a diet rich in fruit and vegetables (5 servings daily) to ensure adequate intakes for magnesium, potassium, vitamin C and vitamin K.[32] Results of a 4-year longitudinal study support the hypothesis that alkaline-producing dietary components contribute to maintenance of bone mineral density in elderly people.[31] Another factor contributing to bone health in a diet rich in fruit and vegetables is vitamin C.

Vitamin C stimulates procollagen, enhances collagen synthesis and stimulates alkaline phosphatase activity, a marker for osteoblast formation. A population-based sample of postmenopausal women found vitamin C supplementation appeared to benefit bone mineral density, especially among postmenopausal women using concurrent oestrogen therapy and calcium supplements.[33] Vitamin C intake ranged from 100 to 5000 mg daily with a mean daily dose of 745 mg over at least 3 years. Another study suggested each 100 mg increment in dietary vitamin C intake was associated with a 0. 017 g/cm² increment in BMD at the femoral neck/hip.[34] These data are consistent with a positive association of vitamin C with BMD in postmenopausal women with dietary calcium intakes of at least 500 mg.

Exercise

Bone density taken alone is a poor predictor of fracture risk. The risk of a fracture is halved when bone mineral density increases by only 8%;[35] on the other hand, even with consistent bone density, the risk of fracture rises 8–10 times between the ages of 45 and 80 years.[36] One explanation for this increase is instability. Sarcopenia, the decline of muscle mass with age, causes impaired gait, disability and falls. Exercise improves gait, coordination, balance, proprioception, reaction time and muscle strength. Muscle performance is an important determinant of functional capacity and quality of life among the elderly and is also involved in the maintenance of balance.[37] Exercise is important both with respect to reducing the risk of falls and protecting bone mass.[38] Physical activity increases bone mass, strength and density and the risk of falling may be reduced by up to 30%. Indeed, the relationship between muscle, bone mass and risk of osteoporosis may largely be mediated through participation in exercise. One study found the prevalence of sarcopenia was 12.5% in premenopausal osteopenic women (t below –1.0); 25% in postmenopausal osteopenic women; and 50% in postmenopausal osteoporotic (t below –2.5).[39] Physical activity, unlike HRT and diet, appears independently related to the relative skeletal muscle mass.[39] Women who used HRT and calcium but did not exercise had no change in BMD.[25]

The relative risk of a fracture is increased about 2.5-fold in persons with decreased bone mineral density and almost as much again in persons with postural instability or in those who need to use their arms when rising from a sitting position.[40] Increased postural sway, particularly in the mediolateral plane, and imbalance appear to be important predictors of falls and fractures in individuals with osteoporosis. In fact, it appears a negative correlation between bone density and self-reported postural unsteadiness may possibly reflect the relationship between bone demineralization and the tendency to fall. One study that explored various biomechanical relationships between exercise and unsteadiness found only an inverse relationship between the level of physical activity and the participants' mediolateral standard deviation and range of sway with their eyes open.[41] This finding is consistent with the reports that not all types of physical activity provide comparable effects on bone health.

Bone mass and strength adapt to the load on bones—and muscle pull rather than body weight is the major determinant of bone strain. Changes in the internal strain in bone, defined as the fractional change in the dimension of a bone in response to a changing load, appear to activate osteocytes altering the balance between bone resorption and formation. Osteogenesis is caused by dynamic, not static, strain. Although greater loads and fewer repetitions of a load result in greater gains in bone mass, exercises that introduce stress to the skeleton through joint-reaction forces such as weight lifting or rowing are also considered potentially more beneficial as they prevent osteoporotic fractures by reducing the risk for falls.[42] Indeed, exercises that do not involve loading are considerably less effective than weight bearing. Brisk walking may only marginally slow rather than prevent bone loss. The osteogenic response to mechanical loading also seems to be site specific. Meta-analysis suggests that exercise programs are effective for preventing spinal bone mineral density loss at the L2–4 level in postmenopausal women over 50 years of age.[43] Isometric back extensor strength appears to be the most significant contributor to the total spinal range of motion.[44] A home-based program of strength and balance retraining exercises effectively reduced falls and injuries in women aged 80 years and older.[45] For those who kept exercising, the benefit continued over a 2-year period. Falls and injuries can be reduced by home based, individually tailored exercise programs. Another study found impact exercise had no effect on bone mineral density; nonetheless, exercise may prevent fall-related fractures in elderly women with low bone mass.[46]

After about 30 years of age, muscle strength decreases and bone remodelling begins to reduce bone mass and strength. Age affects bone architecture by progressive erosion of trabecular bone and reduced rate of bone turnover. Fractures occur when high bone turnover is combined with frequent impact. Padded strong-shield hip protectors may lessen the impact of falls while routine assessment of elderly persons and early intervention for risks attributable to polypharmacy, lower extremity weakness, balance disorders, postural hypotension, cardiovascular impairment, cognitive impairment, visual deficit and other environmental factors may be helpful.[47]

DRUG OPTIONS

With proactive treatment, postmenopausal osteoporosis need no longer be an accepted process of aging.[48] In those at high risk and those who already have had an osteoporotic fracture, pharmaceuticals offer realistic treatment options. Bisphosphonates, hormone replacement therapy, selective oestrogen receptor modulators and calcitonin provide women with an array of alternatives. The efficacy of bisphosphonates (alendronate and risendronate), oestrogen, and selective oestrogen receptor modulators (raloxifene) and calcitonin have been assessed.[4,49–51] Bisphosphonates e.g. alendronate and risedronate, bind permanently to mineralized bone surfaces and inhibit subsequent osteoclastic activity during bone remodelling. They can substantially reduce the risk of both hip and vertebral fractures.[52,53] Alendronate significantly reduces vertebral and non-vertebral fractures. Oestrogen, either alone or with progestin, consistently improves bone density. Side effects are, however, problematic. Teriparatide, an anabolic agent, is a recombinant human parathyroid hormone which reduces the risk of new fractures and is indicated for use in patients with severe osteoporosis.[53] Calcitonin reduces acute pain associated with osteoporotic fractures and has been found useful in treating chronic back pain following vertebral fractures in spinal osteoporosis. It is usually reserved for use in patients who cannot tolerate bisphosphonates. The effectiveness of these therapies may, however, vary between individuals—one bisphosphonate appeared to be effective in subjects with low bone density but not in those at high risk of fall-related risk factors.[54] Tailoring both by drug and non-drug interventions to meet individual patient needs is important.

KEEPING PERSPECTIVE

Osteoporotic fractures represent one of the most important causes of long-standing pain, functional impairment, disability and death among the elderly. Currently, it is estimated that over 200 million people worldwide have osteoporosis and costs to health care are predicted to double by 2050.[55] In the USA alone some 44 million people have osteoporosis and there are around 1.5 million fractures annually.[55] Of the 1 in 3 postmenopausal American women with osteoporosis, some 40% are predicted to have at least one fragility fracture during their remaining lifetime.[55] It is therefore of considerable concern that osteoporosis may be poorly comprehended, underdiagnosed and undertreated.[56]

Regular strength and balance training, minimizing psychotropic medication, and diet supplementation with vitamin D and calcium have all been shown to be effective in reducing the risk of osteoporotic fractures in the elderly.[7] However, management will remain incomplete until such time as the pathogenesis of the condition is better understood. Hypotheses continue to emerge.[57] For example, it has recently been suggested that zinc deficiency may lead to the increase of endogenous heparin, causing degranulation of mast cells and release of endogenous heparin, and an increase in the bone-resorbing effect of prostaglandin E2. Endogenous heparin and prostaglandin E2 are probably cofactors of parathyroid hormone and are postulated to have a role in the pathogenesis of senile osteoporosis by enhancing the action of parathyroid hormone. If correct, zinc replacement by dietary supplementation might aid prevention or treatment of senile osteoporosis. Furthermore, routine vitamin D, calcium and zinc supplementation potentially provides pervasive health benefits in the elderly.[58] The elderly are prone to inadequate intake of these nutrients and in the case of vitamin D there is some epidemiological evidence suggesting supplementation with this vitamin may reduce systolic blood pressure, breast, prostate and colon cancers, and type 2 diabetes in elderly persons with vitamin D insufficiency.

CLINICAL CHALLENGE

A 65-year-old Caucasian female presents with severe pain in the lower thoracic region. The pain is aggravated by movement and relieved by lying down.

She had a smoking history peaking at 40 cigarettes a day but has cut down to 15 a day over the last 20 years. She drinks 6 cups of coffee a day but avoids alcohol. She retired 6 months ago after 40 years as a librarian. She has a dairy intolerance. She had her menopause at 40 years of age.

She reports having had a mastectomy for cancer of the left breast 8 years ago. Subsequent bone scans for secondaries have been negative. Her last scan was 11 months ago.

Questions arising

- What is her working diagnosis?
- What additional information is required before progressing?

Clinical considerations

She could have a pathological fracture due to underlying:

- osteoporosis
- spinal metastases: breast or lung cancer.

On examination she has a dowager's hump and tenderness over T12. Her right breast has no palpable masses. You check her BMI and find she has lost both weight and height. Her BMI is 20.

Questions arising

- Why is she at increased risk of an osteoporotic fracture?
- What investigations could provide a definitive diagnosis?
- How should she be managed?

Clinical considerations

An osteoporotic fracture is likely, given:

- her predisposing factors, including slight Caucasian female, sedentary lifestyle, low calcium intake, early menopause and current age, coffee consumption and smoking habit
- her clinical findings, including loss of height, dowager's hump, pain relieved by lying.

A definitive diagnosis of osteoporotic fracture was confirmed by the following special investigations:

- A spinal X-ray confirmed a vertebral compression fracture.
- Dual photon absorptiometry found her bone mineral density to be 3 standard deviations below the mean.
- Bone scan showed no metastases. Furthermore, pain is also often worst on lying still and somewhat relieved by activity in these cases.

(Bence-Jones proteinuria or protein electrophoresis would confirm the absence of multiple myeloma, another cause of pathological fractures).

Management requires drug treatment. Alendronate, a bisphosphonate, is the drug of choice. Should she be unable to tolerate a bisphosphonate, calcitonin can be used. It reduces pain following vertebral fractures in spinal osteoporosis.

Supplementation with 800 IU daily oral vitamin D3, either alone or combined with 1000 mg calcium may be helpful, but in view of her history of breast cancer HRT should be avoided and caution exercised with respect to phyto-oestrogen intake.

An appropriate exercise program should be developed.

- ◆ The risk of a fracture is related both to bone strength and falling.
  - ◆ Osteoporotic fractures can occur in the absence of trauma or following minimal impact.
- ◆ The most usual occurrence resulting in a fracture of an older adult is a 'simple' fall from standing height or less.
- ◆ Exposing elderly persons to 5–10 minutes of sunlight on 5 days of the week may not meet the RDA for Vitamin D.
- ◆ Elderly people may require a dietary intake of up to 800 IU of vitamin D per day.
- ◆ Calcium supplementation should be combined with vitamin D (calcitriol) to enhance its absorption.
- ◆ Women are at greater risk of osteoporosis than men; nonetheless osteoporosis is a problem in older men.

- ◆ Lifestyle choices such as exercise and nutritional supplementation can reduce the risk of osteoporotic fractures.
- ◆ Exercise reduces the risk of fractures both by its effect on maintenance of bone mass and by improving postural stability and thus decreasing falls.
- ◆ Various drugs are available that can reduce the rate of bone resorption.
- ◆ Oestrogen replacement therapy does reduce the risk of osteoporosis but is best started early in menopause.
- ◆ Women should have their bone mineral density determined within 2 years of menopause in order to ascertain their risk of osteopenia and ractures over the next decade.
- ◆ The relative risk of a fracture is increased 3 times in persons with impaired eyesight!

References

1. Keen RW. Burden of osteoporosis and fractures. Curr Osteoporos Rep 2003; 1(2):66–70.
2. Woolf AD, Pfleger B. Burden of major musculoskeletal conditions. Bull World Health Organ 2003; 81(9):646–656.
3. Brankin E, Mitchell C, Munro R; Lanarkshire Osteoporosis Service. Closing the osteoporosis management gap in primary care: a secondary prevention of fracture programme. Curr Med Res Opin 2005; 21(4):475–482.
4. US Preventive Services Task Force. Screening for osteoporosis in postmenopausal women. Recommendations and rationale. 2002. Online. Available: http://www.ahrq.gov/clinic/3rduspstf/osteoporosis/osteorr.htm#clinical.
5. Siris ES, Brenneman SK, et al. The effect of age and bone mineral density on the absolute, excess, and relative risk of fracture in postmenopausal women aged 50–99: results from the National Osteoporosis Risk Assessment (NORA). Osteoporos Int: 2006 Apr; 17(4):565–574.
6. Long JR, Xiong DH, et al. The genetics of osteoporosis. Drugs Today (Barc) 2005; 41(3):205–218.
7. Kannus P, Uusi-Rasi K, et al. Non-pharmacological means to prevent fractures among older adults.

Ann Med 2005; 37(4):303–310.
8. Pongchaiyakul C, Nguyen ND, et al. Asymptomatic vertebral deformity as a major risk factor for subsequent fractures and mortality: a long-term prospective study. J Bone Miner Res 2005; 20(8):1349–1355.
9. Abrahamsen B, Rejnmark L, et al. Ten-year prediction of osteoporosis from baseline bone mineral density: development of prognostic thresholds in healthy postmenopausal women. The Danish Osteoporosis Prevention Study. Osteoporos Int 2006; 17(2):245–251.
10. Srivastava AK, Vliet EL, et al. Clinical use of serum and urine bone markers in the management of osteoporosis. Curr Med Res Opin 2005; 21(7):1015–1026.
11. Weisman SM, Matkovic V. Potential use of biochemical markers of bone turnover for assessing the effect of calcium supplementation and predicting fracture risk. Clin Ther 2005; 27(3):299–308.
12. Russell RM. New views on the RDAs for older adults. J Am Diet Assoc 1997; 97(5):515–518.
13. Klompmaker TR. Lifetime high calcium intake increases osteoporotic fracture risk in old age. Med Hypotheses 2005; 65(3):552–558.

14. Uenishi K, Ishida H, et al. Calcium requirement estimated by balance study in elderly Japanese people. Osteoporos Int 2001; 12(10):858–863.

15. Hla MM, Davis JW, et al. The relation between lifestyle factors and biochemical markers of bone turnover among early postmenopausal women. Calcif Tissue Int 2001; 68(5):291–296.

16. Krall EA, Dawson-Hughes B. Smoking increases bone loss and decreases intestinal calcium absorption. J Bone Miner Res 1999; 14(2):215–220.

17. Hirani V, Primatesta P. Vitamin D concentrations among people aged 65 years and over living in private households and institutions in England: population survey. Age Ageing 2005; 34(5):485–491.

18. Nowson CA. The significance of vitamin D to health in Australia. Asia Pac J Clin Nutr 2005; 14(Suppl):S17.

19. Francis RM. Calcium, vitamin D and involutional osteoporosis. Curr Opin Clin Nutr Metab Care 2006; 9(1):13–17.

20. Bischoff-Ferrari HA, Willett WC, et al. Fracture prevention with vitamin D supplementation: a meta-analysis of randomized controlled trials. JAMA 2005; 293(18):2257–2264.

21. Grant AM, Avenell A, et al. Oral vitamin D3 and calcium for secondary prevention of low-trauma fractures in elderly people: a randomised placebo-controlled trial. Lancet 2005; 365(9471):1621–1628.

22. Boivin G, Lips P, et al. Contribution of raloxifene and calcium and vitamin D3 supplementation to the increase of the degree of mineralization of bone in postmenopausal women. J Clin Endocrinol Metab 2003; 88(9):4199–4205.

23. Going S, Lohman T, et al. Effects of exercise on bone mineral density in calcium-replete postmenopausal women with and without hormone replacement therapy. Osteoporos Int 2003; 14(8):637–643.

24. Mizunuma H, Shiraki M, et al. Randomized trial comparing low-dose hormone replacement therapy and HRT plus 1alpha-OH-vitamin D(3) (alfacalcidol) for treatment of postmenopausal bone loss. J Bone Miner Metab 2006; 24(1):11–15.

25. Cohen AJ, Roe FJ. Review of risk factors for osteoporosis with particular reference to a possible aetiological role of dietary salt. Food Chem Toxicol 2000; 38(2–3):237–253.

26. Nelson HD, Humphrey LL, et al. Postmenopausal hormone replacement therapy: scientific review. JAMA 2002; 288(7):872–881.

27. Setchell KD, Lydeking-Olsen E. Dietary phytoestrogens and their effect on bone: evidence from in vitro and in vivo, human observational, and dietary intervention studies. Am J Clin Nutr 2003; 78(3 Suppl):593S–609S.

28. Potter SM, Baum JA, et al. Soy protein and isoflavones: their effects on blood lipids and bone density in postmenopausal women. Am J Clin Nutr 1998; 68(6 Suppl):1375S–1379S.

29. Somekawa Y, Chiguchi M, et al. Soy intake related to menopausal symptoms, serum lipids, and bone mineral density in postmenopausal Japanese women. Obstet Gynecol 2001; 97(1):109–115.

30. Rapuri PB, Gallagher JC, Haynatzka V. Protein intake: effects on bone mineral density and the rate of bone loss in elderly women. Am J Clin Nutr 2003; 77(6):1517–1525.

31. Nieves JW. Osteoporosis: the role of micronutrients. Am J Clin Nutr 2005; 81(5):1232S–1239S.

32. Tucker KL, Hannan MT, et al. Potassium, magnesium, and fruit and vegetable intakes are associated with greater bone mineral density in elderly men and women. Am J Clin Nutr 1999; 69(4):727–736.

33. Morton DJ, Barrett-Connor EL, Schneider DL. Vitamin C supplement use and bone mineral density in postmenopausal women. J Bone Miner Res 2001; 16(1):135–140.

34. Hall SL, Greendale GA. The relation of dietary vitamin C intake to bone mineral density: results from the PEPI study. Calcif Tissue Int 1998; 63(3):183–189.

35. Black DM, Cummings SR, et al. Randomised trial of effect of alendronate on risk of fractures in women with existing vertebral fractures. New Eng J Med 1996; 348:1535–1541.

36. Hui SL, Slemenda CW, Johston CC. Age and bone mass as predictors of fracture in a prospective study. J Clin Invest 1988; 81:1804–1809.

37. Sirola J, Rikkonen T. Muscle performance after the menopause. J Br Menopause Soc 2005; 11(2):45–50.

38. Kemmler W, Lauber D, et al. Benefits of 2 years of intense exercise on bone density, physical fitness, and blood lipids in early postmenopausal osteopenic women: results of the Erlangen Fitness Osteoporosis Prevention Study (EFOPS). Arch Intern Med 2004; 164(10):1084–1091.

39. Walsh MC, Hunter GR, Livingstone MB. Sarcopenia in premenopausal and postmenopausal women with osteopenia, osteoporosis and normal bone mineral density. Osteoporos Int 2006 Jan; 17(1):61–67.

40. Ullom-Minnich P. Prevention of osteoporosis and fractures. Amer Family Phys 1999; 60:194–202.

41. Kuczynski M, Ostrowska B. Understanding falls in osteoporosis: the viscoelastic modeling perspective. Gait Posture 2006; 23(1):51–58.

42. Kohrt WM, Ehsani AA, Birge SJ Jr. Effects of exercise involving predominantly either joint-reaction or ground-reaction forces on bone mineral density in older women. J Bone Miner Res 1997; 12(8):1253–1261.

43. Berard A, Bravo G, Gauthier P. Meta-analysis of the effectiveness of physical activity for the prevention of bone loss in postmenopausal women. Osteoporos Int 1997; 7(4):331–337.

44. Miyakoshi N, Hongo M, et al. Factors related to spinal mobility in patients with postmenopausal osteoporosis. Osteoporos Int 2005 Dec; 16(12):1871–1874.

45. Campbell AJ, Robertson MC, et al. Falls prevention over 2 years: a randomized controlled trial in women 80 years and older. Age Ageing 1999; 28(6):513–518.

46. Korpelainen R, Keinanen-Kiukaanniemi S, et al. Effect of impact exercise on bone mineral density in elderly women with low BMD: a population-based randomized controlled 30-month intervention. Osteoporos Int 2005; 17(1):109–118.

47. Morita S, Jinno T, et al. Bone mineral density and walking ability of elderly patients with hip fracture: a strategy for prevention of hip fracture. Injury 2005, 36(9):1075–1079.

48. Miller P, Lukert B, et al. Management of postmenopausal osteoporosis for primary care. Menopause 1998; 5(2):123–131.

49. Miller RG. Osteoporosis in postmenopausal women. Therapy options across a wide range of risk for fracture. Geriatrics 2006; 61(1):24–30.

50. McCarus DC. Fracture prevention in postmenopausal osteoporosis: a review of treatment options. Obstet Gynecol Surv 2006; 61(1):39–50.

51. Reginster JY, Sarlet N. The treatment of severe postmenopausal osteoporosis: a review of current and emerging therapeutic options. Treat Endocrinol 2006; 5(1):15–23.

52. Greenblatt D. Treatment of postmenopausal osteoporosis. Pharmacotherapy 2005; 25(4):574–584.

53. Zizic TM. Pharmacologic prevention of osteoporotic fractures. Am Fam Physician 2004; 70(7):1293–1300.

54. McClung MR, Geusens P, et al. Hip Intervention Program Study Group. Effects of risedronate on the risk of hip fracture in elderly women. New Engl J Med 2001; 344:333–340.

55. Reginster JY, Burlet N. Osteoporosis: a still increasing prevalence. Bone 2006; 38(2 Suppl 1):4–9.

56. Nguyen TV, Center JR, Eisman JA. Osteoporosis: underrated, underdiagnosed and undertreated. Med J Aust 2004; 180(5 Suppl):S18–S22.

57. Atik OS, Uslu MM, et al. Etiology of senile osteoporosis: a hypothesis. Clin Orthop Relat Res 2006; 443:25–27.

58. Mosekilde L. Vitamin D and the elderly. Clin Endocrinol (Oxf) 2005; 62(3):265–281.

PATIENT HANDOUT 8.1 – OSTEOPOROSIS: THE RISK AND HOW TO REDUCE IT[1]

The Facts

- Osteoporosis is a major health problem in elderly persons.
- It is a condition of chronic negative calcium balance; most people over 40 years of age have a net negative calcium balance.
- Imbalance between bone deposition and mineral removal over many years results in porous, light, weak bones.
- Osteoporosis develops insidiously—you don't know you have osteoporosis until you have a fracture.
- Osteoporosis increases with age—fewer than 1 in 6 women between 50 and 59 have osteoporosis, by 80 years of age this increases to 7 out of 10.
- Caucasian women are at greatest risk.
- While inheritance determines up to 75% of an individual's risk of osteoporosis, lifestyle choices can influence the likelihood of fragility fractures.
- The older you are the more important are lifestyle choices in determining your risk.

You can reduce your risk by adopting a healthier lifestyle.
See *www.jamisonhealth.com.au* Handout 21.2

Types of Osteoporosis

There are 2 types of osteoporosis:

- Type 1 or postmenopausal osteoporosis occurs usually 10–15 years after the menopause with fractures of the trabecular-rich bones such as the vertebrae and distal forearm.
- Type 2 or senile osteoporosis, which occurs mainly after 70 years of age, is 2–3 times more prevalent in women than in men, and affects both types of bones.

Check to see if you are at risk

The major predictors of postmenopausal osteoporosis are:

- lower body weight (weight < 70 kg)
- no current use of oestrogen therapy
- older age.

Others include:

- family history
- low calcium and vitamin D intake
- smoking
- weight loss
- decreased physical activity
- alcohol or caffeine use.

Refer to *www.jamisonhealth.com.au* Handout 21.1 to ascertain whether you are at increased risk of osteoporosis.

Consider using *www.jamisonhealth.com.au* Handout 21.5 to improve your bone health. Osteoporotic bones are at increased risk of fracturing.

Reference

1. US Preventive Services Task Force. Screening for osteoporosis in postmenopausal women. Recommendations and rationale. 2002. Online. Available: http://www.ahrq.gov/clinic/3rduspstf/osteoporosis/osteorr.htm#clinical.

PATIENT HANDOUT 8.2 – FRACTURES: IDENTIFYING AND REDUCING THE RISK[1,2]

Osteoporosis is a major risk factor for fractures in the elderly. It is responsible for:

- 1 in 2 postmenopausal woman having a fracture during their lifetime
- 1 in 3 women over 65 years having a vertebral fracture
- 1 in 3 women over the age of 90 having a hip fracture.

Common clinical presentations for osteoporosis include:

- Crush/wedge fracture of the spine
- fracture of the forearm
- hip fractures.

The risk of a fracture is related both to the risk of falling and the strength of the bone.

The risk of an osteoporotic fracture increases over 5-fold in elderly people who:

- smoke
- are thin, have a BMI of less than 23
- have had one previous vertebral fracture.

The risk of a fracture rises almost 12-fold after more than one vertebral fracture.

Refer to *www.jamisonhealth.com.au* Handout 21.3 to self-assess your lifestyle risk of an osteoporotic fracture.

Refer to *www.jamisonhealth.com.au* Handout 21.4 to self-assess the likelihood you have clinically evident osteoporosis.

Tips for the elderly:

- A bone mineral density test can determine whether you have osteoporosis.

- A bone mineral density test within 2 years of menopause can predict your risk over the next 10 years!
- Women 65 years and older should be routinely screened for osteoporosis.
- Women at high risk of an osteoporotic fracture should be screened at 60 years of age.
- Increase vitamin D intake to 700–800 IU/day.
- Exercise regularly—exercise increases bone and muscle strength and improves balance, reducing the risk of falling.
- Treating asymptomatic women who have osteoporosis reduces their risk for fracture.

Internet resources

http://www.niapublications.org/engagepages/osteo.asp
the bone thief

http://www.nof.org/osteoporosis/diseasefacts.htm.
National Osteoporosis Foundation

References

1. Keen RW. Burden of osteoporosis and fractures. Curr Osteoporos Rep 2003; 1(2):66-70.
2. US Preventive Services Task Force. Screening for osteoporosis in postmenopausal women. Recommendations and rationale. 2002. Online. Available: http://www.ahrq.gov/clinic/3rduspstf/osteoporosis/osteorr.htm#clinical.

Chapter 9

Wavering immunity

A 65-year-old man asks whether he should be immunized annually against influenza.

    You urge him to do so.

- Why is annual immunization recommended for elderly persons?
- Are all arms of the immune system equally compromised by age?
- Can immunosenescence be explained?

INTRODUCTION

There is evidence to suggest an association between immune function and longevity. Certainly the elderly are more prone to infection and cancer—both conditions strongly influenced by immune function. Aging is associated with a dramatic reduction in responsiveness as well as functional dysregulation of the immune system. In fact, immunological changes occurring in those who enjoy good health to the maximum life span would appear more closely related to a reshaping rather than to resistance to generalized deterioration of the main immune functions.[1]

IMMUNOSENESCENCE

The aging of the immune system is referred to as immunosenescence. Not all components of the immune system are equally affected. Innate and humoral immunity seem to be relatively unchanged but cellular immunity shows marked age-associated alterations.[2]

Innate immunity functions immediately after birth and manifests little change throughout life. Innate immunity, as measured by macrophage functions, is preserved or even increased during the aging process. Macrophages, granulocytes and natural killer cells, the major components of the innate system, are less affected than T and B lymphocytes which comprise the adaptive systems.

Adaptive immunity, with its humoral and cellular arms, is immature at birth, peaks at puberty and progressively declines thereafter.[2] Despite some changes in humoral immunity, including altered CD5/CD5(+) cell ratios and duration of antibody responses, it is cellular immunity that is most susceptible to the deleterious effects of aging. Age-related changes include a decrease in naive memory T cells with a relative increase in activated/memory T cell phenotypes. Other marked alterations in cell-mediated immunity include the relative proportion of mature to immature T cells and the T-helper 1/T-helper 2 cell ratio.[3,4] The elderly demonstrate decreased responsiveness to T cell receptor stimulation, impaired T cell proliferative capacity, a decline in the frequency of CD4(+) T cells producing IL-2 and a decreased expression in IL-2 receptors.[5,6]

AN IMMUNE RISK PHENOTYPE

Longitudinal studies suggest that immune parameters predominantly related to T cells can be clustered to yield an immune risk phenotype predictive of mortality in the elderly.[7] Clonal expansion is fundamental to adaptive immunity. Replicative senescence is the term used to describe the strict limit on the proliferative potential of normal human somatic cells. In the elderly, clonal expansion of T cells, as predicated by replicative senescence, is limited. Cultures of senescent CD8(+) T cells show resistance to apoptosis, permanent loss of CD28 expression, altered cytokine profiles, reduced ability to respond to stress, and various functional changes. In elderly persons, the presence of high proportions of CD8(+) T cells with characteristics of replicative senescence correlates with reduced antibody responses to vaccines.[8]

Cytomegalovirus (CMV) seropositivity has been associated with many of the same phenotypic and functional alterations to T cell immunity selected as biomarkers of aging.[9] The elderly appear biased towards a more anti-inflammatory response with a reduced capacity to produce gamma-interferon. This cytokine plays an important role in defence against intracellular pathogens and other intracellular viruses. Impaired production is associated with persistent CMV infection.[10,11] This provides the basis for the hypothesis of an 'immune risk phenotype', predicting mortality, associated with CMV seropositivity.[9] Certainly the emerging picture is that senescent CD8(+) T cells may contribute to reduced anti-viral immunity and diverse age-related pathologies.[8]

IS AN ALTERED IMMUNE STATUS ATTRIBUTABLE TO AGE OR DIET?

While the proliferative ability of cellular immunity is apparently lowered in the elderly due to aging, B cell subsets and innate immunity are less affected by aging and more by nutritional status—with respect to both micronutrient status and protein energy malnutrition.[4] In fact, aging and malnutrition appear to have a similar impact on the immune system.[12] In elderly people cell-mediated immune responses are weaker and neither cell-mediated nor humoral responses are as well adapted to antigen stimulation. Likewise, undernutrition induces lower immune responses, particularly with respect to cell-mediated immunity. Protein-energy malnutrition is associated with decreased lymphocyte proliferation, reduced cytokine release and lower antibody response to vaccines. Micronutrient deficits, namely of zinc, selenium, and vitamin B-6, have a similar impact on immune responses. In fact, the influences of aging and undernutrition in humans appear to be cumulative and some changes in immune response that have been attributed to aging may, in reality, be related to nutrition rather than the aging process.[13]

Nutrient deficiencies are frequent in older populations and there is a growing consensus that the use of mixtures containing optimum amounts of essential trace elements and vitamins may enhance immune responses and reduce the occurrence of common infections.[14] There are data to support use of a daily multivitamin or trace-mineral supplement that includes zinc (elemental zinc, >20 mg/day) and selenium (100 µg/day), with additional vitamin E, to achieve a daily dosage of 200 mg/day.[15]

ANTIOXIDANT SUPPLEMENTATION TO BOOST IMMUNE STATUS

Zinc and vitamin E have been shown to increase selected immune responses without any reduction in infectious morbidity.[16] Twelve months supplementation with 200 IU vitamin E daily had no statistically significant effect on lower respiratory tract infections but did appear to have a protective effect on upper respiratory tract infections, particularly the common cold. Furthermore, animal studies suggest vitamin E supplementation may induce a higher differentiation of immature T cells, via increased positive selection by thymic epithelial cells, minimizing the aging-associated decrease in cellular immunity.[17] Ingestion of vitamin E (200 mg daily for 3 months) stimulated lymphoproliferation in the majority of elderly male subjects, but lymphoproliferation was depressed in others.[18] The authors suggested that antioxidants modulated immune function, restoring altered immune function, to more optimum values. In general, daily doses of vitamin E up to 800 IU may enhance, while doses in excess of 800 IU may suppress, immunity. A clinically useful rule of thumb for vitamin E is 800 IU equates to 500 mg. Vitamin E is regarded as safe at levels up to 800 IU/day. While side effects may begin to appear at doses of around 1500 IU/day,[19] even doses of 3200 mg/day have been shown to be without any consistent risk.[20] Vitamin E may enhance the anti-inflammatory effect of aspirin and decrease the dose of anticoagulant, insulin and digoxin required by elderly patients on these medications. Economists estimate a saving of $5–6 billion annually could be achieved if all adults over the age of 50 years took at least 100 IU vitamin E daily.[21]

Vitamin E's mechanisms of action are similar to those of selenium. Animal and human studies have demonstrated that selenium is involved in immunomodulation through enhanced activation and proliferation of B and T lymphocytes[22,23] amongst others. Selenium modulates T lymphocyte mediated immune responses and stimulates peripheral lymphocytes to respond to antigens. It has a narrow safety margin with clinical toxicity reported on daily doses of 1000–2000 µg over a month. The dose for long term use is thought to fall between 100 and 400 µg. As 400 µg daily is probably the upper limit of safety, daily doses of 100–200 µg may be more realistic objectives for inhibiting genetic damage and carcinogenesis in humans.[24] Vitamin E 500 IU daily enhances the efficacy of selenium, and deficiency of one often overlaps with deficiency in the other. Zinc also plays a particularly important role in immunity.[25] While severe zinc deficiency can cause substantial impairment of cellular immunity, the effects of mild zinc deficiency, a common problem in the elderly, may be subtle. Short periods of zinc supplementation have been found to improve immune defence substantially in individuals with diverse diseases.[26] Zinc supplementation can enhance immunity if an underlying deficiency is present and may increase resistance to infection in the elderly through various pathways.[27] Zinc deficiency should be excluded in elderly persons who are lethargic, anorexic, have reduced taste sensation and demonstrate mental slowness. Zinc deficiency affects leukocyte functions, impairing phagocytosis; however its impact is most marked on the adaptive immune system. Zinc deficiency rapidly diminishes antibody- and cell-mediated responses. Impaired immune function due to dietary zinc deficiency is characterized in part by a reduction in the number of lymphocytes and depressed cell-mediated i.e. T lymphocyte function. Zinc deficiency may also possibly be conducive to premature transition from efficient Th1-dependent cellular immune functions to Th2-dependent humoral immune functions.

Immune integrity is tightly linked to zinc status. However, supplementation with zinc as a single nutrient, especially at high doses, can have adverse effects ranging from interference with copper absorption to impairment of immune functions.[28] In fact, high dosages of zinc have negative effects on immune cells, which show alterations similar to those observed with zinc deficiency.[29] Both excessive and inadequate zinc levels can impair immune function! Like vitamin E, dose is important.

There are many more nutrients that affect immunity. Nutrients demonstrated in animal and/or human studies to be required for efficient immune function include essential amino acids, the essential fatty acid linoleic acid, vitamin A, folic acid, vitamin B6, vitamin B12, vitamin C, Cu and Fe.[30] Nutrient deficiencies encountered in the elderly range from zinc, iron, beta-carotene, Vitamins B6, B12, C, D and E to folic acid.[14] A well-balanced diet with supplementation of specific nutrients may be prudent for elderly persons.

DIETARY INTERVENTION TO MODULATE CELL MEMBRANES

Some of the immune effects associated with aging, such as alterations in the viscosity of cell membranes and proteolytic cellular machinery, may be secondary to overall organismic changes.[31] Changes to cellular membranes may contribute to the decreases in the early events of signal transduction, the activation-induced intracellular phosphorylation and cellular proliferative responses to T cell receptor stimulation encountered in the elderly.[6]

Dietary lipids alter cell membrane structure and influence immune status in the elderly. Omega-3-polyunsaturated fatty acids (n-3 PUFA) have immunomodulatory effects but at high dosages (>2 g/day) are known to increase lipid peroxidation. Cell membranes are susceptible to free radical attack. A preliminary study on elderly male rats suggests that dietary supplementation with coenzyme Q10, and enrichment of cell membranes with monounsaturated fatty acids, protects mitochondrial membranes against free radical insult.[32] Moreover, supplementation of healthy elderly people with low doses of n-3 fatty acids (600 mg daily of marine oil containing docosahexaenoate (150 mg) and eicosapentaenoate (30 mg)), modulates the immune responses of elderly subjects with no untoward effect on their antioxidant status.[33] This confirmed an earlier study which found that low doses of n-3 PUFA supplemented with adequate amounts of alpha-tocopherol can be incorporated into blood lipids in elderly subjects without lowering their antioxidant concentrations or increasing lipid peroxidation.[34] Similarly, the age-associated increase in prostaglandin E(2) production that contributes to the decline in T cell-mediated function with age can be modulated by taking blackcurrant seed oil, rich in both gamma-linolenic and alpha-linolenic acids.[35] The clinical importance of such changes requires investigation. Another study in which n-3 PUFAs in doses of up to 1.7 g EPA+DHA/day found no alteration in the functional activity of neutrophils, monocytes, or lymphocytes, despite changes in the fatty acid composition of mononuclear cells.[36]

IMMUNITY AND THE FREE RADICAL THEORY OF AGING

Given the free radical theory of aging which postulates that oxygen-derived free radicals cause oxidative damage, it is possible that antioxidants may be the supplements of choice for retarding immunosenescence.[37] Immune cells, which use free radicals in their functions, may well be particularly prone to suffer senescent deterioration due to their close link with oxidative stress. Vitamin E, selenium and zinc all have antioxidant potential!

Vitamin E protects against lipid peroxidation by acting directly on a number of oxygen radicals, including singlet oxygen, lipid peroxide products and the superoxide radical to form the relatively harmless tocopherol radical.[38] Alpha-tocopherol can, however, act either as an antioxidant to inhibit or as a prooxidant to facilitate lipid peroxidation of low density lipoprotein.

Different antioxidants appear to act synergistically, so supplementation with vitamin E might be more effective if combined with other micronutrients. Combined daily supplementation of vitamins E (200 mg) with C (1000 mg) enhances immunity more than either vitamin alone. Vitamin E also works in conjunction with selenium, a cofactor for glutathione peroxidase, and various enzymes such as superoxide dismutase and catalase. Supplementing selenium may minimize the effect of deficiency of vitamin E. Selenium makes an important contribution to the antioxidant system.

Zinc is another free radical quencher. It also functions as an antioxidant through its protection against vitamin E depletion, stabilization of cell membranes, control of vitamin A release and its contribution to the structure of extracellular superoxide dismutase.[39] Supplementation with an antioxidant enriched drink has been shown to raise plasma levels of enzymatic and non-enzymatic antioxidants in frail elderly people.[40]

In addition to dietary options, a hormone with substantial antioxidant ability deserves particular attention. Melatonin, produced from serotonin by the pineal gland, is a free radical scavenger that stimulates several antioxidative enzymes.[41] Melatonin directly neutralizes hydroxyl radicals, hydrogen peroxide, singlet oxygen, peroxynitrite anion, nitric oxide and hypochlorous acid. It also stimulates superoxide dismutase, glutathione peroxidase and glutathione reductase. Melatonin is a natural antioxidant with significant anti-aging properties and a defined immunomodulatory role.[42]

Melatonin has been proposed as regulating the immune system largely by affecting cytokine production in immunocompetent cells such as granulocyte-macrophage cells, NK cells and lymphocytes. Indeed, there is evidence to suggest that it is this shift in cytokine profile that is largely responsible for triggering immunosenescence.[42] The age-related impairment of the immune system which first appears around 60 years of age coincides with the decrease of plasma melatonin concentration, as do the diurnal and seasonal changes in the immune function with melatonin synthesis and secretion. The loss of amplitude of melatonin rhythm in advanced age appears to be both an indication and cause of age-related disturbances in the circadian pacemaker, leading to chronobiological disorders. Melatonin, along with pituitary growth hormone, adrenal production of dehydro-epiandrosterone and tissue-specific availability of active vitamin D, is one of the hormones whose decline parallels immunosenescence.[43]

BOOSTING IMMUNITY AT SPECIFIC SITES

While boosting general immunity in the elderly is desirable, it is also possible to enhance immunity of specific organs.

The risk of urinary infections can be reduced by good urinary hygiene. This involves a high fluid intake and, in the case of females, care to avoid colonization of the urethra and bladder by gut bacteria. Frequent consumption of fresh juices, especially berry juices, and fermented milk products containing probiotic bacteria decreases the risk of recurrent urinary tract infection.[44] A randomized, double-blind, placebo-controlled trial found 300 mL per day of a commercially available standard cranberry beverage reduced the frequency of bacteriuria in older women.[45] Colonization of the rectum and vagina by live *Lactobacillus acidophilus* may reduce episodes of bacterial vaginosis and urinary infection. Daily consumption of 150 mL of yogurt, enriched with *acidophilus* is recommended.[46]

Probiotics can also reduce the risk of bowel infection. Useful probiotic foods need to provide an adequate number of viable, functional bacteria with a good shelf life. The minimal number of colony forming units considered adequate to maintain a healthy intestinal flora is 1–2 billion. The benefits of probiotic bacteria are diverse, ranging from improved digestion through enhanced production of organic acids, potentially conferring some protection against colon cancer, to vitamin synthesis, e.g. vitamins K, B12, folic acid and biotin. More recently, supplementation with *Bifidobacterium lactis* HN019 has been found to enhance some aspects of cellular immunity in the elderly. A study of 30 elderly people supplemented with *B. lactis* HN019 in a dose 5×10^{10} organisms/day over 3 weeks increased the proportions of total, helper (CD4(+)), and activated (CD25(+))T lymphocytes and natural killer cells.[47]

The efficacy of probiotics can be enhanced by simultaneously consuming prebiotics. Prebiotics are non-digestible food ingredients that selectively stimulate the growth and/or activity of various beneficial probiotic colonic bacterial species such as lactobacilli and bifidobacteria. In addition to providing a probiotic substrate, prebiotics stimulate absorption of several minerals that improve bone mineralization. Prebiotics are non-digestible oligosaccharides and good plant sources are onions, asparagus, wheat and artichoke leaf.

CONCLUDING REMARKS

Immunity, particularly cell mediated immunity, is compromised by aging. Inadequate nutrition aggravates the dysregulation of adaptive immunity. An adequate diet supplemented by antioxidants and functional foods may, to some extent, limit immune inadequacies.

CLINICAL CHALLENGE

Rebecca, a 70-year-old woman, presents complaining of a productive cough. She explains she is prone to frequent colds and bladder infections. She has no appetite and admits to a history of marginal alcohol abuse. She smokes 10 cigarettes a day.

Questions arising

- What is the differential diagnosis?
- How should she be further investigated?

Clinical considerations

The following possibilities need to be explored:

1. Lobar pneumonia needs to be investigated. Request a chest examination, X-ray and sputum culture—treat as necessary.
2. Pyelonephritis needs to be excluded. Send urine for microscopy, culture and sensitivity.
3. Malnutrition needs to be confirmed or excluded. A careful dietary history needs to be taken to exclude/confirm inadequate nutrition—a common problem in the elderly, especially those with an alcohol problem.

Her chest X-ray is clear, her urine culture is negative.

Questions arising

- Has an underlying condition been missed?
- In the absence of any specific current infections what long term intervention would you consider?

Clinical considerations

- Exclude covert disease such as diabetes (do a blood sugar) or leukaemia (do a full blood count).
- Attempt to improve her general immunity by nutritional means.

In the elderly, total energy intake is often inadequate, as is protein. Nutrients most often deficient in the aged include potassium, iron, calcium, magnesium, zinc, folate, vitamin C, vitamin D, vitamin A, pyridoxine and thiamine.

Particular considerations in this patient are:

- zinc deficiency leads to a poor sense of taste and smell and hence appetite.
- energy from alcohol increases the requirement for B vitamins.

Dietary advice:

- Avoid big meals but take care not to miss any meals.
- Eat a diet rich in whole foods—fruit, vegetables and wholegrains.
- Eat an egg—preferably soft boiled each day.
- Be sure to eat meat or fish regularly.
- Supplement the diet with vitamin B complex, vitamin E, zinc and calcium. If long term zinc supplementation is required, consider adding a 2 mg copper supplement each day.

Refer the patient to Patient Handout 9.1 and suggest she consider both the general guidelines and those for urinary hygiene.

PRACTICE GEMS

- Innate immunity is relatively unaffected by aging; adaptive immunity, particularly cell mediated immunity, is somewhat compromised.
- Inadequate nutrition produces changes in the immune system similar to aging.
- Minimize the impact of aging on the immune system by ensuring elderly persons are adequately nourished.
- Supplementation with antioxidants, particularly vitamin E, zinc and selenium, may improve adaptive immunity in elderly persons, particularly if they are deficient in these nutrients.
- Antioxidant supplementation may achieve immunostimulation or –depression depending on the dose.
- Melatonin may emerge as a useful therapy as time progresses—research is ongoing.

References

1. Ginaldi L, De Martinis M, et al. Immunological changes in the elderly. Aging (Milano) 1999; 11(5):281–286.
2. Linton P, Thoman ML. T cell senescence. Front Biosci 2001; 6:D248–D261.
3. Lesourd B, Mazari L. Nutrition and immunity in the elderly. Proc Nutr Soc 1999; 58(3):685–695.
4. Lesourd B. Nutrition: a major factor influencing immunity in the elderly. J Nutr Health Aging 2004; 8(1):28–37.
5. De la Fuente M. Effects of antioxidants on immune system ageing. Eur J Clin Nutr 2002; 56 Suppl 3:S5–S8.
6. Ginaldi L, De Martinis M, et al. The immune system in the elderly: II. Specific cellular immunity. Immunol Res 1999; 20(2):109–115.
7. Pawelec G, Ouyang Q, et al. Pathways to a robust immune response in the elderly. Immunol Allergy Clin North Am 2003; 23(1):1–13.
8. Effros RB, Dagarag M, et al. The role of CD8+ T-cell replicative senescence in human aging. Immunol Rev 2005; 205:147–157.
9. Pawelec G, Akbar A, et al. Human immunosenescence: is it infectious? Immunol Rev 2005; 205:257–268.
10. Ouyang Q, Wagner WM, et al. Dysfunctional CMV-specific CD8(+) T cells accumulate in the elderly. Exp Gerontol 2004; 39(4):607–613.
11. Ouyang Q, Wagner WM, et al. Compromised interferon gamma (IFN-gamma) production in the elderly to both acute and latent viral antigen stimulation: contribution to the immune risk phenotype? Eur Cytokine Netw 2002; 13(4):392–394.
12. Lesourd BM. Nutrition and immunity in the elderly: modification of immune responses with nutritional treatments. Am J Clin Nutr 1997; 66(2):478S–484S.
13. Mazari L, Lesourd BM. Nutritional influences on immune response in healthy aged persons. Mech Ageing Dev 1998; 104(1):25–40.
14. Chandra RK. Impact of nutritional status and nutrient supplements on immune responses and incidence of infection in older individuals. Ageing Res Rev 2004; 3(1):91–104.
15. High KP. Nutritional strategies to boost immunity and prevent infection in elderly individuals. Clin Infect Dis 2001; 33(11):1892–1900.
16. Meydani SN, Leka LS, et al. Vitamin E and respiratory tract infections in elderly nursing home residents: a randomized controlled trial. JAMA 2004; 292(7):828-836.
17. Moriguchi S, Muraga M. Vitamin E and immunity. Vitam Horm 2000; 59:305–336.
18. De la Fuente M, Victor VM. Anti-oxidants as modulators of immune function. Immunol Cell Biol 2000; 78(1):49–54.
19. Pryor WA. Vitamin E and heart disease: basic science to clinical intervention trials. Free Radic Biol Med 2000; 28(1):141–164.
20. Diplock AT, Charleux JL, et al. Functional food science and defence against reactive oxidative species. Br J Nutr 1998; 80 Suppl 1:S77–S112.
21. Bendich A, Mallick R, et al. Potential health economic benefits of vitamin supplementation. West J Med 1997; 166:306–312.
22. Hawkes WC, Kelley DS, Taylor PC. The effects of dietary selenium on the immune system in healthy men. Biol Trace Elem Res 2001; 81(3):189–213.
23. Gazdik F, Horvathova M, et al. The influence of selenium supplementation on the immunity of corticoid-dependent asthmatics. Bratisl Lek Listy 2002; 103(1):17–21.
24. El-Bayoumy K. The protective role of selenium on genetic damage and on cancer. Mutat Res 2001; 475(1-2):123–139.
25. Sprietsma JE. Modern diets and diseases: NO-zinc balance. Under Th1, zinc and nitrogen monoxide (NO) collectively protect against viruses, AIDS, autoimmunity, diabetes, allergies, asthma, infectious diseases, atherosclerosis and cancer. Med Hypotheses 1999; 53(1):6–16.
26. Fraker PJ, King LE, et al. The dynamic link between the integrity of the immune system and zinc status. J Nutr 2000; 130(5S Suppl):1399S–1406S.
27. Mocchegiani E, Muzzioli M, Giacconi R. Zinc and immunoresistance to infection in aging: new biological tools. Trends Pharmacol Sci 2000; 21(6):205–208.
28. Bogden JD. Influence of zinc on immunity in the elderly. J Nutr Health Aging 2004; 8(1):48–54.
29. Ibs KH, Rink L. Zinc-altered immune function. J Nutr 2003; 133(5 Suppl 1):1452S–1456S.
30. Calder PC, Kew S. The immune system: a target for functional foods? Br J Nutr 2002; 88 Suppl 2:S165–S177.
31. Effros RB. Ageing and the immune system. Novartis Found Symp 2001; 235:130–139.
32. Huertas JR, Martinez-Velasco E, et al. Virgin olive oil and coenzyme Q10 protect heart mitochondria from peroxidative damage during aging. Biofactors 1999; 9(2–4):337–343.
33. Bechoua S, Dubois M, et al. Influence of very low dietary intake of marine oil on some functional

aspects of immune cells in healthy elderly people. Br J Nutr 2003; 89(4):523–531.

34. Rodriguez-Palmero M, Lopez-Sabater MC, et al. Administration of low doses of fish oil derived N-3 fatty acids to elderly subjects. Eur J Clin Nutr 1997; 51(8):554–560.

35. Wu D, Meydani M, et al. Effect of dietary supplementation with black currant seed oil on the immune response of healthy elderly subjects. Am J Clin Nutr 1999; 70(4):536–543.

36. Kew S, Banerjee T, et al. Lack of effect of foods enriched with plant- or marine-derived n-3 fatty acids on human immune function. Am J Clin Nutr 2003; 77(5):1287–1295.

37. Meydani M. The Boyd Orr lecture. Nutrition interventions in aging and age-associated disease. Proc Nutr Soc 2002; 61(2):165–171.

38. Clarkson PM, Thompson HS. Antioxidants: what role do they play in physical activity and health? Am J Clin Nutr 2000; 72:637S–646S.

39. DiSilvestro RA. Zinc in relation to diabetes and oxidative disease. J Nutr 2000; 130(5S Suppl):1509S–1511S.

40. Wouters-Wesseling W, Wagenaar LW, et al. Biochemical antioxidant levels respond to supplementation with an enriched drink in frail elderly people. J Am Coll Nutr 2003; 22(3):232–238.

41. Reiter RJ, Tan DX, et al. Actions of melatonin in the reduction of oxidative stress. A review. J Biomed Sci 2000; 7(6):444–458.

42. Srinivasan V, Maestroni G, et al. Melatonin, immune function and aging. Immun Ageing 2005; 2:17.

43. Arlt W, Hewison M. Hormones and immune function: implications of aging. Aging Cell 2004; 3(4):209–216.

44. Kontiokari T, Laitinen J, et al. Dietary factors protecting women from urinary tract infection. Am J Clin Nutr 2003; 77(3):600–604.

45. Avorn J, Monane M, et al. Reduction of bacteriuria and pyuria after ingestion of cranberry juice. JAMA 1994; 271(10):751–754.

46. Shalev E, Battino S, et al. Ingestion of yogurt containing Lactobacillus acidophilus compared with pasteurized yogurt as prophylaxis for recurrent candidal vaginitis and bacterial vaginosis. Arch Fam Med 1996; 5(10):593–596.

47. Gill HS, Rutherfurd KJ, et al. Enhancement of immunity in the elderly by dietary supplementation with the probiotic Bifidobacterium lactis HN019. Am J Clin Nutr 2001; 74(6):833–839.

PATIENT HANDOUT 9.1 – BOOSTING IMMUNITY

General Immunity

Dietary choices

Choose a daily diet that

- Emphasizes whole foods:
  - >4 serves grains/cereals
  - >2 serves fruits* (>270 g)
  - >5 serves vegetables* (>375 g)

(*4 different coloured fruit/vegetables should be selected)

- Favours fat-free or low-fat milk and dairy products
- Includes moderate amounts of
  - lean red meat and poultry
  - fish every third or fourth day
  - beans (especially soybeans), eggs, and nuts
- Is low in saturated fats, *trans* fats e.g. solidified oils, cholesterol
- Limits
  - salt (<4 g)
  - alcohol–1 glass red wine for women, 2 glasses for men.
  - added refined sugars.

Supplementation

Consider taking nutritional supplements such as antioxidants:

- zinc 20 mg/day
- selenium 100 µg/day
- vitamin E 600–800 IU/day plus seeds and nuts.

Food preparation

- Favour microwaving, grilling and steaming
- Avoid frying
- Eat fresh.

Respiratory Hygiene

- Be a non-smoker
- Avoid exposure to cigarette smoke–passive smoking.

Gastro-intestinal Hygiene

General dietary selection

Bowel health is enhanced by a diet rich in:

- fibre, i.e. whole grains, nuts, fruit and vegetables
- brassica: cauliflower, cabbage, Brussels sprouts etc.

Bowel colonization with probiotics

- Functional foods, e.g. yogurt rich in Bifidobacteria along with a diet rich in soybeans, asparagus, onion and wheat
- Probiotic mixtures, e.g. yakult–low sugar variant
- Probiotic tablets–choose a capsule not using heat in its preparation.

To increase the likelihood of a viable culture in probiotics:

- always check use by dates
- store in the fridge
- avoid taking with meals.

1–2 billion bacteria are required for intestinal health!

Urinary Hygiene

- Adequate fluid–drink >2.0 L fluid daily
- Berry drinks–cranberry juice 400–800 mL daily
- Probiotic boost–150 mL of yogurt rich in live *Lactobacillus acidophilus*
- Wipe technique–after defecation wipe backwards, i.e. away from the urethra.

Chapter 10

Fatigue: Faltering energy

CHAPTER CONTENTS

Two elderly women present complaining of persistent fatigue. One has recently recovered from a bad bout of influenza, the other lost her husband a month ago, just 2 weeks after she retired from the workforce.

- Can perturbation of a single biological system explain fatigue in both patients?
- Is exercise likely to benefit either or both women?
- Should coenzyme Q supplementation be considered in either case?

INTRODUCTION

A study of adults aged 60 years and older found every second participant suffered from fatigue.[1] Fatigue is a major source of disablement in patients with significant ill health,[2] and is believed to be under-reported by patients and somewhat overlooked by clinicians.[3]

It is caused by numerous factors and is encountered in many different situations. Patients with anaemia, hypothyroidism and pain rate their fatigue as moderate to high, as may persons with emotional distress or those with disturbed sleep. Elderly patients with conditions as diverse as depression and diabetes, insomnia and chronic renal failure report fatigue. Fatigue may be the presenting symptom of leukaemia, hypercalcaemia and diabetes.

EXPLAINING FATIGUE

Despite its substantial morbidity and prevalence, fatigue lacks a clear pathophysiological explanation.[3] Nonetheless, one plausible postulate which deserves reflection is that stress initiates a sequence of events that produce chronic fatigue. Stress, whether inflammatory, traumatic or psychological in nature, is associated with concurrent activation of the hypothalamic–pituitary–adrenal axis. The hypothalamus sets body tone through its control of the autonomic nervous and endocrine systems. Two major arms of the stress response are the corticotrophin-releasing hormone and the locus ceruleus–norepinephrine/autonomic sympathetic nervous systems.[4] Stress hormones play a key role in mediating both adaptive and maladaptive responses. Cortisol releasing hormone triggers activation of the pituitary–adrenal axis and sympathetic nervous system. The locus ceruleus–norepinephrine system enhances vigilance and increases anxiety centrally, while the sympathetic arm of the autonomic nervous system acts peripherally through the adrenal medulla and peripheral nerves. Stress causes disease when persistent arousal results in tonal exhaustion. The level of arousal is determined by physiological, emotional and cognitive information.

While activation of allostatic mechanisms helps the body adapt to challenges in the short term, persistence of allostatic response mechanisms or exposure to either a single overwhelming stressor or to chronic minor stressors may create an allostatic load.[5] An allostatic load results from sustained or repeated activation of mediators of adaptation.[6] As mental processes and physical functioning are mutually and bidirectionally interactive, both psychosocial and physical stressors may create an allostatic load. As thoughts causally influence the body, and emotions link psyche and soma, social experiences have biochemical repercussions. Psychoneuroimmunology, the discipline studying interrelationships between life events, the neuroendocrine and immune systems, has proposed a plausible explanation for how stress-associated immune modulation may precipitate fatigue in viral infections and chronic fatigue syndrome.[6,7] It has shown how proinflammatory cytokines acting in the brain may cause sickness behaviours, including listlessness, fatigue, malaise and significant changes in sleep patterns.[8,9]

Prolonged activation of the central stress response by cytokines creates an allostatic load. Chronic cytokine stimulation resulting in chronic inflammation is one possible explanation for the decline in physical function associated with aging. Inflammation, measured as high levels of C-reactive protein and interleukins-6 and -1RA, has been shown to be significantly associated with poor physical performance and muscle strength in older persons.[10] Fatigue, increased muscle tenderness and depression appear linked.[11,12] It is thought chronic cytokine elevations engender neuro-endocrine and brain neurotransmitter changes that are interpreted by the brain as stressors which may contribute to the development of these symptoms.[13] Impaired feedback of the hypothalamic–pituitary–adrenal axis, postulated to underlie chronic activation of the immune system, provides a plausible, albeit unproven, explanation for the fatigue characteristic of fibromyalgia, chronic fatigue syndrome and acute onset postviral fatigue.[11,12] An umbrella term, chronic multisymptom illness, has even been proposed to encompass conditions resulting from dysfunction of the stress system in the face of an allostatic load.[14]

DEFINING FATIGUE

In addition to lacking a clear mechanistic explanation, fatigue lacks an objective 'gold standard' means of measurement. Fatigue is a subjective experience. It has variously been defined as an overwhelming sense of tiredness, lack of energy and a feeling of exhaustion, associated with impaired physical and/or cognitive functioning.[2] It differs from depression in that fatigue is not characterized by lack of self-esteem, sadness and despair or hopelessness.[2] Other attempts to define fatigue have used dichotomous approaches: acute versus chronic and physiological versus psychological.[2]

Acute fatigue, with its rapid onset, short duration and clear cause in healthy individuals is perceived as a normal protective event. Acute fatigue is relieved by rest, exercise and/or stress management; chronic fatigue persists despite such restorative attempts. Chronic fatigue is insidious in onset, persistent and has an adverse effect on the quality of life. It is usually multifactorial in aetiology and primarily affects unhealthy persons.

Physiological fatigue, defined either as a loss of maximal force-generating capacity during muscular activity or a failure of the functional organ, may result from diseases e.g. infection, or functional disturbances e.g. insomnia. In contrast, psychological fatigue is a state of weariness related to reduced motivation. Psychological fatigue is associated with intense emotional experiences and may accompany depression and anxiety. In cancer patients there is a correlation between psychological distress, functional disability and fatigue.[15]

Sleepiness and fatigue are two interrelated, but distinct phenomena. In fact, terms regarding fatigue and excessive daytime sleepiness are frequently used interchangeably, or under the general rubric of being 'tired'. Sleepiness is distinguished from fatigue by a presumed impairment of normal arousal mechanism.[2] Sleepiness is a ubiquitous phenomenon, experienced both as a clinical symptom and as a normal physiological state. Sleepiness can be considered abnormal when it occurs at inappropriate times or is excessive. The tendency to fall asleep, or sleep propensity, is the result of the interaction of primary sleep/wakefulness drives determined by circadian and ultradian rhythms and secondary sleep/wakefulness drives influenced by environmental factors, e.g. light, and behavioural factors. Sleepiness, in contrast to fatigue, is caused by an alteration or imbalance in sleep/wake mechanisms—a necessary and sufficient prerequisite. Both fatigue and sleepiness are commonly reported by elderly persons.

MANAGING FATIGUE

The insidious onset of fatigue in the elderly may be a manifestation of conditions as diverse as thyroid disease, malignancy, anaemia, congestive cardiac failure, hypercalcaemia or obstructive sleep apnoea. In each instance when fatigue is clearly related to organic disease, it is somewhat alleviated by specifically treating the underlying disease. Treating disease may aid but not provide sufficient intervention for managing fatigue. A more holistic approach may be required. The potential for fatigue to be but one manifestation of a dysfunctional stress management system leading to a chronic multisymptom type illness should not be overlooked.

Chronic multisymptom illness, the outcome of dysfunction of the stress system, is characterized by otherwise unexplained widespread chronic pain, unremitting fatigue, and cognitive and mood complaints.[14] Organic disease is not a prerequisite to development of these symptoms—healthy individuals stressed by sleep deprivation have been shown to develop muscle tenderness, mood changes and fatigue.[13] Elderly patients complaining of fatigue may well be experiencing a multisymptom illness. Symptom targeted intervention may enhance the quality of life of sufferers. Questionnaires to facilitate identification of individual but overlapping symptoms, such as depression and sleepiness, are available.[16]

APPROACHES TO INTERVENTION

While specific management should always target any organic explanation for fatigue, non-specific interventions that interrupt the development of fatigue may also enhance patient wellbeing. Diverse interventions have been demonstrated to alleviate fatigue. Exercise benefits cancer related fatigue, behavioural modification reduces fatigue in insomniacs while antidepressants improve fatigue in patients with fibromyalgia.[17] In addition to treating any disorders present, fatigued patients may benefit from non-specific interventions that target energy production or interrupt an aberrant stress response system.

Exercise modulation of the stress system

Exercise is known to lead to improvements in pain sensitivity and changes in immune, hypothalamic–pituitary–adrenal and autonomic function. In fact, Glass et al hypothesized that healthy individuals with hypoactive function of their stress response systems unknowingly exercised regularly to augment the function of these systems.[14] A longitudinal study was undertaken to test this postulate. Glass and his co-researchers found that following cessation of their exercise regime a subset of participants experienced fatigue, increased pain and mood disturbances.[14] Fatigue emerged as the most prominent symptom in the susceptible subset of exercise deprived subjects. Exercise may offer a non-specific intervention that reduces fatigue while addressing underlying suboptimal allostasis.

Regular exercise has also been shown to increase longevity.[18] Compared with those who maintained a low physical activity level, moderate and high physical activity increased total life expectancy for men aged 50 years or older by 1.3 and 3.7 years respectively. In women moderate physical activity increased life expectancy by 1.5 years while high physical activity produced a gain of 3.5 years. Survival is inversely related to functional impairment,[19] and physical inactivity is associated with disability. Physical inactivity has emerged as a major determinant of frailty. In fact, inactivity in combination with weight loss has been proposed as a suitable working definition for selecting a frail elderly population among community-dwelling elderly men.[20] Frailty correlates more closely than chronological age with mortality.[21]

Frailty may result from an excess allostatic load on the stress systems. One biochemical explanation for the development of a frailty phenotype incorporates activation of the coagulation and inflammatory pathways. Several studies have shown exposure to severe mental or physical stressors causes excess IL-6 production.[22] Activation of these pathways has been shown to be associated with mortality and decline in function.[23] A cross-sectional study of persons aged 70–79 years found an association between high levels of recreational activity and lower levels of the inflammatory markers IL-6 and CRP.[24] Frailty may be construed as a failure to integrate complex responses to maintain function and be viewed as a set of linked deteriorations affecting many organ systems.[25] Regardless of the precise mechanism, it appears the elderly would benefit from increased physical activity!

In addition to exercise offering an intervention which appears to modulate the stress system, exercise has been shown to benefit various problems prevalent in the elderly. The beneficial effect of physical activity on muscle strength, bone mass and functional independence has repeatedly been demonstrated.[20] Higher fitness achieved over 10 years of regular exercise training in older adults reduced the development of metabolic risk factors for cardiovascular disease—even when the exercise regime was introduced after the age of 65 years.[26] Increased physical activity appears to reduce the risk for breast cancer in postmenopausal women.[27] While physical activity need not be strenuous, the longer the duration of exercise the greater the benefit.[27] Some 10 hours of brisk walking each week are recommended. Daily walking predicts lower costs for hospitalizations and diagnostic testing in elderly persons.[28] A recent study comparing fit and unfit older women found that unfit elderly women demonstrate greater hypothalamic–pituitary–adrenal axis activation in response to a psychological challenge.[29] Arguing that fitness appeared associated with less hypothalamic–pituitary–adrenal axis reactivity in older individuals, the researchers suggested exercise training may be an effective way of modifying some of the neuroendocrine changes associated with aging. Certainly, persons over 68 years of age with the lowest health care costs don't smoke, maintain a desirable body weight and walk every day.[28]

Psychological modulation of the stress system

The stress hypothesis of fatigue accepts that social stimuli may produce prolonged and maladapted physiological arousal. In primary care, patients with chronic fatigue acknowledge psychological factors may be contributing to their tiredness.[30] Given the propensity for beliefs to influence physiology, it seems reasonable to assume that counselling and cognitive behaviour therapy may modulate feelings of fatigue. A randomized trial with parallel group design concluded both counselling and cognitive behaviour therapy were equally effective in managing patients with chronic fatigue in primary care.[31] Of even greater interest is the result of a randomized trial, followed by a prospective cohort study, which concluded short courses of graded exercise therapy were not superior to cognitive behaviour therapy for primary care patients with fatigue of at least 3 months duration.[32]

Chemical modulation of the stress system

Central fatigue is not only the result of psychological factors, it can also be the result of modifications to neurotransmitters induced by chemical or dietary changes. Tryptophan, an amino acid, is the precursor for the neurotransmitter 5-hydroxytryptamine which is involved in fatigue and sleep. In order to boost brain 5-hydroxytryptamine levels, tryptophan must first cross the blood–brain barrier. Tryptophan competes with other neutral and branch chain amino acids to enter the brain. Oral intake of branched chain amino acids may reduce central fatigue by reducing tryptophan levels in the central nervous system.[33] Ingestion of branched chain amino acids has been shown to reduce perceived exertion and mental fatigue during exercise and improve cognitive performance after the exercise.[34] In contrast, to induce sleepiness tryptophan may be combined with a diet rich in carbohydrate and low in protein. Furthermore, a study which compared elderly and young subjects found the elderly were less sensitive to carbohydrate induced sleepiness in the evening.[34] This study also reported a protein meal consumed at breakfast induced more fatigue and sleepiness than an isocaloric carbohydrate meal; this was reversed in the evening when a carbohydrate meal induced more fatigue.[35]

An increase in the plasma concentration ratio of free tryptophan/branch chain amino acids affecting brain serotonin levels is but one metabolic cause of fatigue. Other causes include hypoglycaemia with or without a decrease in the phosphocreatine level, proton accumulation and/or depletion of the glycogen store in muscle.[36] Proton accumulation may be a common cause of fatigue in most forms of exercise and may be an important factor in fatigue in the elderly and chronically physically inactive individuals.

Chronic inactivity decreases aerobic capacity requiring increased ATP to be synthesized by the less efficient anaerobic system. There appears to be some lay support for the energy depletion hypothesis, given the faith a number of fatigued individuals demonstrated in selecting coenzyme Q10 as a self-help intervention.[37] Coenzyme Q10, in addition to its antioxidant effect, facilitates mitochondrial electron transport thereby fuelling energy production. It appears to have a senescence specific protective effect against both aerobic and ischaemic stress.[38] As tissue coenzyme Q10 levels peak at around 20 years of age, there are those who believe everybody over 40 years of age would benefit from taking coenzyme Q10 in doses of 30–60 mg daily. More research is required before routine coenzyme Q10 supplementation can be recommended for older persons.

KEEPING PERSPECTIVE

Fatigue is a universal and a particularly prevalent experience in the elderly. While complaints of fatigue should be thoroughly investigated to identify and treat underlying disease, patients should be made aware of simple measures that may somewhat alleviate the problem. Regular exercise deserves serious consideration in any management regime.

CLINICAL CHALLENGE

An elderly man presents complaining of persistent fatigue. He says he can't take the hot humid weather of summer and asks for a 'pick-me-up'. He says he is sleeping badly and wakes up hot and sweaty at night.

Questions arising

- How can you determine and exclude a serious disease as a cause of fatigue?
- Are there any general measures that may help an elderly patient troubled by fatigue?

Clinical considerations

Fatigue is a symptom of a large number of diseases. A full physical examination is required in any patient complaining of fatigue. Special investigations are helpful for making a definitive diagnosis. Conditions that should be actively excluded with the aid of special investigations include:

- Leukaemia—do a full blood count

- Diabetes—initially a random followed by a fasting blood glucose as indicated. Urinalysis for glucosuria is not helpful in the elderly
- Hypercalcaemia—do blood electrolytes
- Depression—complete a questionnaire
- Anaemia—check the haemoglobin
- Thyroid disease—request thyroid function tests
- Chronic organ failure e.g. cardiac or renal failure—blood electrolytes, urea and creatinine clearance in the latter.

In addition to treating any underlying disease, fatigue patients may benefit from:

- Counselling and behavioural changes e.g. stress and insomnia management programs.
- Regular exercise. Exercise releases endorphins, decreases stress and seems to benefit fatigue, especially if this is associated with a depression.
- Nutritional supplementation. Coenzyme Q10 deserves consideration.

PRACTICE GEMS

◆ Fatigue is a subjective experience related to but distinct from sleepiness, which implies an alteration to sleep/wakefulness.

◆ Always exclude serious organic disease before attributing a patient's fatigue to a functional cause.

◆ Fatigue may be the presenting symptom of diabetes, leukaemia or anaemia attributable to an underlying malignancy.

◆ Fatigue is a major source of disablement and needs to be specifically addressed in patient management.

◆ Fatigue may result from physicochemical or psychosocial factors.

◆ A vicious feedback cycle involving positive feedback of the stress systems may result in persistent arousal and chronic fatigue, even after the initial cause has been eliminated.

◆ Regular exercise may intercept the stress cycle and improve longevity.

◆ Counselling and cognitive behaviour therapy are useful adjuncts and/or alternatives to exercise in fatigue management of elderly patients

◆ Dietary choices may influence the development of fatigue.

◆ Good dietary sources of coenzyme Q10, an antioxidant and mediator of energy production in mitochondiria, are sardines (250 g supplies 30 mg) and peanuts (1250 g supplies 30 mg).

References

1. Sha MC, Callahan CM, et al. Physical symptoms as a predictor of health care use and mortality among older adults. Am J Med 2005; 118(3):301–306.

2. Shen J, Barbera J, Shapiro CM. Distinguishing sleepiness and fatigue: focus on definition and measurement. Sleep Med Rev 2005 Dec 20; [Epub ahead of print]

3. Poluri A, Mores J, et al. Fatigue in the elderly population. Phys Med Rehabil Clin N Am 2005; 16(1):91–108.

4. Tsigos C, Chrousos GP. Hypothalamic–pituitary–adrenal axis, neuroendocrine factors and stress. J Psychosom Res 2002; 53(4):865–871.

5. McEwen BS. Interacting mediators of allostasis and allostatic load: towards an understanding of resilience in aging. Metabolism 2003; 52(10 Suppl 2):10–16.

6. Glaser R, Kiecolt-Glaser JK. Stress-associated immune modulation: relevance to viral infections and chronic fatigue syndrome. Am J Med 1998; 105(3A):35S-42S.

7. Bennett BK, Hickie IB, et al. The relationship between fatigue, psychological and immunological variables in acute infectious illness. Aust N Z J Psychiatry 1998; 32(2):180–186.

8. Kelley KW, Bluthe RM, et al. Cytokine-induced sickness behavior. Brain Behav Immun 2003; 17 Suppl 1:S112–118.

9. Patarca R. Cytokines and chronic fatigue syndrome. Ann N Y Acad Sci 2001; 933:185–200.

10. Goldstein DS, McEwen B. Allostasis, homeostatsis, and the nature of stress. Stress 2002; 5(1):55–58.

11. Cesari M, Penninx BW, et al. Inflammatory markers and physical performance in older persons: the InCHIANTI study. J Gerontol A Biol Sci Med Sci 2004; 59(3):242–248.

12. Moutschen M, Triffaux JM, et al. Pathogenic tracks in fatigue syndromes. Acta Clin Belg 1994; 49(6):274–289.

13. Anisman H, Merali Z, et al. Cytokines as a precipitant of depressive illness: animal and human studies. Curr Pharm Des 2005; 11(8):963-972.

14. Glass JM, Lyden AK, et al. The effect of brief exercise cessation on pain, fatigue, and mood symptom development in healthy, fit individuals. J Psychosom Res 2004; 57(4):391–398.

15. Brown DJ, McMillan DC, Milroy R. The correlation between fatigue, physical function, the systemic inflammatory response, and psychological distress in patients with advanced lung cancer. Cancer 2005; 103(2):377–382.

16. McCall WV. Sleep in the elderly: burden, diagnosis, and treatment. Prim Care Companion J Clin Psychiatry 2004; 6(1):9–20.

17. Pigeon WR, Sateia MJ, Ferguson RJ. Distinguishing between excessive daytime

sleepiness and fatigue: toward improved detection and treatment. J Psychosom Res 2003; 54(1):61–69.

18. Franco OH, de Laet C, et al. Effects of physical activity on life expectancy with cardiovascular disease. Arch Intern Med 2005; 165(20):2355–2360.

19. Pressley JC, Patrick CH. Frailty bias in comorbidity risk adjustments of community-dwelling elderly populations, J Clin Epidemiol 1999; 52:753–760.

20. Chin MJ, Paw A, et al. How to select a frail elderly population? A comparison of three working definitions. J Clin Epidemiol 1999; 52 :1015–1021.

21. Mitnitski AB, Mogilner AJ, et al. The accumulation of deficits with age and possible invariants of aging. The Scientific World Journal 2002; 2:1816–1822.

22. Penninx BW, Kritchevsky SB, et al. Inflammatory markers and depressed mood in older persons: results from the Health, Aging and Body Composition study. Biol Psychiatry 2003; 54(5):566–572.

23. Cohen HJ, Harris T, Pieper CF. Coagulation and activation of inflammatory pathways in the development of functional decline and mortality in the elderly. Am J Med 2003; 114(3):180–187.

24. Reuben DB, Judd-Hamilton L, et al. The associations between physical activity and inflammatory markers in high-functioning older persons: MacArthur Studies of Successful Aging. J Am Geriatr Soc 2003; 51(8):1125–1130.

25. Mitnitski AB, Graham JE, et al. Frailty, fitness and late-life mortality in relation to chronological and biological age. BMC Geriatr 2002; 2:1.

26. Petrella RJ, Lattanzio CN, et al. Can adoption of regular exercise later in life prevent metabolic risk for cardiovascular disease? Diabetes Care 2005; 28(3):694–701.

27. McTiernan A, Kooperberg C, et al. Recreational physical activity and the risk of breast cancer in postmenopausal women: the Women's Health Initiative Cohort Study. JAMA 2003; 290(10):1331–1336.

28. Leigh JP, Hubert HB, et al. Lifestyle risk factors predict healthcare costs in an aging cohort. Am J Prev Med 2005; 29(5):379–387.

29. Traustadottir T, Bosch PR, Matt KS. The HPA axis response to stress in women: effects of aging and fitness. Psychoneuroendocrinology 2005; 30(4):392–402.

30. Darbishire L, Ridsdale L, Seed PT. Distinguishing patients with chronic fatigue from those with chronic fatigue syndrome: a diagnostic study in UK primary care. Br J Gen Pract 2003; 53(491):441–445.

31. Ridsdale L, Godfrey E, et al. Fatigue Trialists' Group. Chronic fatigue in general practice: is counselling as good as cognitive behaviour therapy? A UK randomised trial. Br J Gen Pract 2001; 51(462):19-24.

32. Ridsdale L, Darbishire L, Seed PT. Is graded exercise better than cognitive behaviour therapy for fatigue? A UK randomized trial in primary care. Psychol Med 2004; 34(1):37–49.

33. Newsholme EA, Blomstrand E. Branched-chain amino acids and central fatigue. J Nutr 2006; 136(1):274S–276S.

34. Blomstrand E. Amino acids and central fatigue. Amino Acids 2001; 20(1):25–34.

35. Lieberman HR, Wurtman JJ, Teicher MH. Aging, nutrient choice, activity, and behavioral responses to nutrients. Ann N Y Acad Sci 1989; 561:196–208.

36. Newsholme EA, Blomstrand E, Ekblom B. Physical and mental fatigue: metabolic mechanisms and importance of plasma amino acids. Br Med Bull 1992; 48(3):477–495.

37. Bentler SE, Hartz AJ, Kuhn EM. Prospective observational study of treatments for unexplained chronic fatigue. J Clin Psychiatry 2005; 66(5):625–632.

38. Leong J. Anti-oxidants, cardiac surgery and ageing. J Comp Med 2005; 4(5):88–92.

PATIENT HANDOUT 10.1 – COPING WITH FATIGUE

Fatigue is a common problem in the elderly. It may result from being too busy or from sleeping badly. It may also be an indication of underlying disease that requires treatment. If you find you are always tired tell your doctor.

Persistent fatigue should not be ignored!

Some tips for combating persistent fatigue:

- Exercise regularly. Brisk walking for 1–1.5 hours a day reduces fatigue and increases longevity!
- Eating a breakfast rich in complex carbohydrates may be helpful.
- Check whether your sleep pattern contributes to fatigue. Refer to Patient Handout 7.1 Managing Insomnia: A Self-Care Guide.
- Check whether stress may be contributing to your fatigue. Refer to Patient Handout 2.1 Psychosocial Stress: A Health Risk.
- Consider whether your diet is deficient. Refer to Patient Handout 1.2 for dietary approaches to improving your health and preventing disease.

Chapter 11

Pain: Retirement's killjoy[a]

Mr Jones, a 65-year-old labourer, presents complaining of headache. He has a long history of headaches and backache, worst in the morning and improving as the day goes on. Recently his headaches have worsened; he now finds he is never headache free despite taking paracetamol regularly.

---

[a]Material in this chapter has been adapted with permission from: Jamison JR. *Differential diagnosis for primary practice*. Edinburgh: Churchill Livingstone; 1999; Jamison JR. *Maintaining health in primary care*. Edinburgh: Churchill Livingstone; 2001; Jamison JR. *Clinical guide to nutrition and dietary supplements in disease management*. Edinburgh: Churchill Livingstone; 2003.

On examination you detect limited movement in the region of his neck, lower back and right hip. He is a non-smoker and drinks a couple of glasses of beer most days. His BMI is 28 and his systolic blood pressure is slightly raised.

- Is this a new problem or an acute exacerbation of an underlying condition?
- Can the presentation be explained on the basis of a single pathological process or is multiple pathology present?
- Have any relevant physical examination procedures been omitted or not reported?
- Are there any lifestyle measures that could be helpful?
- Will a single management approach suffice?
- Does he require referral to a pain management centre?

INTRODUCTION

Almost 1 in 3 North Americans is troubled by persistent pain. Compared to younger persons, the elderly experience pain of longer duration, have more comorbidities and receive pain treatment more often.[1] In fact, compared to younger persons, those between 60 and 81 years of age are 31.2% more likely to report chronic pain. Another study recounted the most commonly reported complaints in persons over 60 years of age were musculoskeletal pain (65%), fatigue (55%), back pain (45%), shortness of breath (41%) and difficulty sleeping (38%).[2] Pain is a prevalent problem in the elderly and chronic pain can be incapacitating. Survival appears to be inversely related to functional impairment.[3] Sha et al found a summary score of physical symptoms reported by elderly persons a significant independent predictor of future hospitalization and death—even when controlling for clinical characteristics, chronic medical conditions, self-rated health and affective symptoms.[2] Pain management would appear to be an important consideration in caring for the elderly.

The pain threshold is the point at which a stimulus is perceived as painful. Elderly patients have a raised pain threshold. Pain tolerance is the duration or intensity of pain endured before initiating an overt pain response. Pain tolerance is influenced by the individual's sociocultural background, their learned behaviours and their current physical and psychological state. The source of pain may be somatic, visceral or psychological.

PAIN PRESENTATION BY SOURCE

Psychogenic pain

Psychogenic pain is pain without any apparent physical cause. The patient's experience of the pain is real and distressing. A cardinal feature of psychogenic pain is its indefinite nature and the inconsistency of its symptom pattern with any documented pain pattern for that anatomical area. Pain always has a psychological overlay—in acute pain, this may modify the behavioural response with grimacing or groaning; in chronic pain, management of the psychogenic component of the pain experience may make the difference between successful and unsuccessful intervention.

Somatic pain

The nature and particular presentation of somatic pain varies depending on the source. The skin with its rich supply of sensory nerves presents with well defined sharp pain. On the other hand, pain from muscle and joints is poorly localized and presents as a dull ache. Muscle pain may furthermore be referred to the associated dermatome causing hyperaesthesia in the dermal area sharing a common innervation. In general, somatic pain:

- is aggravated by posture or movement
- is unrelated to visceral activity
- follows injury
- is well localized and fairly intense if superficial, i.e. arising from the skin
- is a poorly defined ache if deep, arising from the musculoskeletal system.

Visceral pain

Visceral pain may result from ischaemia, muscle spasm, chemical irritants or distension of a hollow organ. In contrast to somatic pain, which tends to be constant, visceral pain is intermittent. Individuals seldom become tolerant to visceral pain. Pain adaptation is poor and very slow when it occurs. Pain is often referred and associated with functional disturbance. In general, clinical findings associated with visceral pain are:

- hyperaesthesia due to dermatomal involvement
- muscle spasm due to myotomal involvement
- findings influenced by the organ's pathology, such as
  - obstruction to hollow muscular organs presents with cramping intermittent or colicky pain
  - irritation of organs results in gnawing, burning or boring pain
- disturbed visceral function, including
  - vomiting
  - diarrhoea
  - constipation
  - exaggerated autonomic nervous reflexes such as sweating, vasomotor changes (hypotension, changes in heart rate)
  - nausea
- pain referred to predictable sites.

Pain may be referred according to embryological development:

- Structures arising from the foregut, i.e. lower oesophagus, stomach, duodenum, liver, gall bladder, bile duct and pancreas, refer pain to the epigastrium. Other findings associated with upper abdominal pain suggesting a foregut problem are anorexia, nausea and vomiting.

- Structures arising from the midgut, i.e. small intestine, Meckel's diverticulum, terminal ileum, appendix and caecum, refer pain to the periumbilical region. Anorexia, nausea and vomiting are associated with midgut problems.
- Structures aising from the hindgut, i.e. large bowel, sigmoid colon and rectum, refer pain to the supra-pubic region. Lower abdominal pain associated with blood, mucus and an alteration in bowel habit suggests a hindgut problem.
- The pancreas, kidney/ureter and aorta refer pain to the back. Low backache associated with a vaginal discharge, dyspareunia or a menstrual disorder suggests a lesion of the female genital tract.
- The spleen and gall bladder refer pain to the shoulder.
- The kidney and/or urinary tract may refer pain to the groin or tip of the penis. Pain in the loin, groin or suprapubic area which is associated with frequency, dysuria or haematuria suggests a renal or urinary tract problem.

When inflammation of a viscus spreads to involve the overlying parietal peritoneum, pain moves from its referred site to overlie the involved organ, e.g. the periumbilical pain of acute appendicitis moves to the right iliac fossa. In the case of appendicitis, while autonomic symptoms and the referred pain pattern may be suggestive, the location of the appendix may confuse the clinical presentation. An appendix abutting on the bladder may cause frequency and dysuria; one adjacent to the large bowel may precipitate diarrhoea; one lying on the psoas muscle may trigger spasm resulting in flexion of the right hip or pain when the right hip is hyperextended. An appendix touching the anterior abdominal wall causes abdominal rigidity and guarding in the right iliac fossa. In elderly patients, diagnosis of appendicitis is further complicated as early signs are largely absent.

PAIN PRESENTATION BY CAUSE

The presentation of pain in the elderly may be unusual; however, musculoskeletal pain in the form of persistent low backache followed by myofascial pain syndromes is the most common cause of chronic pain. Musculoskeletal pain may result from a mechanical problem, an inflammatory process or a neoplastic lesion.

Mechanical backache

Mechanical backache may occur with or without a history of overt trauma. Simple backache attributable to ligamentous sprain, muscular strain or a mechanical problem usually lasts for hours, has an ill-defined onset and does not prevent continued exercise. The pain is unilateral and related to posture. Pain is aggravated by movement, sitting, coughing or straining;

and relieved by rest, a change in position or heat. It is worst in the evenings, particularly after physical exertion, and has a long history. The nature of the pain varies with the underlying lesion.

A muscular strain presents as a superficial steady local pain, radicular pain is sharp and stabbing, while facet joint syndrome presents with pain of sudden onset, muscle spasm and protective lateral deviation. Mechanical backache may impair sleep, restrict movement due to muscle spasm and be associated with shooting pains, paraesthesia and/or motor weakness, even foot drop. Referred back pain presents as a diffuse or patchy deep ache. Mechanical back pain due to spinal dysfunction frequently involves the facet joints and/or disruption of an intervertebral disc.

When backache follows trauma, the nature of the injury provides useful diagnostic information. Twisting predisposes to a fractured transverse or spinous process, or a muscular tear with or without apophyseal joint injury. Lifting excessively heavy weights increases the risk of posterior longitudinal ligament, interspinous and/or disc injury. Lifting and twisting with a flexed spine predisposes to intervertebral disc prolapse, whereas direct force predisposes to soft tissue or vertebral injury.

Inflammatory backache

The cardinal sign of inflammatory causes of backache is stiffness. The pain and stiffness of inflammatory backache is insidious in onset, presenting as a localized ache or throb, aggravated by rest and relieved with exercise. It is worst at night and early morning. Morning stiffness is severe and prolonged, persisting for 30 or more minutes after getting up. The erythrocyte sedimentation rate (ESR) may be raised and evidence of immunologically mediated inflammation, e.g. HLA-B27 antigen, rheumatoid factor or antinuclear antibodies, may be present. Continuous pain suggests inflammation associated with infection or malignancy.

Malignancy

Neoplasia causes bone pain which is unremitting and becomes progressively worse. Backache due to neoplasia should be excluded in patients who complain of rapidly increasing, unrelenting pain of insidious onset that is present at night and on waking. The pain is unrelieved by rest and fails to respond to treatment. It is often described as a local boring deep ache that is aggravated by movement. Relentless progression of neurological signs and radicular pain involving more than one nerve root should be regarded with grave concern. Findings such as localized tenderness over a vertebra in a patient with weight loss, fatigue and malaise, fever and a raised alkaline phosphatase are highly suggestive. A positive bone scan confirms the diagnosis.

Bone is a common site for metastases from the lung, breast, prostate, thyroid, kidney/adrenal and melanoma. Bone is a common site for metastases in the elderly. Osteoid osteoma, a benign bone tumour, rather than cancer should be suspected if the associated pain is aggravated by alcohol and relieved by aspirin.

Psychogenic backache

Psychogenic backache tends to present with a pain pattern inconsistent with back problems. Psychogenic backache is vague in onset, indefinite in character, often being bilateral and diffuse with inappropriate radiation, if present. Pain is provoked by any and all movements, aggravated by mood or anxiety and relieved by alcohol and relaxation. Pain seldom, if ever, wakes the sleeping patient and has a degree of severity out of all proportion to any identifiable lesion. Changes in sensation, muscle strength or reflexes are not consistent with an anatomical distribution. Tenderness to palpation is also inconsistent with any recognized lesion. The pain is refractory and commonly associated with anxiety and/or depression.

PRINCIPLES OF PAIN MANAGEMENT

Nociceptors register painful stimuli. They are found in epidermis, subcutaneous tissue, muscles and tendons. Nociceptors are located at the end of small unmyelinated afferent neurons and are sensitive to mechanical, chemical and thermal stimuli. The relative sensitivity of different structures varies with the concentration of nociceptors in various sites. Impulses from these pain receptors are transmitted through small A-delta fibres and C fibres to the spinal cord from where, after a synapse in the dorsal horn cell, they are transmitted to the rest of the central nervous system. C fibres, which transmit sensations of burning and aching, lack a myelin sheath. Their transmission is consequently relatively slow. The larger myelinated A fibres transmit impulses more rapidly and convey well localized, sharp pain sensations. Pain sensations are transmitted to the central nervous system via the spinothalamic tract.

Pain appreciation is mediated centrally by interaction of various systems. The limbic and reticular tracts are involved in arousal and motivational behaviour, the thalamus helps in discrimination and pain localization, while the medulla, hypothalamus and cortex activate various automatic and cognitive coping responses. The relative concentration of various neuromodulators such as substance P, norepinephrine, 5-hydroxytryptamine and calcitonin-gene-related peptide, located in pathways mediating painful stimuli, sets the pain threshold. Substance P lowers while serotonin and endorphins raise the pain threshold. A family of neuropeptides, the endorphins, inhibits pain impulses in the spinal cord and brain. Beta-endorphin, found in the hypothalamus and pituitary, generates a sense of general wellbeing. Endorphins attach to opiate receptors on the plasma membrane of afferent neurons. Pain perception is, however, not solely modified by physiological and chemical measures; it is also affected by psychological factors. Symptomatic relief is influenced by the patient's perceptions.

Management of acute pain focuses on pathophysiological processes; chronic pain management focuses on both changing the underlying pathology and modulating the patient's symptom experience. Management of acute pain targets the site of pain generation; care of patients with chronic pain includes consideration of central and peripheral strategies for pain modification. When managing patients with chronic pain, the clinical consultation is not merely a prescription writing exercise; it is rather an opportunity to undertake cognitive restructuring: 'The experience of chronic pain includes much more than raw physical sensation: pain creates problems of control and meaning-making.'[4]

Central strategies employ psychological and physiological measures; peripheral approaches explore measures to prevent initiation of pain producing processes and modulate pain producing mechanisms e.g. through exercise or drugs. Modifying the patient's perception of their problem and how it can be managed is a fundamental task in the clinical consultation.

CENTRAL CONTROL OF PAIN

Psychosocial approaches to pain management include ascertaining how pain has affected the patient's lifestyle and alerting the patient to measures that can minimize adverse changes. This encompasses consideration of the impact of pain on interpersonal relationships, recreational activities, sleeping and eating patterns, employment and emotional state. Central pain control seeks to alter brain chemistry by diverse mechanisms. Strategies employed when targeting central control of pain are described next.

Physical strategies

There is evidence that regular exercise provides a number of psychological benefits that preserve and even enhance cognitive function, alleviate depression and create a sense of enhanced personal control and self-efficacy.[5] A prospective, longitudinal study found consistent exercise patterns over the long term in physically active seniors are associated with about 25% less musculoskeletal pain than reported by more sedentary controls, either by calendar year or by cumulative area-under-the-curve pain over average ages of 62–76 years.[6] Regular exercise has even been shown to reduce pain in knee osteoarthritis[7] and to help prevent mechanical low back pain.[8] Exercise was associated with significantly lower pain scores over time.[6] On the other hand, physical inactivity is associated with greater pain, increased risk of injury, lower bone density and poorer muscle tone.[9]

The endogenous opiate system is activated during exercise. There are at least four receptors for endogenous opioids in the central nervous system. The delta receptors affect behaviour changes and can cause hallucinations. Epsilon receptors, stimulated by encephalin, cause dysphoria and have psychotic effects. Kappa receptors are stimulated by dynorphin and mediate hypothermia, miosis, sedation and analgesia. The mu receptors are stimulated by beta-endorphin and mediate analgesia, respiratory depression and euphoria. The dose–response relationship between exercise and the opiate system is complicated—plasma levels of beta-endorphin with exercise don't appear to increase proportionally to work intensity.[10]

Results of 34 studies suggest that aerobically fit subjects have a reduced psychosocial stress response when compared to either their baseline values or to control groups.[11] In addition to promoting a sense of wellbeing, regular exercise may reduce symptomatic depression and anxiety. Meta-analysis showed exercise programs for coronary patients had a positive effect on anxiety and depression.[12] Results of three separate studies substantiate the claim that aerobic exercise is associated with reductions in anxiety.[13] Compared to a control group, arthritis patients on a 12-week exercise program showed significant improvement with respect to depression, anxiety, aerobic capacity, 50-foot walking time and physical activity.[14] Furthermore, regular moderate-intensity exercise reduces sleep latency by about 15 minutes and increases sleep duration by about 45 minutes per night.[15] As anxiety, depression and insomnia are barriers to coping with pain, exercise indirectly improves pain management. Exercise is indicated for persons with chronic backache. It is not considered beneficial for treatment of acute back pain.

Chemical modification

Both pharmaceuticals and nutraceuticals can be used.

Pharmaceutical intervention

Morphine, heroin, pethidine and codeine are narcotics that alter the perception of moderate to severe pain by affecting opioid receptors. Opiates relieve pain by enhancing the natural endorphin response. A distinctive feature of the analgesic action of opioids is the blunting of the distressing, affective component of pain without dulling the sensation itself. Enkephalin, a relatively weak analgesic compared to other natural endorphins, is more potent and longer lasting than morphine.

Narcotics should be used with caution in the elderly. Many narcotics stimulate the cough depression centre and the chemoreceptor trigger zone, causing nausea. Moreover, opioid receptors are not restricted to the central nervous system. The gastrointestinal tract is rich in opioid receptors, stimulation of which results in constipation and spasm in the biliary tree.

Although narcotic analgesics are particularly useful for relieving acute back pain, their use should be limited to around 48 hours. Long term use is not recommended in view of the propensity to develop tolerance. Over time, higher doses are required to achieve analgesia and the euphoric effects make regular users prone to addiction. Signs suggestive of addiction are pin point pupils, watery eyes, inattention, anorexia, bradycardia and slow respiration. A narcotic overdose should be suspected in users with cold, clammy skin and slow, shallow respiration. Convulsions and coma are a further complication.

Certain non-narcotic analgesics may also have central and local effects. Prostaglandins are involved in pain transmission in the brain and spinal cord. Non-steroidal anti-inflammatory drugs (NSAIDs) impair prostaglandin synthesis and may have central and local effects. Interference with brain prostaglandins probably explains the mild depression and perceptual disturbances associated with NSAIDs, as does the pain relief experienced by rheumatoid arthritis patients prior to any locally detectable changes in swelling or erythema.

Nutraceuticals

Like pharmaceuticals, some nutrients may alter pain perception by altering the concentration of opioids in the central nervous system. Phenylalanine in high doses can accomplish analgesia by inhibiting the enzyme responsible for the inactivation of encephalin. D-phenylalanine inhibits carboxypeptidase, an enzyme involved in catabolism of opioids in the central nervous system. D-phenylalanine has been used successfully in the management of chronic intractable pain in humans.[16] A therapeutic trial of DL-phenylalanine of 375–750 mg three times a day(tds) is recommended for patients with persistent pain. If after 3 weeks there is no improvement, double the dose and monitor the patient for a further 3 weeks. If no improvement is noted after 6 weeks, discontinue the therapy. In patients who show improvement, establish a minimal schedule by alternating 1 drug week with 2 drug-free weeks. Contraindications to phenylalanine administration are phenylketonuria, malignant melanoma, pregnancy and the use of monoamine oxidase inhibitors, e.g. for the management of depression. As phenylalanine may trigger migraine and aggravate rheumatoid arthritis, caution must be exercised in these patients. Simultaneous administration of vitamin B6 may be helpful.

The other major nutritional strategy for central control of pain is mediated by increased serotonin levels. Tryptophan is converted to serotonin and serotonin in the central nervous system elevates the pain threshold. Tryptophan, 3 g daily, is recommended. In order to enable tryptophan to pass the blood–brain barrier this amino acid should be taken in conjunction with a high carbohydrate, low protein diet. Supplementation with vitamin B3 (to saturate an alternate end product of tryptophan metabolism) and vitamin B6 may also be helpful. Clinically, L-5-hydroxytryptophan can induce a significant decrease of pain in migraine.[17] L-tryptophan is sometimes effective in treating both chronic and acute pain.

While an increased intake of substrate is one option for increasing brain serotonin levels, another is to inhibit serotonin uptake by postsynaptic receptors. The most commonly prescribed antidepressants selectively inhibit serotonin uptake, thereby modulating cerebral neurotransmission. Chronic pain is often accompanied by depression and treatment of depression is a recognized therapeutic option in pain management.

Psychological approaches

Health authorities attending the NIH consensus conference agreed there were a number of well defined behavioural and relaxation interventions effective in the treatment of chronic pain.[18] Their conclusions are supported by evidence from randomized controlled trials, and literature reviews suggest there is a place for mind-body therapies in pain management.[19] Various combinations of stress management, coping skills training, cognitive restructuring and relaxation therapy with appropriate adjunctive treatment are recommended. Cognitive behavioural therapy combined with an educational/informational component is deemed a useful adjunct in the management of both rheumatoid and osteoarthritis; relaxation and thermal biofeedback deserves consideration for recurrent migraine; while relaxation and muscle biofeedback are helpful for recurrent tension headache. Unfortunately, despite their relatively low cost, safety and efficacy in treating chronic pain symptoms, mind body interventions are seldom used by persons with musculoskeletal pain.[20] One possible explanation for this reluctance may be a preference for a passive patient role. Chronic pain is best managed when patients are active participants in management.

The way people perceive events in their life affects their health.[21] 'One of the most consistent findings to emerge from the research on painful stimuli is that patients are better able to cope when they have some feelings of personal control over the situation.'[22] Animal and human studies have confirmed that helplessness or a lack of control is a stressor and causes immunosuppression.[23] On the other hand, there is experimental evidence that coping behaviour leads to the release of endogenous compounds which have brain and behavioural changes similar to those resulting from benzodiazepine administration.[24] Lack of control disturbs the biochemical balance, resulting in increased corticosteroid release which in turn suppresses production of serotonin, dopamine and norepinephrine:

- Serotonin regulates mood, relieves pain, and helps control release of endorphins.
- Dopamine is largely responsible for a sense of reward or pleasure.
- Norepinephrine, when depleted, causes depression. Depression is a common problem encountered by those with chronic pain.

Counselling can enhance self-efficacy and a perception of control. A sense of increased control can be achieved by:[21]

- Gaining information. Information makes outcomes more predictable, creating the perception of better control.
- Being prepared. Positive outcomes are more likely when intellectual strategies such as acquiring better coping skills are coupled with emotional strategies such as positive visualization and encouraging self-talk.

Improved problem solving techniques and adopting a less pessimistic outlook make pain appear more manageable. See Patient Handout 2.2.

Harnessing the placebo response is an integral aspect of chronic pain management. See Box 11.1. More recently, the oft maligned placebo response has achieved recognition as a credible therapeutic outcome. In contrast to specific intervention, which achieves a dramatic response in relatively few clinical situations, non-specific therapy or the placebo response provides a marginal benefit in every clinical encounter. The placebo response is a universal phenomenon. Placebo outcomes are not restricted to a specific personality type. Although placebo intervention can influence almost any symptom, placebos seem to work best and most often to relieve pain, and to modulate disorders of the autonomic nervous or neurohumeral systems. Placebo intervention cannot be used to discriminate between organic and functional ailments.[25]

> **Box 11.1   Capturing the placebo response**
>
> 1. Employ a treatment ritual:
>   a. Predict the responses to therapy.
>   b. Enthusiastically endorse the appropriateness and efficacy of therapy.
>   c. Avoid using placebo interventions without accompanying active treatment.
>   d. Make the patient aware of how therapy changes the course of the condition.
> 2. Use conditioning stimuli:
>   a. Provide continuity of care.
>   b. The clinical consultation is a cue to onset of relief of symptoms.
>   c. Present evidence of being a reputable healer—display qualifications, look professional.
> 3. Enhance desirable outcome expectations:
>   a. Show optimism—verbally and non-verbally.
>   b. Be socioculturally sensitive—suggest non-specific interventions that are credible to the patient.
>   c. Provide patients with coping strategies.

The placebo works through the mind. It relies on 'interactions between the clinician, the treatment process and the patient. The patient's perception of that interaction often ignites the healing/placebo process.'[26] Psychological stimuli to a placebo response encompass hope, faith, credulity, suggestibility, trust, optimism, anxiety, conditioning, expectancy and memory distortion.[27] Biochemical pathways act as psychosomatic linkages and include the endogenous brain systems of opioid, antiopioid and gamma-aminobutyric acid polypeptide transmitters, as well as the neurohumoral systems that release catecholamines and cortisol.[28] In fact, in addition to differences in drug pharmacokinetics, the nature of the pain and the method of drug administration, individual differences in placebo activation of endogenous opioid systems are regarded as an important source of the variability observed in response to pain control.[29]

Expectancy and conditioning appear to underlie the psychological mechanisms responsible for attitudes conducive to analgesia.[30] Expectancy is the perceived likelihood that a procedure or an agent will bring significant pain relief.[27] It can either be produced by previous experiences, as in conditioning, or via verbal information such as the suggestion of pain relief. Classical conditioning occurs through temporal association of a neutral stimulus, e.g. bell, and an unconditioned stimulus, e.g. food. A conditioning response is composed of two components: an unconditioned response caused by the active ingredient and mediated through receptor mechanisms to which it is targeted, and a learned or conditioned response which is usually smaller, more rapid and centrally mediated. When applied to the placebo phenomenon, a neutral, non-active stimulus may acquire an ameliorative effect through repeated association of a stimulus with a proven beneficial effect. Neutral places, persons and things such as therapeutic rituals, when repeatedly associated with effective treatment, may acquire remedial properties. Individuals experience a sense of wellbeing due to the remedial properties of a clinical encounter independently of any benefit attributable to their specific care. It has even been suggested that in certain circumstances 'patient and provider expectations and interactions may be more important than specific treatments'.[31] Placebo analgesia furthermore seems to increase with repeated exposure.[32] Neutral triggers such as the health professional, the clinical environment and the consultation ritual can all potentially acquire potency as non-specific therapy. However, when placebo analgesia was produced by conditioning trials wherein heat-induced experimental pain was surreptitiously reduced in order to test psychological factors of expectancy and desire for pain reduction, the results suggested that conditioning alone was not sufficient for placebo effects.[33] Conditioning appears to be only one ingredient contributing to the placebo response. Relationship skills may be required to optimally enhance the effectiveness of clinical care.

Recent research confirms that the therapeutic consequences of placebo are generated through mental processes in which attitudes are important.[34] Expectation of a therapeutic effect is deemed necessary for placebo outcomes. Although exercise was found to increase fitness in all subjects tested, only those who had been told it would improve psychological wellbeing were found to have significantly improved their self-esteem.[35] Words are not inert—they can trigger placebo outcomes. The attitude and the verbal message conveyed by the health professional influences the clinical outcome. Positive expectations created by enthusiastic endorsement of drug effects have been shown to produce statistically and clinically significant placebo benefits.[36] Furthermore, although there was a strong tendency for positive placebo effects to occur when staff were perceived as friendly and supportive, only the attitude factors obtained statistical significance. Interestingly, the status of the communicator appeared to have little impact. The contribution of the clinic receptionist who enthusiastically endorses the care provided may well extend beyond mere clinic management!

Research suggests that adding a verbal suggestion of pain relief can increase the magnitude of placebo analgesia to that of an active agent.[37] Although a combination of an active agent and the expectation of pain relief created by verbal suggestion failed to increase the analgesic effect beyond either factor given alone, the researchers nevertheless advocated combined use of an active agent and placebo trigger. They postulated that the combination, as it promises a greater chance of benefit than either factor alone, would be more likely to achieve optimal treatment. Indeed, although individual therapeutic encounters that are brief, motivational and provide non-judgemental feedback are necessary for the placebo response, they may be insufficient for a successful outcome.[26] For placebo intervention to be truly successful, conditioning requires that an active therapy is linked with neutral events.[38] Patients who were switched from an active analgesic to placebo had pain relief longer than if the drug was simply stopped; however, in cross-over trials, the placebo response was greater if it was given after the active drug.[39] Furthermore, the efficacy of placebo when used alone decreased over the course of successive administrations.[40] These studies lend support to combining both non-specific or placebo intervention using central pain control measures with specific therapy targeting local changes in the site of pain generation.

PERIPHERAL CONTROL OF PAIN: MODULATING PAIN GENERATION

Elimination of pain triggers provides an optimal pain prevention strategy. When this is not possible, local factors contributing to the generation of pain can be modified by dietary and drug measures.

Eliminating pain triggers

Removing the cause is the most effective strategy for preventing recurrent pain. The difficulty is often to identify the cause. Only 1 in 4 migraine sufferers benefits from elimination of food triggers—in 3 out of 4 cases the pathogenesis of migraine is more complex. When migraine sufferers are exposed to nitrates up to 2 in 3 respond with a headache. Rich sources of nitrates are ham, bacon and corned beef. Over half of the persons diagnosed with migraine have also been found to be sensitive to salicylates, mono-sodium glutamate and various amines. Rich sources of salicylates are fruit, such as oranges, pineapples, kiwifruit and berry fruits, vegetables, especially the nightshade group, honey, licorice, wine and almonds. Amines are equally plentiful in health foods such as avocados, bananas, spinach, tomato, mushrooms and Vegemite® or Marmite®. A migraine attack may be initiated by more than one type of trigger.

Similarly, dietary exclusion of purine rich foods is recommended for patients with gout. The treatment of gout is, however, inadequately addressed by focusing on a single dietary change. While dietary modification may be helpful in long term management of the condition, acute gout requires immediate pain relief. Drugs are required. NSAIDs are recommended. Indometacin (25 mg tds for 48 hours) is the drug of choice. Aspirin may be helpful in high doses but in low doses aggravates the condition due to its impact on the urinary excretion of uric acid. Colchicine is associated with diarrhoea and should be avoided in the elderly. In addition to removing a causal factor, pain relief may be afforded by appreciation of the pathogenesis of a condition.

In the case of peripheral vascular disease, the immediate cause of pain is ischaemia. Resting relieves the pain of intermittent claudication, but never walking is scarcely a solution. In this instance the pain trigger is not the cause of the problem, it is rather a manifestation of the underlying condition. The fundamental problem is hypoxia due to impaired perfusion which may be attributed to various conditions. Interventions such as quitting smoking to reduce vasospasm and carboxyhaemoglobin levels, taking a-tocopheryl-nicotinate (200 mg tds) to encourage vasodilation and persisting with graduated exercise to encourage development of a collateral circulation can together provide a measure of relief. Along similar lines, the pain of muscle spasm may be relieved by muscle relaxants. Cyclo-benzaprine (20–40 mg/day) is sometimes prescribed for cramps but should not be used for longer than 21 days. This may relieve the immediate cause of the pain but fails to address the underlying problem which may be due to a diversity of causes ranging from acid-base imbalance due to hyper-ventilation, through electrolyte disturbances such as hypokalaemia or hypocalcaemia, to chronic musculoskeletal disorders such as fibromyalgia.

In addition to eliminating immediate pain triggers and addressing under-lying conditions, pain may be managed by modifying its pathogenesis.

Modification of pain producing mechanisms

Peripheral pain control is intimately linked with modulating the inflam-matory process. Inflammation is augmented by chemical mediators includ-ing histamine, kinins, eicosanoids, complement and lymphokines. These chemicals enhance inflammation, aid phagocytosis and interact with the specific immune system to achieve cytolysis. They may also be involved in the generation of painful stimuli. One important local mechanism for modifying pain is to reduce the ratio of pro-inflammatory eicosanoids.

Modifying eicosanoid metabolism (see Figs 11.1 and 11.2)

Eicosanoid metabolism may be modified using pharmaceuticals, nutraceu-ticals and/or diet.

Dietary measures

Polyunsaturated fatty acids are eicosanoid precursors. Most eicosanoid products from omega-6 fatty acid metabolism tend to augment inflam-mation and hence the generation of pain mediating chemicals; those from

Figure 11.1   Nutrient modulation of eicosanoid production. Jamison, J. 2004 Clinical guide to nutrition and dietary supplements in disease management. Churchill Livingstone: Edinburgh.

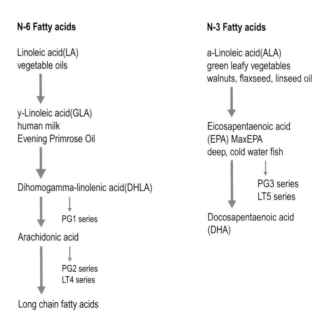

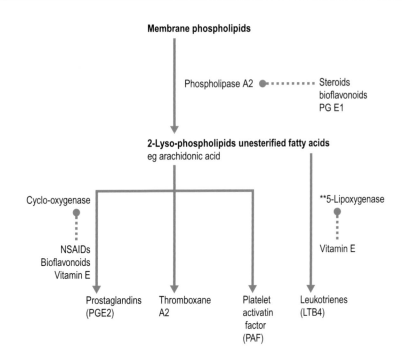

Figure 11.2 Inflammation and arachidonic acid metabolism. Jamison, J. 2004 Clinical guide to nutrition and dietary supplements in disease management. Churchill Livingstone: Edinburgh.

omega-3 fatty acids do not. The omega-6 fatty acids that enhance pain are predominantly derived from arachidonic acid, the precursor of the prostaglandin (PG) 2 series and the leukotriene 4 series. Ranked from highly inflammatory to non-inflammatory are leukotriene 4 series, leukotriene 3 series, PG 2 series, PG 3 series and the non-inflammatory PG 1 series. Omega-6 fatty acid consumed as linoleic acid in vegetable oils is the precursor of the PG 1 series. Omega-3 fatty acids consumed as alpha-linolenic acid in green leafy vegetables, walnuts and linseed oil and as eicosapentaenoic acid (EPA) in deep cold water fish are the dietary precursors of the PG 3 series and the leukotriene 5 series.

Meat and eggs are a rich source of preformed arachidonic acid. Dietary modification to dampen the inflammatory response therefore focuses on a vegetarian diet that avoids animal products with the exception of fish. Fish rich in the eicosanoid precursors of PG 3, EPA and docosahexaeonic acid (DHA) include kippers, mackerel, pilchards, Atlantic salmon, trout, blue grenadier, herring, sardines, tuna, yellowtail and perch. Plant sources that are good sources of alpha-linolenic acid (18:3n-3) which can be converted after ingestion to EPA (20:5n-3) are flaxseed oil, spinach and walnuts. By replacing meat, meat products, eggs and lard in the diet with fish, spinach, walnuts, soy products, canola and linseed oil, the composition of cell membrane can be changed. Over time, this dietary change produces a less pro-inflammatory state. At least one meal of fish (100 g) each week is recommended for everybody. Persons hoping to get their omega-3 fatty acids from alpha-linolenic acid probably require a daily intake of 2 g or 1% of their total energy intake.[41]

Nutraceuticals

While dietary change is recommended, it may not alone achieve a discernible clinical change in the short or even medium term. Taking fish oil capsules provides an alternative option. Ingestion of dietary supplements of omega-3 fatty acids has consistently been shown to reduce both morning stiffness and the number of tender joints in patients with rheumatoid arthritis.[42] Clinical benefits were only apparent after 12 or more weeks of supplementation. A minimum daily dose of 3 g EPA and DHA was necessary to achieve a significant reduction in the release of leukotriene B4 from stimulated neutrophils and of interleukin 1 from monocytes. An earlier randomized, controlled, double-blind study found that rheumatoid arthritis patients on 10 g per day of fish oil reported a significantly decreased consumption of NSAIDs at 3 and 6 months.[43]

Pharmaceuticals

Non-narcotic analgesics frequently achieve relief of mild pain by modifying eicosanoid production. Although analgesics were mainly taken when needed, a Finnish study found 70% of elderly people were taking at least one analgesic.[44] In this study less than 1 in 5 persons took any analgesics regularly. The most commonly used analgesics were non-steroidal anti-inflammatory drugs (51%) and acetaminophen (23%). Opioid use became more common with increasing age, reaching16% in patients 85 years and older.

The analgesic and anti-inflammatory effects of NSAIDs are dose dependent, rapid in onset and reversible. Popular choices are ibuprofen (200–400 mg 4 times daily (qid), maximum dose 3200 mg daily) and diclofenac (25–50 mg bd or tds). NSAIDs should be taken with food or after meals. The clinical effectiveness of NSAIDs is influenced by:[45]

- the ability to concentrate the drug in an area of inflammation.
- the dose of the drug used.

NSAIDs concentrate in areas of relative acidity e.g. inflamed joints, the renal medulla and gastric mucosa.

Aspirin dose is a determinant of both clinical efficacy and toxic effect. The dose of aspirin for analgesia is between 300 and 600 mg/day and peaks between 2.0 and 5.0 g/day. The analgesic effect lasts for about 4 hours. An anti-inflammatory effect is achieved between 900 and 3600 mg/day and lasts much longer than the analgesic effect.[46] A plasma level of 1.1 mmol/L–2.2 mmol/L (150–300 mg/L) is the optimal range for the anti-inflammatory actions of aspirin and other salicylates. As hepatic metabolism of salicylate is induced by continual aspirin usage, dose adjustments may be necessary.

The clinical effects of NSAIDs are attributed to inhibition of cyclo-oxygenase, lipoxygenase, polymorph functions and the activity of NF-kappa B.[47]

- Cyclo-oxygenase is the enzyme which converts arachidonic acid to prostaglandins. By inhibiting prostaglandin production at the site of tissue injury, NSAIDs impede potentiation of pain producing chemicals (kinins, e.g. bradykinin and kallidin) by prostaglandins. Locally, PGE2 is an important inflammatory mediator in the joints of rheumatoid patients. At low concentrations PGE2 causes erythema and enhances the pain and oedema mediated by bradykinin and histamine. Local synovial production of prostaglandins causes inhibition of T-suppressor cells and the production of rheumatoid factor assisted by T-helper cells proceeds unopposed. PGE2 is believed to mediate bone resorption by increasing osteoclast numbers, stimulating collagenase secretion by macrophages and inhibiting proteoglycan production by synoviocytes and articular chondrocytes. However, despite alleviating symptoms, NSAIDs do not appear to substantively modify the progression of rheumatoid arthritis; periarticular bony lesions develop in patients on these drugs.

- Lipoxygenase is the enzyme involved in formation of the inflammatory leukotrienes.
- Polymorph functions include the release of free radicals, lysosomal enzymes and polymorph migration.
- NF-kappa B is a factor needed for transcription of some genes associated with inflammation.[48]

Aspirin and NSAID toxicity is strongly dose related.[49] The toxicity index for aspirin is 1.37 compared with 1.87–2.90 for selected NSAIDs. In the case of aspirin, toxicity is 0.73 for a dose of 651–2600 mg/day; 1.08 for 2601–3900 mg/day; and 1.91 for more than 3900 mg daily.[49] Aspirin shows greater gastrointestinal toxicity than other NSAIDs due to its prolonged binding to the stomach wall. Toxicity is also influenced by the type of aspirin used: toxicity for plain aspirin is 1.36; for buffered aspirin 1.1; and for enteric coated aspirin 0.92. In general, low dose long term therapy is considered relatively safe. The adverse effects of NSAIDs may be attributed to the physiological consequences of prostaglandin synthetase inhibition, resulting in impaired prostaglandin production increasing susceptibility to gastric ulceration and potentially compromising renal and hepatic function.
General guidelines for the use of NSAIDs and other drugs are:[50,51]

- Avoid the use of particular drugs in persons at increased risk of toxic side effects from that drug.
- Start therapy with a low initial dose.
- Use the lowest feasible maintenance dose. Aspirin in doses below 300 mg/day is rarely associated with toxicity. When larger doses are required for analgesia, the therapeutically effective dose of NSAIDs may be reduced by the judicious use of fish oil.[43,52]
- Minimize the risks of toxicity by not combining drugs with similar toxicity and avoiding behaviours that potentiate toxic effects, e.g. smoking cigarettes and drinking alcohol while on NSAIDs.

Extra caution with the use of NSAIDs in the elderly is warranted in view of the high incidence of cardiovascular and gastrointestinal disease, the age-related decline in renal function and the propensity for polypharmacy in this age group.[53] Particular care should be taken when using NSAIDs for patients on anticoagulants. With aspirin this problem is exacerbated as salicylates (80 mg/day) irreversibly modify cyclo-oxygenase (COX). In patients contemplating surgery, COX-2 specific inhibitors are preferred as they do not affect platelet aggregation or bleeding time.

The newer COX-2-specific inhibitors have comparable efficacy to traditional dual inhibitor NSAIDs but have a demonstrably better gastrointestinal safety profile.[53] Coxib should be considered for patients who have severe pain and/or signs of inflammation, especially if the patient is at increased risk for serious adverse upper gastrointestinal events from a traditional NSAID. It should, however, be noted that Vioxx and Celebrex, popular COX-2 inhibitors, were recently removed from the market due to their long term toxicity.[54] In view of the many adverse reactions, interactions, and contraindications to NSAIDs in elderly patients, it is not surprising that there are those who regard acetaminophen (paracetamol) as the over-the-counter analgesic drug of choice.[55]

While acetaminophen is more efficacious than placebo for treating mild to moderate pain and is generally considered to be safe and well tolerated, it is not as efficacious as NSAIDs for pain management and in doses of 2 or more grams daily may carry the same magnitude of risk for serious upper gastrointestinal adverse events as NSAIDs.[55] Such confusion is not entirely unexpected as, although there is considerable evidence that the analgesic effect of paracetamol is central due to activation of descending serotonergic pathways, it is believed that paracetamol's primary site of action remains inhibition of prostaglandin synthesis.[56] In summary, current thinking suggests using paracetamol unless there is good evidence that NSAIDs are more effective in a particular patient. Certainly in patients with chronic pain, paracetamol can reduce the dose of NSAID required, with resultant benefits in terms of both reduced adverse effects and cost savings.[57] Similarly, paracetamol has been demonstrated to improve pain and wellbeing without major side effects in patients with cancer and persistent pain despite a strong opioid regimen.[58]

Herbal remedies

Herbal remedies may also have a role. Some arthritis suffers seem to get a degree of pain relief from taking up to 6 teaspoons of ginger daily. The symptomatic relief reported by some arthritis and fibromyalgia patients may be due to ginger inhibiting prostaglandin and leukotriene biosynthesis from arachidonic acid. An effective dose is 100–1000 mg/day as tablets, or 50 g of lightly cooked or 5 g of raw ginger.[59] Although animal experiments with eugenol caused significant suppression of both paw and joint swelling,[60] a controlled, double blind, double dummy, cross-over study comparing ginger extract to placebo in osteoarthritic patients failed to report significant benefit.[61]

Feverfew is another herb that inhibits eicosanoid production from arachidonic acid and the release of serotonin and lysosomal enzymes. Despite its popular lay use in rheumatoid arthritis, a random placebo controlled trial in symptomatic rheumatoid arthritis found no apparent benefit from 6 weeks of dried chopped feverfew (70–86 mg).[62]

Bromelain, derived from the stem of pineapples, modulates prostaglandin synthesis, blocks mobilization of arachidonic acid by phospholipases and blocks bradykinin. Bradykinin enhances vasodilation, vascular permeability and pain. Bromelain and feverfew are often combined with antioxidant vitamins and minerals in over-the-counter pain formulas.

Free radical control

Modification of eicosanoid metabolism is not the only local mechanism that may be altered in a bid to control pain. Free radicals generated by the inflammatory process boost inflammation and the resultant pain experience. Produced as a result of oxidative phosphorylation, free radicals are increased in circumstances of tissue destruction and phagocytosis. Once an inflammatory process has been initiated, free radicals contribute to a self-propagating system of cellular damage. Efforts to neutralize free radicals attempt to interrupt this vicious cycle. This is most easily achieved by taking antioxidants such as vitamins C, E, the carotenes and flavonoids. Minerals such as zinc and selenium have an antioxidant action both by sparing vitamin E and as a component of glutathione peroxide, the enzyme that prevents generation of free radicals that destroy polyunsaturated fatty acids in cell membranes.

Although it has not been directly identified as having a role in pain relief, vitamin C is the major aqueous phase antioxidant defence acting directly with superoxide, hydroxyl radicals and singlet oxygen. It also spares vitamin E. However, depending on the environment, vitamin C may exhibit either reducing or oxidizing activity.[63] At lower concentrations, ascorbic acid displays its antioxidant property; at higher concentrations, its prooxidant action emerges. Nonetheless, megadoses of vitamin C (10–50 g daily) may reduce moderately severe pain while 1 g tds appears to reduce delayed onset muscle soreness following strenuous exercise.

Vitamin E is another vitamin that may be considered in pain management. Vitamin E neutralizes nitric oxide and other free radicals.[64] Nitric oxide activates cyclo-oxygenase and lipoxygenase, leading to the production of physiologically relevant quantities of PGE2 and leukotrienes.[65] Vitamin E has an inhibitory effect on both cyclo-oxygenase and lipoxygenase activity. This property may well explain how vitamin E further decreased pro-inflammatory cytokine and eicosanoid activity and achieved significant clinical improvement in rheumatoid arthritis patients already on gamma-linolenic acid and fish oil.[66,67]

Flavonoids are a group of free radical scavengers that dampen inflammation by diverse metabolic interactions.[68,69] Bioflavonoids have an inhibitory effect on the release of arachidonic acid from cell membranes and consequently limit its availability as a substrate for cellular oxygenase enzymes. They also have an inhibitory effect on cyclo-oxygenase. The pain and swelling of acute inflammation is reported to be reduced by taking 400 mg of quercetin, a potent flavonoid, 20 minutes before meals three times a day. Quercetin is also reputed to reduce swelling resulting from hard contact sports when taken in doses of 0.6–1.8 g before playing.

Modulating neural transmission of pain

The gate control theory of pain transmission proposed by Melzack and Wall[70] suggests that painful stimuli are transmitted from skin nociceptors to the spinal cord through large A and small C fibres. Interaction between these small and large afferent fibres when they converge on the dorsal horn neurons affects pain transmission to higher centres. Various techniques of pain control, including transcutaneous electrical nerve stimulation (TENS) and capsaicin, employ this construct. Capsaicin, an ingredient in red peppers, acts selectively on a subpopulation of primary sensory neurons which generate pain sensations and participate in neurogenic inflammation.[71] On first exposure, topically applied capsaicin elicits pain and a local inflammatory effect. With repeated exposures, the neurons become insensitive to all further stimulation. Randomized studies suggest capsaicin cream can be used to advantage in patients with osteo- but not rheumatoid arthritis.[72] TENS, a relatively non-invasive physical treatment, alters the body's ability to receive or perceive pain signals. Similarly, as recorded on electromyography, movements of acupuncture needles cause depolarization of innervated single or grouped muscle fibre discharges.[73] In high frequency electroacupuncture a non-opioid 'gate' mechanism is but one mechanism believed to operate.[74,75] In acupuncture, analgesia nociceptive information may be inhibited by stimulation of opiate receptors located presynaptically on primary afferent neurons coupled with tonic inhibition from the descending 5-hydroxytryptamine system. In contrast, Western medicine achieves temporary nerve blocks by injecting local anaesthetic e.g. lidocaine.

IN PERSPECTIVE

Chronic pain is a common complaint amongst elderly patients. Chronic pain is a psychophysiological phenomenon and is best managed holistically using diverse approaches

A 75-year-old female with a history of arthritis presents complaining of joint pain, dizziness, epigastric discomfort, anorexia, bloating and occasional tinnitus. She had a stroke 3 years ago and gradually improved and is now 'doing nicely'. On examination her blood pressure and pulse are normal for her age group. She has evidence of chronic obstructive airways disease, and demonstrates widespread and symmetrical joint tenderness, swelling and deformity, especially of the fingers and wrists. Joint pain is somewhat relieved by activity while stiffness is worsened by rest. You note some bilateral muscle weakness and on laboratory investigation she returns a positive rheumatoid factor, raised ESR and C-reactive protein. She is currently taking 1.25 g aspirin four times a day to manage her arthritis. She has a history of smoking and currently smokes 15 cigarettes a day.

Her X-ray shows fusiform soft tissue swelling; periarticular osteopenia, diffuse loss of interosseous space and marginal erosion of bone were noted.

Questions arising

- What is this patient's definitive diagnosis?
- Why has she presented now?
- Could she have an iatrogenic disease complication?
- How should she be managed?

Clinical considerations

The patient with longstanding rheumatoid arthritis presents with the side effects of high dose aspirin therapy.

Additional investigations were undertaken.

Her haemoglobin was low. Her barium swallow suggested, and gastroscopy confirmed, peptic ulceration.

Intervention

Reduce the required dose of NSAIDs to minimize side effects without exacerbation of the arthritis.

Aspirin action: Reduce her aspirin dose and ensure she has enteric coated aspirin and/or consider using another NSAID. The peak analgesic effect of aspirin is between 2.0 and 5.0 g per day. The analgesic effect lasts for about 4 hours while the anti-inflammatory effect lasts much longer. Most toxicity from aspirin and other NSAIDs is dose related. Toxicity is highest for plain aspirin (1.36), decreasing for buffered (1.1) and enteric coated (0.92) aspirin.

Lifestyle changes:

- Regular exercise
- Stop smoking or cut down on the number of cigarettes smoked.

Dietary changes:

1. Reduce animal fats but eat 200 g or more of deep sea fish daily.
2. Avoid gluten, dairy, soy, yeast, eggs, red meat.
3. Favour a vegetarian diet but avoid the nightshade family: tobacco, tomatoes, potatoes, peppers, aubergine.
4. Avoid food additives: benzoates, sulphite, nitrate, glutamates, artificial colourings.
5. Use garlic and ginger (100 mg/tds).
6. Use plant seed oil, e.g. flaxseed oil, olive oil.

Nutritional supplements:

1. Lactobacillus acidophilus
2. Fish oil 2 g tds, eicosapentaeonic acid(EPA) around 3.0-4.5 g/day, docosahexaenoic acid(DHA) 1-2 g/day
3. Gamma-linolenic acid 1g tds—evening primrose oil or starflower oil
4. Vitamin E—400 mg tds/500 IU bd.

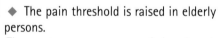

Mr Jones is a 65-year-old labourer. He presents complaining of headache. He has a long history of headaches and backache—both of which are worst in the morning and improve as the day goes on. Recently his headaches have got worse. He now finds he is never headache free even though he has started taking paracetamol regularly.

On examination you detect limitation of movement in the region of his neck, lower back and right hip. He is a non-smoker and drinks a couple of glasses of beer most days. His BMI is 28 and his systolic blood pressure is slightly raised.

On further direct questioning Mr Jones reports he has recently started vomiting but is not nauseous. His headache is aggravated when he coughs, bends down and lifts loads at work. He has no history of trauma. On further examination he is found to have papilloedema. No cranial nerve lesions were detected.

Questions arising

■ What is his differential diagnosis?

■ What is his working diagnosis?
■ Does he require referral for further investigations and treatment?

Clinical considerations

His differential diagnosis includes:

■ Spinal dysfunction
■ Cervical spondylosis
■ Subdural haematoma
■ Subarachnoid haemorrhage
■ Cerebral tumour or metastasis.

His working diagnosis is raised intracranial pressure. He needs to be referred for a computerized axial tomography(CAT) scan and magnetic resonance imaging(MRI).

Caution: Never do a lumbar puncture in patients with raised intracranial pressure.

Red flags:

■ The patient's chronic condition changed – be alert to multiple pathology, especially in elderly patients.
■ The headache ceased to respond to paracetamol - use of analgesics may mask and delay diagnosis of serious underlying pathology.

◆ The pain threshold is raised in elderly persons.

◆ The most common causes of chronic pain are persistent low backache and myofascial syndromes – however, cancer should also be excluded as a cause of chronic pain in the elderly.

◆ Pain may be classified as somatic/physical, visceral or psychogenic in origin.

◆ Psychogenic pain, despite lacking a recognizable physiological basis, is real to the patient and requires active intervention.

◆ Acute pain is predominantly a pathophysiological phenomenon that begins suddenly and is often relieved by chemical mediators.

◆ Chronic pain is a psychophysiological phenomenon and requires a more comprehensive or holistic approach to management.

◆ Lifestyle management of chronic pain includes changing the individual's perception of the problem, enhancing coping skills and modifying central and peripheral pain mediating chemicals.

◆ Nutritional intervention in pain management is most successful when a dietary trigger can be eliminated; however, dampening local inflammatory processes at the level of eicosanoid production and free radical neutralization is helpful.

◆ Depression should be actively considered and treated when detected in patients with chronic pain.

References

1. Rustoen T, Wahl AK, et al. Age and the experience of chronic pain: differences in health and quality of life among younger, middle-aged, and older adults. Clin J Pain 2005; 21(6):513–523.

2. Sha MC, Callahan CM, et al. Physical symptoms as a predictor of health care use and mortality among older adults. Am J Med 2005; 118(3):301–306.

3. Pressley JC, Patrick CH. Frailty bias in comorbidity risk adjustments of community-dwelling elderly populations. J Clin Epidemiol 1999; 52:753–760.

4. Kelinman A, Brodwin PE, et al. Pain as human experience: an introduction. In: Good MD, Brodwin PE, et al. eds. Pain as human experience: an anthropological perspective. Berkeley: University of California Press; 1992: 8.

5. American College of Sports Medicine Position Stand. Exercise and physical activity for older adults. Med Sci Sports Exerc 1998; 30(6):992–1008.

6. Bonnie B, Fries JF, Lubeck DP. Aerobic exercise and its impact on musculoskeletal pain in older adults: a 14 year prospective, longitudinal study. Arthritis Research & Therapy 2005, 7:R1263–R1270.

7. Brady TJ, Kruger J, et al. Intervention programs for arthritis and other rheumatic diseases. Health Educ Behav 2003; 30:44–63.

8. Vuori I. Exercise and physical health: musculoskeletal health and functional capabilities. Res Q Exerc Sport 1995; 66:276–285.

9. Taimela S, Diederich C, et al. The role of physical exercise and inactivity in pain recurrence and absenteeism from work after active outpatient rehabilitation for recurrent or chronic low back pain: a follow-up study. Spine 2000; 25:1809–1816.

10. Farrell PA. Exercise and endorphins—male responses. Med Sci Sports Exerc 1985; 17(1):89–93.

11. Crews DJ, Landers DM. A meta-analytic review of aerobic fitness and reactivity to psychosocial stressors. Med Sci Sports Exerc 1987; 19(5 Suppl):S114–S120.

12. Kugler J, Seelbach H, Kruskemper GM. Effects of rehabilitation exercise programmes on anxiety and depression in coronary patients: a meta-analysis. Br J Clin Psychol 1994; 33(Pt 3):401–410.

13. Petruzzello SJ, Landers DM, et al. A meta-analysis on the anxiety-reducing effects of acute and chronic exercise. Outcomes and mechanisms. Sports Med. 1991; 11(3):143–182.

14. Minor MA, Hewett JE, et al. Efficacy of physical conditioning exercise in patients with rheumatoid arthritis and osteoarthritis. Arthritis Rheum 1989; 32(11):1396–1405.

15. King AC, Oman RF, et al. Moderate-intensity exercise and self-rated quality of sleep in older adults. A randomized controlled trial. JAMA 1997; 277(1):32–37.

16. Ehrenpreis S. Pharmacology of enkephalinase inhibitors: animal and human studies. Acupuncture and Electrotherapeutics Res Int J 1985; 10:203–208.

17. Nicolodi M, Sicuteri F. L-5-hydroxytryptophan can prevent nociceptive disorders in man. Adv Exp Med Biol 1999; 467:177–182.

18. Richmond J, Berman BM, et al. Integration of behavioral and relaxation approaches into the treatment of chronic pain and insomnia. NIH Technol Statement Online http://odp.od.nih.gov/consensus/ta/017/017_sta tement.htm 1995 Oct 16–18 [cited 2005/1/15]. 1–34.

19. Astin JA. Mind-body therapies for the management of pain. Clin J Pain 2004; 20(1):27–32.

20. Tindle HA, Wolsko P, et al. Factors associated with the use of mind body therapies among United States adults with musculoskeletal pain. Complement Ther Med 2005; 13(3):155–164.

21. Hafen BQ, Karren KJ, et al. Mind/body health: the effect of attitudes, emotions, and relationships. Needham Height, Massachussetts: Simon & Schuster; 1996:475.

22. Kaplan RM. Coping with stressful medical examinations. In: Friedman HS, DiMatteo MR, eds. Interpersonal issues in health care. New York : Academic Press; 1982; 187–208.

23. Bolletino RC. Cancer: the roots of mind-body treatment of cancer patients. In: Watkins A, ed. Mind-body medicine. New York: Churchill Livingstone; 1997; 87–111.

24. Drugan RC, Basile AS, et al. The protective effects of stress control may be mediated by increased brain levels of benzodiazepine agonists. Brain Research 1994; 661:127–136.

25. Brody H. Placebos and the philosophy of medicine. Chicago: University of Chicago Press; 1980.

26. Bootzin RR, Caspi O. Explanatory mechanisms for placebo effects: cognition, personality and social learning. In: Guess HA, Kleinman A, et al, eds. The science of the placebo. London: BMJ Books; 2002:108–132.

27. Vase L, Robinson ME, et al. The contributions of suggestion, desire, and expectation to placebo effects in irritable bowel syndrome patients. An empirical investigation. Pain 2003; 105(1–2):17–25.

28. Oh VM. Magic or medicine? Clinical pharmacological basis of placebo medication. Ann Acad Med Singapore. 1991; 20(1):31–7.

29. Amanzio M, Pollo A, et al. Response variability to analgesics: a role for non–specific activation of endogenous opioids. Pain 2001; 90:205–215.

30. Brody H. The placebo response. Recent research and implications for family medicine. J Fam Pract 2000; 49:649–654.

31. Vernon H. Chiropractic: a model of incorporating the illness behavior model in the management of low back pain patients. J Manipulative Physiol Ther 1991; 14(6):379–389.

32. Kirsch I. Specifying nonspecifics: psychological mechanisms of the placebo response. In: Harrington A, ed. The placebo effect. Cambridge, MA: Harvard University Press; 1997:166–186.

33. Price DD, Milling LS et al. An analysis of factors that contribute to the magnitude of placebo analgesia in an experimental paradigm. Pain 1999; 83:147–156.

34. Norheim AJ, Fonnebo V. Attitudes to the contribution of placebo in acupuncture—a survey. Complement Ther Med 2002; 10(4):202–209.

35. Desharnais R, Jobin J, et al. Aerobic exercise and the placebo effect: a controlled study. Psychosom Med 1993; 55(2):149–154.

36. Gryll SL, Katahn M. Situational factors contributing to the placebos effect. Psychopharmacology. 1978; 57(3):253–261.

37. Verne GN, Robinson ME, et al. Reversal of visceral and cutaneous hyperalgesia by local rectal anesthesia in irritable bowel syndrome (IBS) patients. Pain 2003; 105(1–2):223–230.

38. Suchman AL, Ader R. Classic conditioning and placebo effects in crossover studies. Clin Pharmacol Ther 1992; 52(4):372–377.

39. Thompson WG. Placebos: a review of the placebo response. Am J Gastroenterol 2000; 95(7):1637–1643.

40. Siegel S. Explanatory mechanisms for placebo effects: Pavlovian conditioning. In: Guess HA, Kleinman A, et al, eds. The science of the placebo. London: BMJ Books; 2002:133–157.

41. de Deckere EA, Korver O, et al. Health aspects of fish and n-3 polyunsaturated fatty acids from plant and marine origin. Eur J Clin Nutr 1998; 52(10):749–753.

42. Kremer JM, Lawrence DA, et al. Effects of high-dose fish oil on rheumatoid arthritis after stopping nonsteroidal antiinflammatory drugs. Clinical and immune correlates. Arthritis Rheum 1995; 38:1107–1114.

43. Lau CS, Morley KD, Belch JJ. Effects of fish oil supplementation on non-steroidal anti-inflammatory drug requirement in patients with mild rheumatoid arthritis—a double-blind placebo controlled study. Br J Rheumatol 1993: 32(11):982–989.

44. Hartikainen SA, Mantyselka PT, et al. Balancing pain and analgesic treatment in the home-dwelling elderly. Ann Pharmacother 2005; 39(1):11–16. (Epub 2004 Dec 14).

45. Brooks P, Girgis L. Nonsteroidal anti-inflammatory drugs. Current Therapeutics 1995; 36: 31–39.

46. Hung J, Joyce DA. An aspirin a day. Current Therapeutics 1994; 35:11–15.

47. Day RO. Mode of action of non-steroidal anti-inflammatory drugs. Med J Aust 1988; 148:195–199.

48. Kopp E, Gosh S. Inhibition of NF-kappa B by sodium salicylate and aspirin. Science 1994; 265:956–958.

49. Fries JF, Ramey DR, et al. A reevaluation of aspirin therapy in rheumatoid arthritis. Archives of Internal Medicine 1993; 153:2465–2471.

50. Australian Gastroenterolgy Institute, Arthritis Foundation of Australia & Australian Rheumatology Association Joint Statement. Nonsteroidal anti-inflammatory drugs (NSAIDs) and the upper gut. Modern Medicine Aust 1992; July: 105–107.

51. Chapman GD. Therapeutic usage of the non-steroidal anti-inflammatory drugs. Med J Aust 1988; 149:203–213.

52. Skoldstam L, Borjesson O, et al. Effect of six months of fish oil supplementation in stable rheumatoid arthritis. A double-blind, controlled study. Scand J Rheumatol 1992; 21:178–185.

53. Peterson GM. Selecting nonprescription analgesics. Am J Ther 2005; 12(1):67–79.

54. Various authors. Discontinuation of Vioxx. Lancet 2005; 365(9453):24–27.

55. Hochberg MC, Dougados M. Pharmacological therapy of osteoarthritis. Best Pract Res Clin Rheumatol 2001; 15(4):583–593.

56. Graham GG, Scott KF. Mechanism of action of paracetamol. Am J Ther 2005; 12(1):46–55.

57. Nikles CJ, Yelland M, et al. The role of paracetamol in chronic pain: an evidence-based approach. Am J Ther 2005; 12(1):80–91.

58. Stockler M, Vardy J, et al. Acetaminophen (paracetamol) improves pain and well-being in people with advanced cancer already receiving a strong opioid regimen: a randomized, double-blind, placebo-controlled cross-over trial. J Clin Oncol 2004; 22(16):3389–3394.

59. Srivastava KC, Mustafa T. Ginger (Zingiber officinale) in rheumatism and musculoskeletal disorders. Med Hypotheses 1992; 39(4):342–348.

60. Sharma JN, Srivastava KC, Gan EK. Suppressive effects of eugenol and ginger oil on arthritic rats. Pharmacology 1994; 49(5):314–318.

61. Bliddal H, Rosetzsky A, et al. A randomized, placebo-controlled, cross-over study of ginger extracts and ibuprofen in osteoarthritis. Osteoarthritis Cartilage 2000; 8(1):9–12.

62. Pattrick M, Heptinstall S, Doherty M. Feverfew in rheumatoid arthritis: a double blind, placebo controlled study. Ann Rheum Dis 1989; 48(7):547–549.

63. Sakagami H, Satoh K, et al. Apoptosis-inducing activity of vitamin C and vitamin K. Cell Mol Biol (Noisy-le-grand) 2000; 46(1):129–143.

64. Schwenke DC. Does lack of tocopherols and tocotrienols put women at increased risk of breast cancer? J Nutr Biochem 2002; 13(1):2–20.

65. McCann SM, Licinio J, et al. The nitric oxide hypothesis of aging. Exp Gerontol 1998; 33(7–8):813–826.

66. Calder PC, Zurier RB. Polyunsaturated fatty acids and rheumatoid arthritis. Curr Opin Clin Nutr Metab Care 2001; 4(2):115–121.

67. Tidow-Kebritchi S, Mobarhan S. Effects of diets containing fish oil and vitamin E on rheumatoid arthritis. Nutr Rev 2001; 59(10):335–338.

68. Yochum LA, Folsom AR, Kushi LH. Intake of antioxidant vitamins and risk of death from stroke in postmenopausal women. Am J Clin Nutr 2000; 72:476–483.

69. Miller AL. The etiologies, pathophysiology, and alternative/complementary treatment of asthma. Altern Med Rev 2001; 6(1):20–47.

70. Melzack R, Wall P. Pain mechanisms: a new theory. Science 1965; I5O:171–179.

71. Fusco BM, Giacovazzo M. Peppers and pain. The promise of capsaicin. Drugs 1997; 53(6):909–914.

72. Keitel W, Frerick H, et al. Capsaicin pain plaster in chronic non-specific low back pain. Arzneimittelforschung 2001; 51(11):896–903.

73. Chu J. The local mechanism of acupuncture. Zhonghua Yi Xue Za Zhi (Taipei) 2002; 65(7):299–302.

74. Hole K, Berge OG. Regulation of pain sensitivity in the central nervous system. Cephalalgia 1981 Mar; 1(1):51–59.

75. Ma SX. Neurobiology of acupuncture: toward CAM. Evid Based Complement Alternat Med 2004; 1(1):41–47.

PATIENT HANDOUT 11.1 – PAIN SELF-CARE: THE ANALGESIC OPTION

Pain is the body's warning system. Over-the-counter analgesics relieve pain but may mask a serious cause of pain. If pain persists, always seek medical advice.

All drugs have side effects—the higher the dose the greater the risk. Reduce your risk of side effects from analgesics by:

- taking the lowest dose that gives pain relief
- reducing the dose required by simultaneously using different methods to relieve pain, e.g. taking fish oil and/or avocado/soybean unsaponifiables reduces the amount of NSAIDs needed to relieve the pain of rheumatoid arthritis
- choosing analgesics with fewer side effects—aspirin is safer than NSAIDs
- not combining drugs with similar side effects
- avoiding behaviours that aggravate side effects
    —don't smoke and take NSAIDs at the same time
    —avoid alcohol when taking NSAIDs
- consulting a doctor before taking analgesics if you have kidney or liver disease.

ASPIRIN

Aspirin can provide most people with pain relief at a dose of 300–600 mg/day.
Choose the safest form available - most safe is enteric coated aspirin, followed by buffered aspirin. Plain aspirin has most side effects. Start at the lowest dose and increase this as needed. The analgesic effect lasts for about 4 hours so it may help to divide your daily dose into 6 portions.

A warning: There is no additional benefit from taking more than 2.0–5.0g of aspirin daily. There are just additional side effects!

- Beware of taking aspirin if you are on anticoagulants. At 80 mg/day aspirin slows clotting.
- Aspirin may cause stomach problems that range from indigestion to bleeding ulcers. At 900 mg/day bleeding is common. The chance of a chronic gastric ulcer is increased over 16 times by self-medication with aspirin.

NSAIDs (Non-steroidal anti-inflammatory drugs)

- Stop taking analgesics as soon as pain permits. The longer you take analgesics the greater your risk of stomach problems - 2% of patients who take NSAIDs for 3 months have problems, this doubles at 12 months.
- Avoid behaviours that increase the risk of side effects. The chance of a chronic gastric ulcer is increased 4.7 times in a non-smoker on NSAIDs; it increases 6.9 times for cigarette smokers.

A warning:
- NSAIDs may cause kidney damage—avoid prolonged use of high doses.
- NSAIDs may cause liver damage.

Lower doses are recommended for patients with liver or kidney disease. Extra precautions are advisable for elderly persons and pregnant women.

A tip: Drugs are not the only option. If you are troubled by chronic pain consider other options such as:

- exercise
- muscle relaxation
- mental strategies.

SECTION 2 PATHOLOGIES PREVALENT IN OLD AGE

SECTION CONTENTS

Chapter **12**

Obesity

CHAPTER CONTENTS

An overweight 68-year-old woman presents complaining of fatigue. She has a history of weight fluctuations. Her BMI is 27.5, her blood pressure is raised as is her blood glucose.

- Is being overweight a health hazard?
- Would encouraging her to maintain her current weight comprise less health risk than continued weight cycling?
- Which management considerations may reduce weight fluctuations?

INTRODUCTION

We are in the grips of an obesity epidemic. The prevalence of obesity and overweight increased in the United States between 1978 and 1991 and the trend continued in 1999–2000.[1] A later study examining trends in obesity among the 'baby boom' (born 1946–1965) and 'silent' (born 1926–1945) generations confirmed the baby boomers were more obese, and became so at younger ages than their predecessors.[2] A consistent trend of increasing waist circumference, i.e. abdominal obesity, has also been observed for both sexes in aging Americans.[3] Abdominal adiposity is an important component of the insulin resistance syndrome, and this syndrome is associated with hypertension, hyperinsulinaemia, impaired glucose tolerance, increased blood triglycerides and LDL cholesterol, and decreased HDL cholesterol. A Canadian study examining trends in the health status of the entire population 65 years or older confirmed the prevalence of diabetes and hypertension increased substantially over the 14-year period studied.[4] These trends are not confined to North America, they are a global phenomenon. Demographic health surveys from the Middle East report the prevalence of obesity increases with age from an average of 6% in healthy children to 20% in adolescent males to 32% in elderly patients.[5] We are in the grips of an obesity pandemic.

ADDRESSING THE PROBLEM

Obesity is a modern lifestyle disorder. As a buffer against nutrient scarcity, natural selection would appear to have favoured genotypes with a thrifty metabolism.[6] However, genetic factors, which contribute to differences among patients in the resting metabolic rate and in weight gain in response to overeating, account for no more than 40% of the variance in body weight. A sedentary lifestyle with excess caloric intake combined with obesity susceptibility genes has produced the current obesity/overweight pandemic. Furthermore, there is increasing evidence to suggest obesity is not simply a problem of will power or self-control but a complex disorder involving appetite regulation and energy metabolism that is associated with a variety of comorbid conditions.

Obesity in adulthood is an undeniable health risk. Obesity and overweight are preventable causes of death and disease. Adult obesity is associated with excess mortality and excess risk of coronary heart disease, hypertension, hyperlipidaemia, diabetes, gallbladder disease, certain cancers, and osteoarthritis.[7] Waist circumference has proved an even better predictor of cardiovascular and coronary artery disease than body mass index (BMI),[8] and the group with the largest waist circumferences are 60–69 years of age.[3] Weight control is germane regardless of advancing age. Diet, exercise, behavioural interventions, pharmaceuticals and even surgery are options used for weight management. Unfortunately, long term success is limited and no single weight-loss option is without its pitfalls.[9]

THE DIETARY OPTION

When energy intake exceeds energy output weight increases. If the situation persists, overweight and obesity are inevitable. Dietary choice plays a major role. The energy density of macronutrients varies. One gram of fat, regardless of whether it is animal or vegetable in origin, provides 39 kJ (9 Cal/g). The energy density of alcohol is 29 kJ/g (7 Cal/g), of carbohydrates 16 kJ/g (4 Cal/g) and of protein 17 kJ/g (4 Cal/g). A 12 year follow-up study found the crude risk of becoming overweight ranged from 22% in women who ate a lower-fat, nutritionally varied healthy heart diet to 41% in women who ate a diet rich in sweets and fats with fewer servings of nutrient-dense fruits, vegetables, and lean foods.[10]

Two particularly popular dietary options are the low carbohydrate and low fat diets.

Low carbohydrate diets

Low carbohydrate diets, by reducing circulating insulin levels, are postulated to enhance lipolysis and lipid oxidation and reduce fat storage. Obese participants on a low carbohydrate diet (<30 g/day) were found to have a more favourable overall outcome at 1 year than those on a conventional diet.[11] Another study reported significantly greater weight loss on low carbohydrate diet (< 10% calories from carbohydrates) despite higher caloric intake (1855 kcal/day) compared to a high carbohydrate diet (60% calories from carbohydrates) with lower caloric intake (1562 kcal/day).[12] This diet also achieved preferential loss of fat in the trunk region. A low carbohydrate diet may consequently offer a particularly desirable option for type 2 diabetics.[13] Similarly, a randomized controlled trial over 12 months found subjects on the Atkins diet had greater weight loss than those on a conventional low energy diet for the first 6 months, but not significantly so at 1 year.[14]

The popular Atkins diet derives around 53% of its energy from fat, stressing a very low carbohydrate intake and dietary elimination of white flour and sugar. Despite the high fat content of these low carbohydrate diets, atherogenic dyslipidaemia and glycaemic control were more favourable in the low carbohydrate diet than the conventional control diets with less than 30% fat. More specifically, although low-density lipoprotein (LDL) and total cholesterol levels were similar, subjects on the low carbohydrate diet had greater rises in high-density lipoprotein (HDL) cholesterol and greater falls in serum triglycerides.[15] Nonetheless, as low carbohydrate diets inevitably tend to be higher fat diets, the type of dietary fat bears consideration.

Saturated fatty acids tend to increase LDL cholesterol levels, whereas monounsaturated and polyunsaturated fatty acids tend to decrease LDL cholesterol levels with the long chain omega-3 fatty acids, eicosapentaenoic acid and docosahexaenoic acid, decreasing triglyceride levels in hyper-triglyceridaemic patients. Trans-fatty acids increase LDL cholesterol levels. Obese persons on a low carbohydrate diet should consequently also consider selecting monounsaturated and polyunsaturated fatty acids, especially long chain omega-3 fatty acids, and limiting saturated and trans-fatty acids. Certainly one study found trans-10, cis-12 conjugated linoleic acid, a fat included in some weight loss supplements, increased insulin resistance and lipid peroxidation in obese men.[14] Another study reported a diet lower in total carbohydrates but higher in monounsaturated fat, complex carbohydrates and protein than that recommended by the US National Cholesterol Education Program achieved greater weight loss and better lipid levels.[16]

Low fat diets

Diets high in fat are postulated to lead to accumulation of fat stores. Fat is the most energy dense food and oxidation of fat fails to adjust rapidly to acute increases in dietary fat. Obese persons have a decreased capacity to oxidize fat in the postprandial state. A low fat diet would seem a logical approach to weight loss. Meta-analyses of intervention trials do suggest fat-reduced diets achieve a 3–4 kg greater weight loss than normal-fat diets.[17] A 10% reduction in dietary fat can cause a 4–5 kg weight loss in individuals with an initial BMI of 30. A randomized intervention trial of postmenopausal women found weight loss was greatest among women who decreased their percentage of energy from fat.[18] On the other hand, an energy unrestricted, very low carbohydrate diet has been shown to achieve better short term weight loss than a calorie restricted diet with 30% of the calories as fat.[19] Furthermore, there is no convincing evidence to suggest dietary fat intake promotes the development of obesity under isoenergetic conditions more than other macronutrients.[20] The lack of convincing evidence may be linked to different fats having diverse effects. Monounsaturated fatty acids may be more fattening than polyunsaturated and saturated fats,[17] while docosahexaenoate, a long chain fatty acid of the omega-3 series (22:6n–3) may increase basal fat oxidation and encourage weight loss.[21] However, a randomized trial comparing energy restricted diets found that the diet fashioned to decrease carbohydrate levels (<10% of energy) achieved a better outcome than a low fat diet (% carbohydrate:fat:protein = ~60:25:15%).[12] Moreover, results of trials lasting one or more years suggest fat consumption within the range of 18–40% of energy appears to have little if any effect on body fatness.[22] Nonetheless, dietary fat does increase the energy density of foods; fat is efficiently stored and data from the National Weight Control Registry suggest that moderating dietary fat intake is a key strategy for long term management of body weight in individuals who have successfully maintained a substantial weight loss.[23]

Dietary adherence

Long term dietary adherence is a crucial consideration in weight management. A single-centre randomized trial compared adherence rates and the effectiveness of four popular diets.[24] The Atkins diet represented the carbohydrate restricted option, the Zone diet the macronutrient balance (40% carbohydrate:30% fat:30% protein by energy) option, Weight Watchers the calorie restricted diet and the Ornish diet the fat restriction alternative. Each diet significantly reduced the LDL:HDL cholesterol ratio by approximately 10% with no significant effects on blood pressure or glucose at 1 year. The amount of weight loss in each diet reflected self-reported dietary adherence level. While each popular diet modestly reduced body weight and several cardiac risk factors at 12 months, overall dietary adherence rates were low.

As long term dietary adherence has emerged as a barrier to successful weight control, mention should perhaps therefore be made of a 'culturally' determined diet with weight loss potential. A randomized, prospective 18 month trial in a free-living population found the Mediterranean diet achieved weight loss and favourably modified cardiovascular risk factors.[25] Recent studies consistently suggest that the Mediterranean diet, based on virgin olive oil, is compatible with a healthier aging and increased longevity.[26] This diet improves lipoprotein profile, blood pressure and glucose metabolism, and positively modulates the antithrombotic profile, endothelial function, inflammation and oxidative stress. In addition to being rich in virgin olive oil, the Mediterranean dietary pattern consists of:[27]

- daily consumption of non-refined cereals and products (whole grain bread, pasta, brown rice, etc.), vegetables (2–3 servings/day), fruits (6 servings/day), olive oil (as the main added lipid) and dairy products (1–2 servings/day)
- weekly consumption of fish (4–5 servings/week), poultry (3–4 servings/week), olives, pulses and nuts (3 servings/week), potatoes, eggs and sweets (3–4 servings/week) and
- monthly consumption of red meat and meat products (4–5 servings/month).

The Mediterranean diet enjoys superior long term participation and adherence.

Hunger and satiety

While overeating is often habitual and socially influenced, physiological factors may play a role. Appetite regulation involves an interplay between hunger and satiety signals. Hunger signals generated in peripheral organs and produced in the hypothalamus are expressed during states of energy deficiency. Satiety signals act by inhibiting or blunting the expression of hunger signals and produce feelings of fullness. Feel 'full' is postulated to influence ad libitum food intake. Palatable foods up-regulate the expression of both hunger and satiety signals but blunt the response to satiety signals.[28]

Food groups can also influence appetite. Protein is more satisfying and thermogenic than carbohydrate, hence replacing some carbohydrate with protein is a potential option for enhancing weight loss.[29] Trials comparing low fat high protein with standard or low protein low fat diets confirmed both dietary patterns achieved net weight loss and improvements in cardiovascular risk factors.[30,31] Furthermore, one study reported greater reductions in total and abdominal fat mass and LDL cholesterol in subjects on the high protein diet.[31] Although high protein diets tend to be more palatable and satisfying, and achieve greater weight loss initially due mainly to reduced high water and glycogen storage,[32] adherence is poor on high protein diets![30]

In view of the association between leptin levels, body weight and serum insulin it has been suggested that leptin is a satiety hormone that reduces appetite.[33] One human trial found that a carbohydrate meal induced higher postprandial leptin levels than an isoenergetic fat meal.[34] However, although 3 weeks of supplementation with non-fermentable fibre (methylcellulose 27 g/day) enhanced satiety compared with fermentable fibre (pectin, β-glucan 27 g/day), neither diet altered body weight.[35]

Another attempt to enlist the aid of carbohydrate to decrease appetite compared the effects of equal energy portions of 7 different breads.[36] The mean 'satiety index score' used in this study ranged from 100% to 561%, with regular white bread having the lowest score. Ironically, the strongest predictor of the breads' satiety index scores was portion size and energy density. Advising individuals to eat portions of low energy dense foods has nonetheless been found to be a more successful weight loss strategy than fat reduction coupled with restriction of portion sizes.[37] Several studies have demonstrated that eating low energy dense foods (such as fruits, vegetables and soups) maintains satiety while reducing energy intake. Furthermore, as aging is associated with resistance to the effects of leptin on food intake and energy homeostasis,[38] weight loss in older persons may be better served by attention to a balanced diet favouring satisfying portions of low energy, nutrient dense foods.

Food selection

Food selection can also be used as a tool to reduce energy intake. A reduction in energy intake with unchanged physical activity predictably results in weight loss. By maintaining portion size and avoiding energy dense foods, energy intake may be reduced. Energy dense foods include butter, oil, nuts; moderately energy dense food are a boiled egg or rice, grilled lean meat, bread and fried fish; and low energy dense foods include pumpkin, broccoli, carrot, skimmed milk and clear soup. When energy intake is reduced, care must be taken to ensure adequate nutrition. Without changing portion size and by selecting nutrient dense foods, nutrient intake can be maintained. Nutrient dense foods include eggs, green leafy and yellow vegetables, liver, milk and oysters. In contrast, butter, sugar, alcohol and soft drinks have a low nutrient density and should be limited or avoided.

An alternative option is sugar substitution. Low joule foods and soft drinks using artificial sweeteners have lower energy content than their sucrose equivalents. Artificial sweeteners are considerably sweeter than sugar but their taste profile is not as pleasing. Eating certain foods may provide an additional advantage. Isocaloric substitution of yogurt (calcium content 1100 mg/day) for other foods may augment fat loss and reduce central adiposity during energy restriction.[39] Analysis of six observational studies and three controlled trials in which calcium intake was the independent variable revealed a consistent relationship between higher calcium intakes, lower body fat and/or body weight plus reduced weight gain at midlife.[40] Each 300 mg increment in regular calcium intake was associated with approximately 2.5–3.0 kg lower body weight in adults. As bone loss caused by weight loss may be greater in overweight than obese women, an additional consideration for overweight postmenopausal women is to increase their calcium intake to 1.7 g/day during active weight loss.[41] One explanation for the antiobesity effect of dietary calcium may be suppression of calcitriol levels, resulting in reduced adipocyte intracellular $Ca2+$ and, consequently, a coordinated increase in lipid utilization and a decrease in lipogenesis.[42] However, as calcium supplementation may counter this process, the efficacy of dairy-specific dietary calcium may stem from or require the presence of other dairy components such as angiotensin converting enzyme inhibitory peptides or conjugated linoleic acid.

While dairy foods are a realistic option, other 'special' weight loss foods are more suspect. A number of popular lay remedies are more folklore than fact. Grapefruit, although an excellent low calorie food, does not possess any particular enzyme which enhances catabolism. Kelp (seaweed), although a natural source of iodine, does not stimulate thyroid hormone production in euthyroid subjects. In fact, excess doses of iodine in such persons may suppress thyroxine production. Cider vinegar may not mix with oil in a bottle but its consumption has little relevance to cellular metabolism.

Weight loss supplements

In addition to lay remedies, more than 50 individual over-the-counter dietary supplements and more than 125 commercial combination products are available for weight loss.[43] Commercial products for weight loss incorporate various individual items, each of which is believed to enhance weight loss by diverse means: e.g. 5-hydroxytryptophan may decrease appetite, green tea is thought to increase the 24-hour energy expenditure, chromium is believed to promote fat rather than lean tissue loss, carnitine and conjugated linoleic acid may increase fat oxidation, hydroxycitrate may inhibit hepatic lipogenesis while ephedrine and pyruvate may increase the metabolic rate.[44]

Despite the array of options currently available, no weight loss supplements meet the criteria for recommended use, either because evidence of efficacy is lacking or untoward effects are unacceptable.[43] For example, there is evidence of modest weight loss secondary to ephedra-caffeine ingestion, but potentially serious adverse effects have led the US Food and Drug Administration to ban the sale of these products. Like Ephedra sinica, ephedrine containing supplements appear to be effective but unsafe due to an increased risk of adverse events. The long term safety and efficacy of chromium, another popular weight loss supplement, is also uncertain.

Guar gum and chitosan appear to be ineffective. Evidence of efficacy is insufficient or conflicting with respect to conjugated linoleic acid, ginseng, glucomannan, green tea, hydroxycitric acid, L-carnitine, psyllium, pyruvate and St John's wort.[43] Analysis of five systematic reviews and meta-analyses of 25 additional trials involving chitosan, chromium picolinate, Garcinia cambogia, glucomannan, guar gum, hydroxy-methylbutyrate, plantago psyllium, pyruvate, yerba mate and yohimbe failed to provide evidence beyond a reasonable doubt that any of these dietary supplements was effective for reducing body weight.[45] The reviewers felt none of the above dietary supplements justified a recommendation for over-the-counter use. Another report examined conjugated linoleic acid, ephedra, ephedrine, chromium, Garcinia cambogia, hydroxycitric acid, chitosan and pyruvate. The reviewers concluded pyruvate was promising, conjugated linoleic acid hopeful, ephedra effective but high risk and Garcinia and chitosan unhelpful.[46]

The nutritional option in a nutshell

An average weight-loss goal of 10% is recommended for an obese patient. Studies have shown:[47]

- A diet that is individually planned to help create a deficit of 500 to 1000 kcal/day should be part of any program aimed to achieve a weekly weight loss of 0.5–1 kg (1–2 lbs).
- Low energy diets are effective, reducing waist circumference and total body weight by an average of 8% over a period of 6 months.
- Reducing both dietary fat and carbohydrate facilitates calorie reduction.
- Overall, herbal products and dietary supplements promoted for weight loss currently lack sufficient supporting efficacy and safety data for any to be recommended.

THE EXERCISE OPTION

The American Dietetic Association specifies that 'successful weight management … takes a lifelong commitment to healthful lifestyle behaviors emphasizing sustainable and enjoyable eating practices and daily physical activity'.[48] It has, moreover, been postulated that weight loss is facilitated by emphasizing positive rather than negative or restrictive messages.[49] One positive message is to eat breakfast. Skipping breakfast is associated with increased prevalence of obesity,[50] and eating breakfast a characteristic common to successful weight loss maintenance.[51] Another positive message is to take regular exercise.

In elderly men, leisure time physical activity is inversely associated with body fat and BMI, but positively associated with appendicular fat free mass,[52] and exercise-induced weight loss is associated with a preferential reduction in abdominal fat and a corresponding maintenance of fat free mass.[53] It has been reported that the surgeon general suggested that '… an increase in daily expenditure of approximately 150 kilocalories per day is associated with substantial health benefits and the activity does not need to be vigorous to achieve benefit…'.[54] Walking slowly for 90 minutes daily or 45 minutes briskly could expend the desired additional 150 kcals.[55] Walking less than 30 minutes per day is associated with a 2.7 times greater probability of being obese!

Exercise both reduces disease risk and, by aiding retention of lean body mass during active weight loss, protects against regaining weight lost. Lean body mass is an important determinant of basal metabolic rate (BMR), a measure of the energy required at rest. Although being fit does not completely reverse the increased risk associated with excess adiposity,[56] it encourages both weight loss and health. Data from most weight loss studies suggest that 60–75 minutes of moderate intensity activity (e.g. walking) or 35 minutes of vigorous activity (e.g. jogging) daily is needed to maintain long term weight loss. In previously inactive patients, an initial exercise program should be of short duration, 10 minutes daily, and then gradually increase to 30 minutes of low intensity activity.[57] Exercise increases the gap between energy expenditure and food intake.[54]

High intensity exercise also suppresses appetite immediately after exercise, increases basal metabolism rate by 5–15% for 24–48 hours and improves long term eating behaviour. High intensity activities expending at least 4 BMR, include gardening activities (digging, carrying loads, 4.1 BMR), brisk walking (4.5 BMR), climbing up stairs (6 BMR), heavy construction work (7 BMR), and most sports (6–12 BMR). Although high intensity exercises may be required for weight control, moderate intensity activities may be able to prevent deaths from all causes and from coronary heart diseases.[55] Moderate intensity activities that expend 3–3.9 BMR encompass most household chores and professional activities such as that of locksmith, handyman or electrical worker. Low intensity activities that increase basal metabolism less than 3 fold (<3 BMR) include seated office work, reading, watching television and walking slowly.

Exercising and losing weight benefit health even in people who remain overweight. Weight loss and exercise improve the dyslipidaemia related to obesity even when individuals fail to normalize their body weight.[58] Increased physical activity coupled with dietary change to a low-fat high-fibre diet improves the obesity-associated pro-thrombotic risk profile.[59] In addition to exercise expending energy, it favourably modulates cardio-vascular and other disease risk factors. On the other hand, lack of exercise itself is believed to contribute to overweight and obesity. A dramatic decrease in energy expenditure consistent with a sedentary lifestyle may explain the diverging trend in energy consumption (falling) and obesity prevalence (rising) observed in many economically developed countries.[60]

Exercise in a nutshell

While a lower BMI is the strongest predictor of remaining metabolically normal, higher levels of physical activity and/or lower levels of cigarette smoking are both independently associated with being metabolically normal in men.[61] Any physical activity is useful in weight control. There are basically two approaches:[47]

- Programmed exercise. Patients can implement a regular exercise regime of walking, swimming or cycling. In general, 30–45 minutes of exercise 3–5 days each week is recommended, although more exercise and greater intensity afford additional benefits.
- Lifestyle exercise. Patients increase their overall physical activity; for example, by using the stairs rather than an elevator and avoiding the use of a car for short distances. Three 10 minute periods of activity have about the same benefit as one 30 minute period. Lifestyle activities, such as climbing stairs or walking rather than taking a car, have been shown to be as effective as structured exercise in maintaining weight loss.

THE PHARMACEUTICAL OPTION

Lifestyle modifications are the preferred management approach to weight control. However, when these interventions fail pharmacological and surgical options are available.[62] Drugs evaluated for weight loss include ephedrine, the antidepressants fluoxetine and bupropion, and the anti-epileptics topiramate, zonisamide, sibutramine and orlistat.[63]

However, the only drugs the US Food and Drug Administration (FDA) has approved for long term obesity control are sibutramine and orlistat.[62] With the exception of raised diastolic blood pressure in the case of sibu-tramine, addition of these drugs to a weight loss program generally decreases risk factors.[64] Metformin use has been associated with decreased mortality after 10 years in obese people with type 2 diabetes.[64]

Despite some benefits, drugs may be associated with untoward effects. For example, by reducing dietary fat absorption orlistat may impair assimilation of fat soluble vitamins. Despite orlistat therapy significantly reducing antioxidative capacity without affecting oxidative stress, exercise training of patients on this drug shows significantly decreased lipid peroxidation.[65]

Patients on drug therapy should simultaneously be following lifestyle weight management options.

THE BEHAVIOURAL OPTION

Lifestyle management is the mainstay of weight control. The issue of weight control is at least as much one of long term commitment to behaviour change as it is of determining a desirable dietary composition or exercise schedule. Psychosocial and behavioural variables, which include diet and exercise, appear useful pretreatment predictors of possible success or attrition[66] and self-efficacy for specific behaviour changes has emerged as a fundamental determinant of successful weight loss.[67]

The most useful behavioural modification lies in planning and self-monitoring. Behavioural changes leading to successful weight loss are more likely when individuals are provided with the tools to help them realize desirable changes. Patient education and motivation is an integral part of successful weight loss. See the Handout 3.1 at *www.jamisonhealth.com*. In order to change eating and exercise behaviours, it is important to change environmental cues and reinforcers that control these behaviours. No single method or combination of behavioural methods has proved to be clearly superior. Various strategies include:[47]

- Self-monitoring. Keeping a food and exercise diary improves insight into personal behaviour, making patients aware of unhealthy habits. Self-monitoring through lifestyle diaries provides a record of success and may motivate patients to maintain their weight loss.[68]
- Stress management. Stress can trigger dysfunctional eating patterns. Coping strategies, meditation and relaxation techniques can be learned.
- Stimulus control. Once high risk situations have been identified using a

food diary, controlling strategies such as eating before shopping, buying only healthy food, keeping high calorie foods out of the house, limiting the times and places of eating, and consciously avoiding situations in which overeating occurs, can be initiated.

- Problem solving. By actively engaging in and self-correcting problem behaviours/situations, patients can take responsibility for their weight loss program.
- Contingency management. Rewarding beneficial changes in behaviour can motivate patients.
- Social support. A strong system of social support facilitates weight reduction.

Cognitive behavioural therapy, which includes cognitive restructuring and relapse prevention training, has also been helpful. Cognitive restructuring involves modifying negative thoughts, creating realistic goals and correcting inaccurate beliefs about weight loss. Relapse prevention training focuses on helping patients acquire skills to overcome setbacks and cope with problems.

Behavioural intervention, typically delivered in 15–26 weekly group sessions, produces a mean weekly weight loss of approximately 0.4 kg during treatment followed by a mean post-treatment weight loss of approximately 8.5 kg. Prolonged behavioural therapy sessions with reassessments over a year achieve greater weight loss with a substantial percentage of participants maintaining their initial weight loss. This compares very favourably with dietary/exercise weight loss programs in which the 5 year success rate may approximate zero.

Behavioural options in a nutshell

'Behavioural treatment' does not refer to the specific diet or exercise plan that is adopted, but rather to the principles and techniques used to change behaviour and habits.[47] To achieve sustained weight loss, individuals must learn specific skills to facilitate a long term change in eating behaviour and increased energy expenditure.

Meta-analyses have found behaviour therapy results in significantly greater weight reductions than placebo when assessed as a stand-alone weight loss strategy (about –2.5 kg).[69] Furthermore, compared with diet/exercise alone, a combination of diet, exercise and behaviour therapy or cognitive behaviour therapy achieves even greater weight loss. For successful long term weight loss a combined approach including dietary, exercise and behavioural or cognitive behavioural strategies appears the most effective alternative.

A STING IN THE TAIL

It is generally accepted that weight management is a challenging problem. Over 70% of older adults in the United States are overweight or obese, and if the rate of increase in obesity reported over the last decade continues, it is likely one third of the US will be obese in 9 years, and 50% may be obese in 16 years.[70] To make matters worse, physicians in an American survey rated the treatment of obesity as significantly less effective than therapies for 9 of 10 chronic conditions.[71] Moreover, a study of persons between the ages of 50 and 76 found that of 7 serious diseases, 23 medical conditions, and 11 health complaints, only osteoporotic fractures and prolonged constipation were less prevalent in overweight and obese persons.[72]

While it is generally accepted that obesity affects mortality and evidence that being overweight affects risk factors, the effect on life expectancy of being overweight is unproven.[70] In fact, aggregated data suggest that those who are overweight, but not obese, live about the same amount of time as those who are 'normal' weight. After adjusting for age, gender, smoking and exercise, while obese subjects appeared to have quality of wellbeing scale scores that were 0.046 lower than those of normal weight, the health-related quality of life for overweight people did not differ significantly from those of normal weight.[70] Results are inconsistent across studies. What makes this uncertainty frustrating are:

- Studies such as the retrospective cohort analysis of the longitudinal Study of Aging which suggest obesity may be protective compared with thinness or normal weight in older community-dwelling Americans![73]
- The finding that overweight participants had better cognitive performance in terms of reasoning and visuospatial speed of processing than normal weight participants.[74]
- Links between frailty and being overweight. Frailty is more closely associated with mortality than with chronological age. Markers of frailty are weakness, slowness, weight loss, low physical activity and exhaustion. Prefrailty, the presence of 1 or 2 of these markers, is associated with being overweight.[75]

Adding to the conundrum is the finding that in the absence of a universal definitive long term weight loss protocol, weight cycling has become a substantial problem. Weight cycling is associated with greater weight gain, less physical activity, and a higher prevalence of binge eating.[76] This study found that over an 8 year period mild yo-yo dieters gained an average of 6.7 pounds and severe cyclers gained approximately 10.3 lbs. Another longitudinal study reported weight fluctuation was associated with a higher risk of all-cause and cardiovascular disease mortality, even after adjusting for pre-existing disease, initial BMI and excluding subjects who were in poor health or incapacitated.[77] A cross-sectional study suggested frequent intentional weight loss may have long-term effects on immune function.[78] Loss of 10 or more pounds on more than one occasion predictably resulted in decreased natural killer cell (NK) cytotoxicity. In contrast, prolonged recent weight stability is an independent predictor of higher NK cytotoxicity. As immunosenescence is a recognized phenomenon, the question arises as to whether weight loss may be particularly hazardous for elderly people. A longitudinal observational cohort study of persons 65 years and over found weight loss but not weight gain of 5% or more over a 3 year period was associated with an increased risk of mortality, even in the absence of serious illness in the period of weight change.[79] The authors concluded that even modest decline in body weight was an important and independent marker of risk of mortality in older adults.

KEEPING PERSPECTIVE

Health risk is decreased by maintaining an ideal body weight. While obesity is a substantial health hazard, the relationship between being overweight and mortality is less clear. For overweight persons the objective should perhaps be a healthy lifestyle conducive to sustained weight loss rather than temporary adherence to a weight loss regime.

CLINICAL CHALLENGE

Jim, a large framed 65-year-old man, asks for your help in developing a weight loss program. His height is 180 cm, his weight 90 kg and his BMI 27.78. His waist circumference is 99 cm. He has a moderately active lifestyle.

Questions arising

- How do you determine how much weight he needs to lose?
- To what extent is his health compromised by his current body weight?
- What are the steps involved in developing a weight loss program suited to this patient?

Clinical considerations

Step 1: Identify the problem
Jim's actual BMI is 27.78, but his ideal BMI would be 23, giving an ideal weight of 74.5 kg. His actual weight is 90 kg. Weight loss goal = 90 kg – 74.5 kg = 15.5 kg.

Step 2: Identify the increased health risks and discuss the cost–benefit of change ratio
The costs—for example:

- Identify and list the health risks associated with being obese/overweight.
- Discuss the problems associated with yo-yo dieting, i.e. cycles of weight loss followed by

weight gain are associated with progressive loss of lean body mass. The basal metabolic rate (BMR) is determined by lean body mass and consequently yo-yo dieting exacerbates the problem by reducing BMR.

The increased health risk for an overweight man for the following conditions is:[72]

- History of serious diseases: coronary artery disease 1.1×; congestive heart failure 1.1×; pulmonary embolism 1.6×; deep vein thrombosis 1.3×.
- Cardiovascular disease risk factors: hypercholesterolaemia 1.5×; hypertension 1.8×.
- Other medical conditions: depression 1.0×; gastroesophageal reflux disease 1.3×; diabetes 1.6×; gallbladder removal 1.3×; pancreatitis 1.1×; kidney stones 1.1×; osteoarthritis 1.2×.
- Health complaints: knee replacement 1.5×; hip replacement 1.1×; neck, back or joint pain 1.1×; fatigue/lack of energy 1.1×; depressed/anxious 1.1×; chronic insomnia 1.2×; indigestion 1.3×; impotence 1.3×.

The benefits—for example:

- Improved blood lipid and thrombogenic profiles and consequently reduced risk of ischaemic heart disease.
- Decreased risk of diabetes, osteoarthritis etc.
- Improved body image.

Step 3: Identify energy intake required to lose weight safely

A rule of thumb estimation is that the energy intake permitted for weight loss is 90 kJ/kg of desired body weight. The energy intake Jim requires to reach his ideal body weight is 74.5 kg × 90 kJ = 6705 kJ.

The rate of weight loss will be influenced by the daily energy intake. Weight loss will be quicker if the rule of thumb estimation is applied. As Jim is moderately active and has a large frame, his basal energy intake is higher than that determined by the rule of thumb estimation. Whatever approach is chosen, it is important to appreciate that the minimum energy required to achieve adequate nutrition is 2500 kJ and a safe weight loss target is 0.5–1.0 kg/week

Step 4: List strategies for achieving desired weight loss

Food choices must fall within permitted energy range for weight loss.

Dietary options

- Option 1: a low carbohydrate diet
- Option 2: a low fat diet
- Option 3: selection of nutrient dense and avoidance of energy dense foods
- Option 4: converting to a vegetarian i.e. plant-based diet
- Option 5: smaller portions of usual diet within permitted energy consumption range
- Option 6: modify usual diet but eliminate or limit high energy choices, e.g. chocolates, fried foods, alcohol, fat spread and only purchase low fat and/or low kilojoule packaged food varieties
- Option 7: eat any foods but use a calorie counter to ensure remaining within permitted energy range.

Behavioural strategies

- No eating between meals.
- Always eat breakfast.
- Only eat when seated at the table and do not do other things, e.g. watch television, read, while eating.
- Eat slowly; put the knife/fork/spoon down between mouthfuls, chew food well.
- Don't shop when hungry.
- Be wary of eating as a therapy for emotional distress.

Exercise options

- Walk slowly for 90 minutes daily or 45 minutes briskly to use 630 kJ.
- High-intensity activities are most effective for enhancing weight loss, e.g. brisk walking, jogging, climbing up stairs, tennis etc.
- Weight bearing exercise helps to maintain lean body mass.
- Exercise helps to retain coordination and mobility.

Appetite suppression

- High satiety foods may be helpful—consider protein, foods with a low glycaemic index, e.g. apples, peaches, baked beans, lentils, bran cereals, low fat milk or yogurt.

Pharmacological and/or surgical options

- These should only be considered in selected cases.

Step 5: Prepare a personalized weight management program

Successful weight management requires a lifestyle change. Patients should therefore select a combination of strategies best suited to their lifestyle. Selection should be guided by:

1. energy intake that does not exceed permitted kilojoules
2. food selection that ensures adequate nutrition
3. some form of exercise should always be included
4. specific consideration given to dietary changes in individuals at high risk of particular diseases, e.g. waist circumference in excess of 94 cm (males) or 80 cm (females) increases risk of metabolic syndrome i.e. ischaemic heart disease, diabetes.

Step 6: Implement the program

- Set up a monitoring system/diary that includes interim target weights and deadlines.

- Include rewards for successful weight loss.
- Provide options for managing failures.

Step 7: Maintain weight loss

When the target weight has been achieved, gradually increase energy intake to permitted level. Weight maintenance requires 110–140 kJ per kilogram of desired body weight. Jim is permitted 74.5 × 120 = 9680 kJ per day once he reaches his desired body weight. Continue to monitor weight and adapt energy intake as required.

Remember: Energy intake calculations are mere guidelines. The acid test is maintaining a desirable body weight!

Remind patients: Successful weight management is a lifetime task.

◆ Long term successful weight loss requires a lifestyle change.

◆ When energy intake exceeds energy output weight increases, and vice versa.

◆ In all weight loss diets care must be taken to eat nutrient dense foods to ensure adequate nutrition.

◆ Low carbohydrate diets appear to reduce weight more effectively than conventional low energy, low fat diets and may be the option of choice for type 2 diabetics.

◆ Long term compliance is poor and behavioural measures combined with diet and exercise achieve the best result.

◆ Selection of low energy nutrient dense foods is conducive to healthy weight loss.

◆ A moderate decrease in caloric intake (500–1000 kcal/day) will result in a slow but progressive weight loss (1–2 lb/week, or 0.45–0.90 kg/week).

◆ For most patients, weight loss diets should supply 1000–1200 kcal/d for women and 1200–1600 kcal/day for men.

◆ Exercise is an essential component of any weight loss regime: exercise 60 minutes daily to prevent weight gain and 90 minutes daily to lose weight.

◆ Convincing evidence of the efficacy and/or safety of herbal and nutritional supplements for weight loss is lacking.

◆ A weight loss program that utilizes feasible lifestyle changes acceptable to the individual enhances the likelihood of success.

◆ Strategies associated with successful long term weight loss include eating a diet low in calories (around 1400 kcal/day) and fat (24% of the total energy intake), frequently monitoring body weight, and participating in regular physical activity (equivalent to 2800 kcal/week, or about 60 minutes of moderate activity per day).

◆ Persons who successfully maintain weight loss reduce their portion sizes, avoid snacking, have breakfast daily, eat meals away from home no more than 3 times a week and spend less than 3 hours a week watching television.

◆ While overweight patients should be encouraged to lose weight, both the propensity for an individual to be a weight cycler and their overall risk factor status should be considered when preparing a management protocol.

References

1. Flegal KM, Carroll MD, et al. Prevalence and trends in obesity among US adults, 1999–2000. JAMA 2002; 288(14):1723–1727.

2. Leveille SG, Wee CC, Iezzoni Ll. Trends in obesity and arthritis among baby boomers and their predecessors, 1971–2002. Am J Public Health 2005; 95(9):1607–1613.

3. Okosun IS, Chandra KM, et al. Abdominal adiposity in U.S. adults: prevalence and trends, 1960–2000. Prev Med 2004; 39(1):197–206.

4. Menec VH, Lix L, et al. Trends in the health status of older Manitobans, 1985 to 1999. Can J Aging 2005; 24 (Suppl 1):S5–S14.

5. Elabbassi WN, Haddad HA. The epidemic of the metabolic syndrome. Saudi Med J 2005; 26(3):373–375.

6. Damcott CM, Sack P, Shuldiner AR. The genetics of obesity. Endocrinol Metab Clin North Am 2003; 32(4):761–786.

7. Ogden CL, Carroll MD, Flegal KM. Epidemiologic trends in overweight and obesity. Endocrinol Metab Clin North Am. 2003; 32(4):741–760, vii.

8. Welborn TA, Dhaliwal SS, Bennett SA. Waist-hip ratio is the dominant risk factor predicting cardiovascular death in Australia. Med J Aust 2003; 179(11–12):580–585.

9. Strychar I. Diet in the management of weight loss. CMAJ 2006; 174(1):56–63.

10. Quatromoni PA, Copenhafer DL, et al. Dietary patterns predict the development of overweight in women: The Framingham Nutrition Studies. J Am Diet Assoc 2002; 102(9):1239–1246.

11. Stern L, Iqbal N, et al. The effects of low-carbohydrate versus conventional weight loss diets in severely obese adults: one-year follow-up of a randomized trial. Ann Intern Med 2004; 140(10):778–785.

12. Volek J, Sharman M, et al. Comparison of energy-restricted very low-carbohydrate and low-fat diets on weight loss and body composition in overweight men and women. Nutr Metab (Lond) 2004; 1(1):13.

13. Arora SK, McFarlane SI. The case for low carbohydrate diets in diabetes management. Nutrition & Metabolism 2005; 2:16.

14. Foster GD, Wyatt HR, et al. A randomized trial of a low-carbohydrate diet for obesity. N Engl J Med 2003; 348(21):2082–2090.

15. Riserus U, Vessby B, et al. Effects of cis-9, trans-11 conjugated linoleic acid supplementation on insulin sensitivity, lipid peroxidation, and proinflammatory markers in obese men. Am J Clin Nutr 2004; 80(2):279–283.

16. Aude YW, Agatston AS, et al. The national cholesterol education program diet vs a diet lower in carbohydrates and higher in protein and monounsaturated fat: a randomized trial. Arch Intern Med 2004; 164(19):2141–2146.

17. Astrup A. The role of dietary fat in obesity. Semin Vasc Med 2005; 5(1):40–47.

18. Howard BV, Manson JE, et al. Low-fat dietary pattern and weight change over 7 years: the Women's Health Initiative Dietary Modification Trial. JAMA 2006; 295(1):39–49.

19. Brehm BJ, Seeley RJ, et al. A randomized trial comparing a very low carbohydrate diet and a calorie-restricted low fat diet on body weight and cardiovascular risk factors in healthy women. J Clin Endocrinol Metab 2003; 88(4):1617–1623.

20. Seidell JC. Dietary fat and obesity: an epidemiologic perspective. Am J Clin Nutr 1998; 67(3 Suppl):546S–550S.

21. Kunesova M, Braunerova R, et al. The influence of n-3 polyunsaturated fatty acids and very low calorie diet during a short-term weight reducing regimen on weight loss and serum fatty acid composition in severely obese women. Physiol Res 2006; 55:63–72.

22. Willett WC. Is dietary fat a major determinant of body fat? Am J Clin Nutr 1998; 67(3 Suppl):556S–562S.

23. Peters JC. Dietary fat and body weight control. Lipids 2003; 38(2):123–127.

24. Dansinger ML, Gleason JA, et al. Comparison of the Atkins, Ornish, Weight Watchers, and Zone diets for weight loss and heart disease risk reduction: a randomized trial. JAMA 2005; 293(1):43–53.

25. McManus K, Antinoro L, Sacks F. A randomized controlled trial of a moderate-fat, low-energy diet compared with a low-fat, low-energy diet for weight loss in overweight adults. Int J Obes Relat Metab Disord 2001; 25(10):1503–1511.

26. Perez-Jimenez F. International conference on the healthy effect of virgin olive oil. Eur J Clin Invest 2005; 35(7):421–424.

27. Polychronopoulos E, Panagiotakos DB, Polystipioti A. Diet, lifestyle factors and hypercholesterolemia in elderly men and women from Cyprus. Lipids Health Dis 2005; 4:17.

28. Erlanson-Albertsson C. How palatable food disrupts appetite regulation. Basic Clin Pharmacol Toxicol 2005; 97(2):61–73.

29. Astrup A, Astrup A, et al. Low-fat diets and energy balance: how does the evidence stand in 2002? Proc Nutr Soc 2002; 61(2):299–309.

30. Brinkworth GD, Noakes M, et al. Long-term effects of a high-protein, low-carbohydrate diet on weight control and cardiovascular risk markers in obese hyperinsulinemic subjects. Int J Obes Relat Metab Disord 2004; 28(5):661–670.

31. Parker B, Noakes M, et al. Effect of a high-protein, high-monounsaturated fat weight loss diet on glycemic control and lipid levels in type 2 diabetes. Diabetes Care 2002; 25(3):425–430.

32. Pannowitz D. High-protein diets. J Comp Med 2005; 4:84–86.

33. Heini AF, Lara-Castro C, et al. Association of leptin and hunger-satiety ratings in obese women. Int J Obes Relat Metab Disord 1998; 22(11):1084–1087.

34. Romon M, Lebel P, et al. Leptin response to carbohydrate or fat meal and association with subsequent satiety and energy intake. Am J Physiol 1999; 277(5 Pt 1):E855–E861.

35. Howarth NC, Saltzman E, et al. Fermentable and nonfermentable fiber supplements did not alter hunger, satiety or body weight in a pilot study of men and women consuming self-selected diets. J Nutr 2003; 133(10):3141–3144.

36. Holt SH, Brand-Miller JC, Stitt PA. The effects of equal-energy portions of different breads on blood glucose levels, feelings of fullness and subsequent food intake. J Am Diet Assoc 2001; 101(7):767–773.

37. Ello-Martin JA, Ledikwe JH, Rolls BJ. The influence of food portion size and energy density on energy intake: implications for weight management. Am J Clin Nutr 2005; 82(1 Suppl):236S–241S.

38. Muzumdar RH, Ma X, et al. Central resistance to the inhibitory effects of leptin on stimulated insulin secretion with aging. Neurobiol Aging 2005 Aug 22; [Epub ahead of print].

39. Zemel MB, Richards J, et al. Dairy augmentation of total and central fat loss in obese subjects. Int J Obes Relat Metab Disord 2005; 29(4):391–397.

40. Heaney RP, Davies KM, et al. Calcium and weight: clinical studies. J Am Coll Nutr 2002; 21(2):152S–155S.

41. Riedt CS, Cifuentes M, et al. Overweight postmenopausal women lose bone with moderate weight reduction and 1 g/day calcium intake. J Bone Miner Res 2005; 20(3):455–463.

42. Parikh SJ, Yanovski JA. Calcium intake and adiposity. Am J Clin Nutr 2003; 77(2):281–287.

43. Saper RB, Eisenberg DM, Phillips RS. Common dietary supplements for weight loss. Am Fam Physician 2004; 70(9):1731–1738.

44. Bell SJ, Goodrick GK. A functional food product for the management of weight. Crit Rev Food Sci Nutr 2002; 42(2):163–178.

45. Pittler MH, Ernst E. Dietary supplements for body-weight reduction: a systematic review. Am J Clin Nutr 2004; 79(4):529–536.

46. Lenz TL, Hamilton WR. Supplemental products used for weight loss. J Am Pharm Assoc 2004; 44(1):59–67.

47. Lang A, Froelicher ES. Management of overweight and obesity in adults: behavioral intervention for long-term weight loss and maintenance. Eur J Cardiovasc Nurs 2006 Jan 5; [Epub ahead of print].

48. Position of the American Dietetic Association. Weight management. J Am Diet Assoc 2002; 102:1145–1155.

49. Rolls BJ, Ello-Martin JA, Tohill BC. What can intervention studies tell us about the relationship between fruit and vegetable consumption and weight management? Nutr Rev 2004; 62(1):1–17.

50. Ma Y, Bertone ER, et al. Association between eating patterns and obesity in a free-living US adult population. Am J Epidemiol 2003; 158(1):85–92.

51. Wyatt HR, Grunwald GK, et al. Long-term weight loss and breakfast in subjects in the National Weight Control Registry. Obes Res 2002; 10(2):78–82.

52. Di Francesco V, Zamboni M, et al. Relationships between leisure-time physical activity, obesity and disability in elderly men. Aging Clin Exp Res 2005; 17(3):201–206.

53. Mayo MJ, Grantham JR, Balasekaran G. Exercise-induced weight loss preferentially reduces abdominal fat. Med Sci Sports Exerc 2003; 35(2):207–213.

54. Bernstein MS, Costanza MC, Morabia A. Association of physical activity intensity levels with overweight and obesity in a population-based sample of adults. Prev Med 2004; 38(1):94–104.

55. Morabia A, Costanza MC. Does walking 15 minutes per day keep the obesity epidemic away? Simulation of the efficacy of a populationwide campaign. Am J Public Health 2004; 94(3):437–440.

56. Stevens J, Cai J, et al. Fitness and fatness as predictors of mortality from all causes and from cardiovascular disease in men and women in the lipid research clinics study. Am J Epidemiol 2002; 156(9):832–841.

57. Klein S, Sheard NF, et al. Weight management through lifestyle modification for the prevention and management of type 2 diabetes: rationale and strategies. A statement of the American Diabetes Association, the North American Association for the Study of Obesity, and the American Society for Clinical Nutrition. Am J Clin Nutr 2004; 80(2):257–263.

58. Howard BV, Ruotolo G, Robbins DC. Obesity and dyslipidemia. Endocrinol Metab Clin North Am 2003; 32(4):855–867.

59. De Pergola G, Pannacciulli N. Coagulation and fibrinolysis abnormalities in obesity. J Endocrinol Invest 2002; 25(10):899–904.

60. Heini AF, Weinsier RL. Divergent trends in obesity and fat intake patterns: the American paradox. Am J Med 1997; 102:259–264.

61. Hayes L, Pearce MS, Unwin NC. Lifecourse predictors of normal metabolic parameters in overweight and obese adults. Int J Obes (Lond) 2006 Jan 17; [Epub ahead of print].

62. Joyal SV. A perspective on the current strategies for the treatment of obesity. Curr Drug Targets CNS Neurol Disord 2004; 3(5):341–356.

63. Ioannides-Demos LL, Proietto J, McNeil JJ. Pharmacotherapy for obesity. Drugs 2005; 65(10):1391–1418.

64. Avenell A, Broom J, et al. Systematic review of the long-term effects and economic consequences of treatments for obesity and implications for health improvement. Health Technol Assess 2004; 8(21):iii–iv, 1–182.

65. Ozcelik O, Ozkan Y, et al. Exercise training as an adjunct to orlistat therapy reduces oxidative stress in obese subjects. Tohoku J Exp Med 2005; 206(4):313–318.

66. Teixeira PJ, Going SB, et al. A review of psychosocial pre-treatment predictors of weight control. Obes Rev 2005; 6(1):43–65.

67. Krummel DA, Semmens E, et al. Stages of change for weight management in postpartum women. J Am Diet Assoc 2004; 104(7):1102–1108.

68. Reynolds LR, Anderson JW. Practical office strategies for weight management of the obese diabetic individual. Endocr Pract 2004; 10(2):153–159.

69. Shaw K, O'Rourke P, et al. Psychological interventions for overweight or obesity. Cochrane Database Syst Rev 2005 Apr 18; (2):CD003818.

70. Groessl EJ, Kaplan RM, et al. Body mass index and quality of well-being in a community of older adults. Am J Prev Med 2004; 26(2):126–129.

71. Foster GD, Wadden TA, et al. A. Primary care physicians' attitudes about obesity and its treatment. Obes Res 2003; 11(10):1168–1177.

72. Patterson RE, Frank LL, et al. A comprehensive examination of health conditions associated with obesity in older adults. Am J Prev Med 2004; 27(5):385–390

73. Grabowski DC, Ellis JE. High body mass index does not predict mortality in older people: analysis of the Longitudinal Study of Aging. J Am Geriatr Soc 2001; 49(7):968–979.

74. Kuo HK, Jones RN, et al. Cognitive function in normal-weight, overweight, and obese older adults: an analysis of the advanced cognitive training for independent and vital elderly cohort. J Am Geriatr Soc 2006; 54(1):97–103.

75. Blaum CS, Xue QL, et al. The association between obesity and the frailty syndrome in older women: the Women's Health and Aging Studies. J Am Geriatr Soc 2005; 53(6):927–934.

76. Field AE, Manson JE, et al. Association of weight change, weight control practices, and weight cycling among women in the Nurses' Health Study II. Int J Obes Relat Metab Disord 2004; 28(9):1134–1142.

77. Diaz VA, Mainous AG 3rd, Everett CJ. The association between weight fluctuation and mortality: results from a population-based cohort study. J Community Health 2005; 30(3):153–165.

78. Shade ED, Ulrich CM, et al. Frequent intentional weight loss is associated with lower natural killer cell cytotoxicity in postmenopausal women: possible long-term immune effects. J Am Diet Assoc 2004; 104(6):903–912.

79. Newman AB, Yanez D, et al. Cardiovascular Study Research Group. Weight change in old age and its association with mortality. J Am Geriatr Soc 2001; 49(10):1309–1318.

PATIENT HANDOUT 12.1 – WEIGHT MANAGEMENT

You can formulate your own weight management program by following a few simple steps.

Step 1: Determining target weight. See Patient Handout 12.2.
Step 2: Determining energy needs. See Patient Handout 12.3.
Step 3: Select and implement a combination of dietary and exercise options. See Patient Handout 12.4.

A warning: If you are overweight it is less of a health risk to maintain a stable weight than to do yo-yo dieting, i.e. repeatedly lose and regain weight.

PATIENT HANDOUT 12.2 – DETERMINING IDEAL WEIGHT

Step 1—Am I overweight?

Determine if you have a weight problem by calculating your body mass index (BMI).

BMI = weight (kg)/height (m)^2
Overweight BMI = 25 – 30
Obese BMI = >30

For example: Sally is a 45-year-old medium framed female, weight 70 kg, height 165 cm. BMI = 70/1.65 × 1.65 = 25.7
Sally is overweight.

- If your BMI is over 25 you need to lose weight.
- Your health risk increases the more your BMI exceeds 25.

I AM ☐ OBESE ☐ OVERWEIGHT ☐ IDEAL WEIGHT

Step 2—What is my health risk?

See Chapter 3 handouts at *www.jamisonhealth.com*.

For more information on increased risk relative to overweight and obesity in persons over 50 years of age refer to: Patterson RE, Frank LL, Kristal AR, White E. *A comprehensive examination of health conditions associated with obesity in older adults.* Am J Prev Med 2004 Dec; 27(5):385–390.

I AM AT INCREASED RISK OF: (please insert)

....
....
....

Step 3—What is my ideal body weight?

Depending on body type, ideal body weight ranges from a BMI of 20 for those with small bones up to 25 for big boned, muscular individuals.

To determine your ideal weight:
1. Evaluate your body frame by encircling your wrist using your middle finger and thumb. If the thumb and finger:
   - overlap you have a small body frame and your BMI should be just over 20
   - meet you have a medium body frame and your BMI should be close to 22.5
   - fail to meet you have a large body frame and your BMI should be just under 25.
2. Calculate your ideal i.e. target body weight by inserting your height and ideal BMI into the following formula: Ideal weight (kg) = ideal BMI × height (m)^2.
3. Ascertain your desired weight loss using the following formula: Current weight – target/ideal weight = desired weight loss (kg).
   Sally's ideal weight (kg) = 22.5 × 2.72 = 61.2 kg. Sally needs to lose:
   70 – 61.2 = 8.8 kg.

MY IDEAL WEIGHT IS:.. kg

PATIENT HANDOUT 12.3 – DETERMINING ENERGY NEEDS

What is my ideal energy intake, i.e. how much food measured as calories may I eat? There are two easy methods for calculating your required energy intake.

A quick estimation

For weight maintenance, take in 138 kJ (33 kcal) per kilogram of desired body weight.
To lose weight, take in 92 kJ per kilogram of desired body weight.
To reach her ideal weight, Sally is permitted 61.2 × 92 = 5630 kJ/day.
To maintain her ideal weight Sally is permitted 61.2 × 138 = 8445 kJ/day.

The adjusted calculation

Determine your basal energy requirement (BER):

- Basal energy requirement (BER) (kilojoules) = 100 × ideal body weight for females.
- Basal energy requirement (BER) (kilojoules) = 110 × ideal body weight for males.

Example: Sally's BER is 100 × 61.2 = 6120 kJ.

Adjust the basal energy requirement for:

- age
  −45 years old—BER × 1.0
  −65 years old—BER × 0.8
- body frame
  −small–boned persons—BER reduced by 10%
  −medium frame—BER
  −large–boned individual—BER increased 10%
- activity level
  −strenuous—BER +100%
  −moderate—BER +50%
  −sedentary—BER +30%

For example, Sally is 45 years old, with a medium frame and leads a sedentary lifestyle. To maintain her ideal body weight, Sally's adjusted BER = (6120 × 1 × 1) + (6120 × 0.3) = 6120 + 1836 = 7956 kJ. (Note this is slightly lower than that permitted with the other method!) If she undertakes a moderate exercise lifestyle, she can increase her basal energy requirement by 50%, i.e. her

permitted intake will be 9180 kJ (BER = (6120 × 1 × 1) + (6120 × 0.5) = 6120 + 3060 = 9180.

When Sally reaches the age of 65, to maintain her ideal weight she will need to have reduced her energy intake to 4896 kJ (BER × 0.8 = 6120 × 0.8 = 4896 kJ). This can be increased depending on her level of activity.

TO MAINTAIN MY IDEAL BODY WEIGHT I REQUIRE .... kJ daily

How much weight should I aim to lose each week?

- The recommended rate of weight loss is 0.5–1.0 kg per week.
- This requires a daily reduction of up to 4600 kJ (1100 kcal).

To lose weight, in theory Sally could decrease her energy intake by up to 4600 kJ each day.
To get adequate nourishment, however, she always needs to eat a minimum of 2750 kJ daily.
For active weight loss, Sally can eat around 5630 kJ/day. In order to obtain adequate nourishment Sally should not reduce her energy intake below 2750 kJ. Sally would lose weight if she ate less than the permitted 5630 kJ daily but successful weight loss requires a change of lifestyle and Sally may be able to retain her weight loss if she acquires new eating and exercise habits while gradually losing weight. Once Sally has reached her ideal weight she can increase her energy intake to at least 7956 kJ daily (depending on the calculation used).

TO REACH MY IDEAL BODY WEIGHT I AM PERMITTED .... kJ daily

How much can I eat to lose this weight?

- A minimum of 2500 kJ (600 kcal) of nutritious food is required daily.
- The energy equivalent of 1 calorie is 4.186 kilojoules.

You have reached your ideal weight loss target when your waist circumference is 94 cm (males) or 80 cm (females) or less!

PATIENT HANDOUT 12.4 – OPTIONS FOR WEIGHT LOSS

How can I lose weight?

By reducing your energy intake (food) to the daily energy intake permitted, and by increasing your energy expenditure (exercise) you will lose weight.

What should I eat?

- Eat low energy, nutrient dense foods: see *www.jamisonhealth.com* Handouts for Chapter 23.
- Find out about portion size: see *www.health.gov/dietaryguidelines/dga2005/ document/html/appendixA.htm*
- For details about the energy and nutrient content of various foods refer to *http://www.nal.usda.gov/fnic/foodcomp/search/* and/or *http://nat.crgq.com/mainnat.html.*

How much should I exercise?

To use up 100 kcals you need to walk slowly for 60 minutes or briskly for 30 minutes. The Handouts for Chapter 23 at *www.jamisonhealth.com* provide information on the energy consumed by various activities.

High intensity exercise such as brisk walking, climbing stairs or running suppresses appetite immediately after the exercise, increases basal metabolism rate and aids weight loss. Moderate intensity activities such as household chores improve cardiovascular health. Exercise helps to retain lean body mass which protects against regaining lost weight, i.e. as occurs with yo-yo dieting.

Every weight loss program should include exercise!

Internet resources

Dietary guidelines for Americans can be viewed at: *www.health.gov/dietaryguidelines/dga2005/document/.*

Consult the food pyramid to select a healthy diet and modify energy intake and exercise to achieve weight loss at: *http://www.mypyramid.gov/.*

Chapter 13

Osteoarthritis

A 59-year-old man presents with knee pain. Pain is worst at the end of the day, particularly on those days he is required to walk a lot. He also reports joint stiffness which improves with movement but recurs after rest. On examination the knee appears normal. Ultrasound detects early cartilage loss.

- Which risk factors may be modified to impede progression of the disease?
- Can cartilage be restored or further destruction limited?
- Do analgesic anti-inflammatories halt or hasten progression of pathology?
- What causes functional limitation and how may it be minimized?

INTRODUCTION

Osteoarthritis leads to pain and loss of function, primarily in the knees and hips. It affects 9.6% of men and 18% of women over 60 years of age.[1]

Increased life expectancy in an aging population is predicted to make osteoarthritis the fourth leading cause of disability in developed nations by the year 2020. In fact, knee osteoarthritis is already regarded as the single greatest cause of chronic disability among community dwelling older adults.

Age is the most powerful risk factor for osteoarthritis in the United States—68% of individuals over 55 years are estimated to have radiographic evidence of osteoarthritis and by 2020 it is predicted 59.4 million persons in the US will be sufferers.[2] About 1 in 6 Americans have arthritis, and most are older than 45 years.

Osteoarthritis or degenerative joint disease represents joint failure. It represents a net loss of articular cartilage. The earliest change is a relative decrease in the concentration of mucopolysaccharide and chondroitin sulphate in the cartilage matrix. The ability of the matrix to hydrostatically dissipate biomechanical stresses is impaired and collagen fibres are subjected to excessive flexural and torsional stresses leading to rupture and the lesions characteristic of osteoarthritis.[3] The natural history of this disease encompasses genetic, mechanical, inflammatory and metabolic considerations.

DISEASE PATHOGENESIS

For many decades the mechanical hypothesis held sway with respect to the development of osteoarthritis. Today experts believe osteoarthritis is the result of at least two distinct processes.

Biomechanical distortions

Cartilage is an avascular tissue. Chondrocytes depend on diffusion for nutrition and cyclic loading induced by everyday activities produces deformations and pressure gradients and aids fluid flow. While moderate to strenuous joint loading appears to have no adverse effects and may promote the health of normally congruent joints, a single traumatic event or repetitive high impact events may lead to joint degeneration. Osteoarthritis is attributed to a disproportion between the load applied to the articular cartilage and the quality of the cartilaginous matrix.

Obese persons are at increased risk. In fact, osteoarthritis of the knee has been shown to increase fourfold in men with a current BMI of 23–25 compared to men with BMI of less than 23.[4] In women the increase is 1.6 times.[4] Whereas obesity increases overall loading of the knee, limb malalignment concentrates that loading on a focal area, predisposing cartilage at that site to damage. In fact, BMI only influences the progression of osteoarthritis in knees with moderate malalignment (2–7 degrees).[5] The pathogenesis of osteoarthritis in knees with neutral (0–2 degrees) or severe malalignment (> or =7 degrees) is unaffected by weight. Joint laxity, observed to be related to joint space narrowing and malalignment, further corroborates the importance of biomechanical factors in degeneration of the knee joint.[6]

The progression of disease and/or degree of disability in knee osteo-arthritis, in addition to being provoked by biomechanical factors such as passive knee laxity, knee alignment, quadriceps inhibition or activation failure and obesity, is also influenced by psychological concerns such as fear of physical activity and self efficacy.[7]

Inflammatory changes

The structural changes in knee osteoarthritis, previously believed to result from non-inflammatory deterioration of the articular cartilage due to biome-chanical distortion, are now also recognized to result from interactive bio-chemical processes in cartilage, synovial membrane and subchondral bone.[8]

Osteoarthritis is now considered a polygenic disease and genes encoding for cytokines have been linked to joint susceptibility.[8,9] Cytokines, such as interleukin-1 (IL-1) and tumour necrosis factor, and nitric oxide and metallo-proteases all promote inflammation and contribute to the clinical mani-festations of this disease.[8] IL-1 is a potent cartilage catabolic factor. Nitric oxide can induce chondrocyte death, reduce anabolism of cartilage by inhibiting the synthesis of collagen and proteoglycan, increase activity of cyclo-oxygenase-2 and consequently prostaglandin production, as well as stimulate the synthesis and activities of metalloproteases. Gelatinase, a metalloenzyme, contributes to cartilage degradation.

CLINICAL PRESENTATION

Assessment of patients with osteoarthritis includes history and exami-nation, self-reports and performance assessments, ultrasound and X-ray evaluations. Patients experience mild early morning stiffness and stiffness following periods of rest. They complain of pain that worsens with pro-longed joint use and is relieved by rest. The more marked the inflammatory response, the greater the likelihood pain is present at rest and persists at night. Pain in the osteoarthritic knee may result from several causes includ-ing loss of articular cartilage, microfractures or mechanical compression of either the medial or lateral knee compartment. Other joints frequently involved are the thumb, hips, lumbar and cervical spine.

Self-reports and performance measures assess distinct aspects of mobility in knee osteoarthritis.[10] Self-reported measures largely relate to impairment and pain. Performance measurements provide information on perceived self-efficacy for mobility i.e. the level of confidence for completing a specific task. Perceived self-efficacy, rather than reflecting a skill, represents the individual's belief about their ability. One exercise study reported self-efficacy was the most influential variable among osteoarthritic patients, determining commitment to a plan for exercise.[11] Self-efficacy accounted for 53% of the variance in that study! Consequently, both self-reports and performance measures provide useful information when formulating suitable intervention.

The findings on joint examination depend on the stage of the disease. Over time, joint examination may detect local tenderness, soft tissue swelling, joint crepitus, bony swelling and restricted mobility. Ultrasound detects cartilage loss early,[12] while radiology shows more advanced osteoarthritic joints to have irregular loss of cartilage, sclerosis of subchondral bone, subchondral cysts, marginal osteophytes and variable degrees of synovial inflammation.

INTERVENTION

Pain and impaired function are major complaints resulting in impaired mobility, a major determinant of disability. Mobility is influenced by a wide variety of pathophysiological and personal factors. Pathophysiological changes interrupt normal physiological processes or structures, resulting in impairment due to pain, stiffness and functional limitation, i.e. an inability to perform an action consistent with normal function. Muscle strength, an important biomechanical factor, appears to be related to all mobility outcome measures. In knee osteoarthritis quadriceps strength predicts function. Pain, along with quadriceps weakness, limits the range of motion of the knee joint. On the other hand, restricted knee flexion is a strong risk factor for disability, limiting daily activities such as walking, climbing stairs, getting up and sitting down in a chair.

Improving joint stability, limiting cartilage loss and pain management would seem to be important therapeutic goals. While drug intervention focuses primarily on relieving pain, exercise, joint protection and stress reduction also provide symptom relief with few side effects. The latter are particularly important considerations in older adults in whom the risk of side effects and interactions between medications is of concern.[13]

Limiting cartilage loss/damage

Limiting further joint damage focuses on avoiding trauma, minimizing any malalignment and staying mobile while augmenting cartilage and connective tissue repair. As articular joints are avascular, movement improves nutrient diffusion and appropriate weight bearing exercise is recommended. The goal of exercise is to maintain range of motion and muscle strength.[14] In the case of knee osteoarthritis, quadriceps strengthening exercises reduce instability, while swimming, walking or other low impact aerobic exercise provide an additional psychological benefit, decreasing anxiety and depression. Low impact exercise does not accelerate damage to osteoarthritis joints.[15] Risk can further be reduced by walking rather than jogging, wearing appropriate soft-soled shoes or inserting foam rubber inner soles and avoiding obesity.

Obese persons, especially those who perform more than 3 hours of heavy physical activity daily, are at increased risk of knee osteoarthritis.[16] Risk may be minimized by using specifically tailored exercise regimes coupled with a weight loss program. Although it has yet to be demonstrated that weight loss improves symptoms in persons with knee osteoarthritis, men with a BMI of over 25, who lose 5 kg (2 BMI units) reduce their likelihood of developing the condition by 25%.[17] Furthermore, each pound of weight lost in obese and overweight persons results in a fourfold reduction in the load exerted on the knee per step during daily activities.[18]

While appropriate exercise may help to control weight and enhance cartilage perfusion, only dietary supplementation may provide the nutrients necessary for healthy cartilage. Recent reports suggest there is strong evidence that glucosamine sulphate, in doses of 1500 mg/day, is effective for treating mild to moderate osteoarthritis of the knee and good evidence it helps osteoarthritis elsewhere.[19,20] Two 3-year, randomized, placebo-controlled, prospective independent studies showed no joint space narrowing in postmenopausal woman on glucosamine sulphate, whereas participants in the placebo group experienced a narrowing of 0.33 mm.[21] Glucosamine is a substrate and stimulant for synthesis of proteoglycans, and may inhibit cartilage degradation. Although considered safe, glucosamine is contraindicated in patients with a hypersensitivity to glucosamine sulphate. Persons with shellfish allergy should inquire about the source of the glucosamine sulphate and as the oral formulation contains aspartame it should be avoided by patients with phenylketonuria. Persons on anticoagulants require blood coagulation monitoring. Despite some concerns, chondroitin does not appear to alter glucose metabolism significantly in patients with type-2 diabetes.[22] Although the long term benefits of glucosamine have been questioned, as has its ability to aid cartilage regeneration, glucosamine is a popular natural remedy used alone or in conjunction with other nutriceuticals. Oral administration of two 250 mg glucosamine tablets or capsules is recommended three times daily, preferably with meals. Treatment should be continued for at least 6 weeks.

Chondroitin sulphate is often used in conjunction with glucosamine. In general, the effect size of this combination seems to be of slightly lower magnitude than that seen for NSAIDs, and although it takes 4–6 weeks before symptomatic improvement, benefit is maintained after stopping the treatment for periods of 4–8 weeks.[23] Chondroitin sulphate is postulated to have anti-inflammatory activity and a chondroprotective action by modifying the structure of cartilage.[24] Although intermittent administration at doses of 800 mg/day for 3 months twice annually may modify symptoms in patients with osteoarthritis,[25] there are currently insufficient data from clinical trials to support the use of chondroitin sulphate in symptomatic treatment of osteoarthritis.[26]

The concentration of sulphur in arthritic cartilage is lower than that in healthy cartilage. Another combination therapy for osteoarthritis that may achieve faster and more complete pain relief than when either drug is taken alone is glucosamine sulphate and methyl sulphonyl methane (MSM). MSM is the isoxidised form of dimethyl sulphoxide. MSM has been shown to benefit arthritis suffers. The toxicity of MSM is reputed to be similar to that of water.[27]

Another nutriceutical which may protect cartilage is S-adenosylmethionine (SAMe). SAMe functions as a methyl donor and up-regulates the proteoglycan synthesis of chondrocytes.[28] In vitro studies have shown that SAMe stimulates the synthesis of proteoglycans by human articular chondrocytes. IL–1, when it targets synovial cells, liberates prostaglandin E2, proteases, collagenases and glycosidases and decreases SAMe levels in chondrocytes. Supplementation with SAMe appears to reverse this situation. Meta-analysis has confirmed that SAMe appears to be as effective as NSAIDs in reducing pain and improving functional limitation in osteoarthritic patients—without the adverse effects often associated with NSAID therapies;[29] nonetheless, in view of the 'uncertain risk profile' of SAMe, there is some hesitation in definitively recommending this intervention.[30]

Despite all providing some symptomatic relief, the nutriceutical that holds the greatest promise to repair and restore cartilage is glucosamine sulphate.

Managing pain

Compared to nutraceuticals, pharmaceuticals achieve symptomatic relief with greater predictability and efficacy. Nonetheless, the relative role of acetaminophen (paracetamol or Tylenol) and non-steroidal anti-inflammatory drugs (NSAIDs) as first line pharmacological therapy in osteoarthritis is disputed.[31]

In 2000, American and European authorities recommended acetaminophen as first line oral therapy for patients with mild to moderate lower limb pain due to osteoarthritis.[32] This recommendation was made in view of acetaminophen's greater safety in doses of 1.0 g six times per day. Unfortunately, acetaminophen at high dose (>2 g/day) may carry a similar risk to NSAIDs for serious upper gastrointestinal problems. Although acetaminophen and NSAIDs have a similar impact on function, NSAIDs more effectively relieve moderate to severe levels of pain.[31] However, NSAIDs, particularly aspirin, may impair chondrocyte production of proteoglycan and inhibit bone repair. Certainly subjects receiving diclofenac for over 6 months had a 2.4-fold increased risk of progression of hip and a 3.2-fold increased risk of knee osteoarthritis on X-ray.[32] Whether this reflected NSAID-induced accelerated progression of hip and knee osteoarthritis or resulted from excessive mechanical loading permitted by effective pain relief is uncertain. Despite such concerns, in the presence of significant synovitis, NSAIDs may yet have a protective role by inhibiting synovial production of interleukin-1. Interleukin-1 induces the synthesis and release of matrix degrading proteinases from chondrocytes.

NSAIDs warrant consideration in patients who have severe pain and/or signs of inflammation. Newer cyclo-oxygenase (COX)-2 specific inhibitors (coxibs) appear to carry less risk for serious gastrointestinal problems than older dual acting NSAIDs.[33] They are of particular interest for those patients with rest and/or nocturnal pain, warm, tender joints and joint effusion, who are at increased risk for serious upper gastrointestinal adverse events or contemplating surgery. However, while COX-2 specific inhibitors do not affect platelet aggregation or bleeding time, their renal and cardiovascular toxicity remains a potential problem. Two coxibs, Vioxx and Celebrex, were removed from the market in 2004 due to their long term toxicity.

Compared to NSAIDs, glucosamine is considerably less toxic, more protective of cartilage and potentially provides as effective symptom relief, albeit slower in onset.[34] In addition to oral preparations, glucosamine is available as a topical cream containing glucosamine sulphate, chondroitin sulphate and camphor. A randomized, placebo-controlled trial found this topical preparation effectively relieved knee pain in patients with osteoarthritis within 4 weeks of starting treatment.[35]

Another effective topical remedy is capsaicin, the most pungent ingredient in red peppers. Capsaicin acts selectively on a subpopulation of primary sensory neurons that generate pain sensations and participate in neurogenic inflammation.[36] Topically applied capsaicin induces the release of substance P, a neurotransmitter, from sensory C–fibres. In addition, there is a specific blockade of transport and de novo synthesis of substance P. On first exposure, capsaicin has an intense orthodromic i.e. pain sensation and antidromic i.e. local inflammatory effect. With repeated exposure, the neurons become insensitive to all further stimulation, including that from capsaicin. The desensitizing effect is fully reversible. Randomized studies suggest a role for capsaicin cream in managing patients with osteoarthritis.[37]

Animal studies suggest that New Zealand green-lipped mussel (Lyprinol) has significant anti-inflammatory activity.[38] A multicentre trial of patients with symptomatic osteoarthritis of the knee and hip concluded that patients who received Lyprinol at a dose of two capsules twice a day achieved improved joint function and experienced pain relief after 4 weeks of treatment.[39] After 8 weeks of treatment, even more substantial improvements were recorded.

Much of the anti-inflammatory activity of Lyprinol is associated with omega-3 fatty acids and natural antioxidants e.g. carotenoids. Omega-3 polyunsaturated fatty acid supplementation, unlike other fatty acid supplements, decreases both degradative and inflammatory aspects of chondrocyte metabolism in a dose-dependent manner.[40] Omega-3 fatty acids specifically reduce endogenous and IL-1-induced release of proteoglycan metabolites from articular cartilage explants and abolish endogenous aggrecanase and collagenase proteolytic activity.

Another nutriceutical worthy of comment is niacinamide. A placebo-controlled randomized trial using 3 g niacinamide daily in 6 doses of 500 mg for 12 weeks achieved improved joint flexibility, reduced inflammation, and allowed for reduction in standard anti-inflammatory medications when compared to placebo.[41] It has been hypothesized that niacinamide, by suppressing cytokine-mediated induction of nitric oxide synthase, may blunt the impact of IL-1 in osteoarthritis.[42]

Bromelain, an enzyme with anti-inflammatory and analgesic properties when used alone, has also been reported to ameliorate knee pain of less than 3 months duration in a dose-dependent fashion.[43] When used in combination with trypsin and rutosid in a 6 week randomized, double-blind, parallel group trial, the enzyme-rutosid combination afforded levels of safety, pain relief and functional improvement to patients with knee osteoarthritis similar to diclofenac.[44]

More recently, a review of viscosupplementation in the treatment of knee osteoarthritis provides further encouragement. The reviewers concluded hyaluronan and hylan derivatives appear to have comparable efficacy to NSAIDs and provide longer lasting benefit than intra-articular corticosteroids.[45] Few adverse events were reported but product variability made prognosis difficult. The reviewers felt viscosupplementation was an effective treatment for knee osteoarthritis, benefiting pain, function and patient global assessment at different post injection periods but especially at the 5th to 13th week. Nutriceuticals are not the only alternative therapies worth considering in the management of symptomatic osteoarthritis. Clinical trials suggest acupuncture is worthy of further investigation.[46,47]

Improving joint stability

While total hip and total knee replacement surgery are both the most effective treatment and the most cost effective interventions for the management of lower limb osteoarthritis, exercise and strength training for knee osteoarthritis are also highly cost effective.[48] Therapeutic exercise may prevent accelerated degeneration resulting from disuse, without causing further degeneration and pain as a consequence of joint deformity or incongruence.[9] A systematic review concluded there was evidence that exercise therapy benefited both osteoarthritis of the hip and the knee.[49,50] In the case of knee osteoarthritis, high and low intensity aerobic exercise appear to be equally effective in improving a patient's functional status, gait, pain and aerobic capacity;[51] aerobic walking and home based quadriceps strengthening exercise reduce pain and disability;[52] and land-based therapeutic exercise reduces knee pain and improves physical function.[53] Unfortunately, there are insufficient data to provide useful guidelines on the optimal amount or type of exercise required and it remains unclear whether exercise for those with osteoarthritis should be weight-bearing or non-weight-bearing.[12]

Nonetheless, the ratio of quadriceps to hamstring muscle strength is clearly important for knee stability, hence appropriate muscle strengthening exercises are beneficial. Isotonic or isometric exercise appear most effective for initial strengthening in patients with exercise knee pain, followed later by isokinetic exercise for improving joint stability and walking endurance.[54] Although isokinetic strengthening exercise most effectively diminishes disability, improves muscular strength and ambulation in patients with knee osteoarthritis, it does induce knee pain and compliance is problematic. Despite conflict surrounding the efficacy of using low level laser,[55] use of ultrasound, particularly pulsed ultrasound, does improve exercise compliance.[9] Specifically designed exercise programs have been shown to increase joint mobility and strength and enhance sports performance.

When formulating a treatment strategy for an individual with 'early' osteoarthritis, both the risk of toxicity from prolonged exposure to pharmaceuticals and the possibility of retarding the rate of disease progression require consideration. In addition to sociobehavioural interventions such as weight optimization and exercise, orthotics may prove helpful. Orthotics can be used to minimize malalignment.[56] A review concluded braces and orthoses provided some, albeit limited benefit.[57] A fitted knee brace may help knee osteoarthritis, as may a foot lift ease hip osteoarthritis. The usefulness of physical aids is determined by the needs of individual cases.[58] Certainly, in some patients, bracing significantly reduces pain, increases function and reduces excessive loading to the damaged compartment.[59] Although changes in angulation are relatively minimal, braces have been shown to load share and thus reduce the stresses in the degenerated medial compartment of the knee. Other diverse non-invasive methods have positive reports. Successful interventions range from occupational therapy, which plays a central role in the management of hip osteoarthritis with functional limitations,[60] to guided imagery with progressive muscle relaxation.[61]

Despite attempts to provide evidence-based recommendations,[62] there is as yet no single definitive treatment for osteoarthritis. Nonetheless, 10 key recommendations have been made for the treatment of hip osteoarthritis.[63] This study group commented on 21 interventions including paracetamol, NSAIDs, symptomatic slow acting disease modifying drugs, opioids, intra-articular steroids, non-pharmacological treatment, total hip replacement and osteotomy.

IN CONCLUSION

Osteoarthritis is a debilitating condition characterized by chronic pain. As both the course of the disease and the patient's requirements change over time, periodic review and readjustment of therapy rather than the rigid continuation of a single treatment is advisable.[64] Until such time as gene therapy is able to reverse the disease process or some injectable compound is able to mimic healthy synovial fluid or surgical intervention,[65] education to prevent joint damage would seem indispensable.

CLINICAL CHALLENGE

A 78-year-old woman presents with pain in the buttocks, thighs and calves. The pain is precipitated by walking and prolonged standing and is relieved by resting for 30 or more minutes. She has been troubled by back and neck pain for many years. She has a 20 year history of osteoarthritis.

On examination, spinal movement is restricted, her thighs and calves are not tender. Pedal pulses are present. Her erythrocyte sedimentation rate (ESR) is raised.

Questions arising

- What is the working diagnosis?
- How may the development of her symptoms be explained?

Clinical considerations

Neurogenic claudication is present in a patient with spinal osteoarthritis.

Pressure on the spinal cord due to lumbar spinal stenosis may be encountered in persons with osteoarthritis. Hypertrophy of the ligamentum flavum, apophyseal joints and vertebral body narrows the spinal canal and pressure on the spinal cord or cauda equina causes discomfort or weakness in the calf, thigh and buttock.

A 68-year-old man presents with groin pain. On examination his hernial orifices are intact and he has no local swelling. You notice the patient has an antalgic gait. On closer questioning he reports that the pain in his groin is worst on moving.

He also reports that for some years he has had morning stiffness and backache. His mobility improves after he has been up for half an hour or so but the stiffness recurs after he has been sitting for a while.

His vital signs are normal and his BMI is 29.

Questions arising

- What is his working diagnosis?
- How should the patient be counselled?

Clinical considerations

A working diagnosis of hip osteoarthritis can be confirmed on finding loss of joint space on X-ray. Spinal X-ray may also show osteophytes and narrowed disc spaces in the lumbar region.

In the interim, the patient should be advised to lose weight, avoid prolonged standing, walk regularly, consider analgesics/anti-inflammatories (paracetamol or COX-2 NSAIDs) and glucosamine sulphate. Capsaicin cream with glucosamine may also provide some short term relief. Hip replacement provides the only long term solution.

PRACTICE GEMS

- Both self-reports and performance measures should be included in assessment of osteoarthritis—the former reflects pain, knee strength, and depression, and the latter self-efficacy.
- Weight loss reduces the risk of lower limb osteoarthritis, but only if malalignment is present.
- Walking enhances cartilage nutrition and helps retain muscle strength—do at least 30 minutes of moderate intensity exercise on most days of the week.
- Muscle weakness contributes to mechanical pathology of the knee joint.

- Specific knee exercises that restore an appropriate balance between quadriceps and hamstring muscles can increase joint stability.
- The most effective treatment of lower limb osteoarthritis is surgical replacement of the affected joint.
- Chondroitin sulphate may preserve cartilage.
- Paracetamol and COX-2 NSAIDs are the pharmaceuticals of choice for this condition.
- Viscosupplementation may have efficacy comparable to NSAIDs and provide longer term benefits than intra-articular steroids.

References

1. Woolf AD, Pfleger B. Burden of major musculoskeletal conditions. Bull World Health Organ 2003; 81(9):646–656. Epub 2003 Nov 14.
2. Elders MJ. The increasing impact of arthritis on public health. J Rheumatol Suppl 2000; 60:6–8.
3. Huang MH, Lin YS, et al. Use of ultrasound to increase effectiveness of isokinetic exercise for knee osteoarthritis. Arch Phys Med Rehabil 2005; 86(8):1545–1551.
4. Holmberg S, Thelin A, Thelin N. Knee osteoarthritis and body mass index: a population-based case-control study. Scand J Rheumatol 2005; 34(1):59–64.
5. Felson DT, Goggins J, et al. The effect of body weight on progression of knee osteoarthritis is dependent on alignment. Arthritis Rheum 2004; 50(12):3904–3909.
6. van der Esch M, Steultjens M, et al. Structural joint changes, malalignment, and laxity in osteoarthritis of the knee. Scand J Rheumatol 2005; 34(4):298–301.
7. Fitzgerald GK. Therapeutic exercise for knee osteoarthritis: considering factors that may influence outcome. Eura Medicophys 2005; 41(2):163–171.
8. Pelletier JP. Rationale for the use of structure-modifying drugs and agents in the treatment of osteoarthritis. Osteoarthritis Cartilage 2004; 12 Suppl A:S63–S68.
9. Pola E, Papaleo P, et al. Interleukin-6 gene polymorphism and risk of osteoarthritis of the hip: a case-control study. Osteoarthritis Cartilage 2005 Sep 28; [Epub ahead of print].
10. Maly MR, Costigan PA, Olney SJ. Determinants of self-report outcome measures in people with knee osteoarthritis. Arch Phys Med Rehabil 2006; 87(1):96–104.
11. Shin YH, Hur HK, et al. Exercise self-efficacy, exercise benefits and barriers, and commitment to a plan for exercise among Korean women with osteoporosis and osteoarthritis. Int J Nurs Stud 2006; 43(1):3–10.
12. Amin S, Lavalley MP, et al. The relationship between cartilage loss on magnetic resonance imaging and radiographic progression in men and women with knee osteoarthritis. Arthritis Rheum 2005; 52(10):3152–3159.
13. Burks K. Osteoarthritis in older adults: current treatments. J Gerontol Nurs 2005; 31(5):11–19; quiz 59–60.
14. Manek NJ, Lane NE. Osteoarthritis: current concepts in diagnosis and management. Am Fam Physician 2000; 61(6):1795–1804.
15. Rogers LQ, Macera CA, et al. The association between joint stress from physical activity and self-reported osteoarthritis: an analysis of the Cooper Clinic data. Osteoarthritis Cartilage 2002; 10(8):617–622.
16. McAlindon TE, Wilson PW, et al. Level of physical activity and the risk of radiographic and symptomatic knee osteoarthritis in the elderly: the Framingham study. Am J Med 1999; 106(2):151–157.
17. Meisler JG, St Jeor S. Foreward. Am J Clin Nutr 1996; 63(suppl): 409S–411S.
18. Messier SP, Gutekunst DJ, et al. Weight loss reduces knee-joint loads in overweight and obese older adults with knee osteoarthritis. Arthritis Rheum 2005; 52(7):2026–2032.
19. Ulbricht C, Basch E, et al. An evidence based systemic review of glucosamine. J Comp Med & Integrative Med 2005; 2(1):1. Online. Available: http://www.bepress.com/jcim/vol2/iss1/1/
20. Morelli V, Naquin C, Weaver V. Alternative therapies for traditional disease states: osteoarthritis. Am Fam Physician 2003; 67(2):339–344.
21. Bruyere O, Pavelka K, et al. Glucosamine sulfate reduces osteoarthritis progression in postmenopausal women with knee osteoarthritis: evidence from two 3-year studies. Menopause 2004; 11(2):134–135.
22. Scroggie DA, Albright A, Harris MD. The effect of glucosamine-chondroitin supplementation on glycosylated hemoglobin levels in patients with type 2 diabetes mellitus: a placebo-controlled, double-blinded, randomized clinical trial. Arch Intern Med 2003; 163(13):1587–1590.
23. Hochberg MC, Dougados M. Pharmacological therapy of osteoarthritis. Best Pract Res Clin Rheumatol 2001; 15(4):583–593.
24. Volpi N. The pathobiology of osteoarthritis and the rationale for using chondroitin sulfate for its treatment. Curr Drug Targets Immune Endocr Metabol Disord 2004; 4(2):119–127.
25. Uebelhart D, Malaise M, et al. Intermittent treatment of knee osteoarthritis with oral chondroitin sulfate: a one-year, randomized, double-blind, multicenter study versus placebo. Osteoarthritis Cartilage 2004; 12(4):269–276.
26. Wang Y, Prentice LF, et al. The effect of nutritional supplements on osteoarthritis. Altern Med Rev 2004; 9(3):275–296.
27. Parcell S. Sulfur in human nutrition and applications in medicine. Altern Med Rev 2002; 7:22–44.

28. Gaby AR. Natural treatments for osteoarthritis. Altern Med Rev 1999; 4(5):330–341.

29. Soeken KL, Lee WL, et al. Safety and efficacy of S-adenosylmethionine (SAMe) for osteoarthritis. J Fam Pract 2002; 51(5):425–430.

30. Fetrow CW, Avila JR. Efficacy of the dietary supplement S-adenosyl-L-methionine. Ann Pharmacother 2001; 35(11):1414–1425.

31. Towheed TE, Judd MJ, et al. Acetaminophen for osteoarthritis. Cochrane Database Syst Rev 2003; (2):CD004257.

32. Reijman M, Bierma-Zeinstra SM, et al. Is there an association between the use of different types of nonsteroidal antiinflammatory drugs and radiologic progression of osteoarthritis? The Rotterdam study. Arthritis Rheum 2005; 52(10):3137–3142.

33. Hochberg MC, Dougados M. Pharmacological therapy of osteoarthritis. Best Pract Res Clin Rheumatol 2001; 15(4):583–593.

34. Matheson AJ, Perry CM. Glucosamine: a review of its use in the management of osteoarthritis. Drugs Aging 2003; 20(14):1041–1060.

35. Cohen M, Wolfe R, et al. A randomized, double blind, placebo controlled trial of a topical cream containing glucosamine sulfate, chondroitin sulfate, and camphor for osteoarthritis of the knee. J Rheumatol 2003; 30(3):523–528.

36. Fusco BM, Giacovazzo M. Peppers and pain. The promise of capsaicin. Drugs 1997; 53(6):909–914.

37. Keitel W, Frerick H, et al. Capsaicin pain plaster in chronic non-specific low back pain. Arzneimittelforschung 2001; 51(11):896–903.

38. Halpern GM. Anti-inflammatory effects of a stabilized lipid extract of Perna canaliculus (Lyprinol). Allerg Immunol (Paris) 2000; 32(7):272–278.

39. Cho SH, Jung YB, et al. Clinical efficacy and safety of Lyprinol, a patented extract from New Zealand green-lipped mussel (Perna Canaliculus) in patients with osteoarthritis of the hip and knee: a multicenter 2-month clinical trial. Allerg Immunol (Paris) 2003; 35(6):212–216.

40. Curtis CL, Rees SG, et al. Pathologic indicators of degradation and inflammation in human osteoarthritic cartilage are abrogated by exposure to n-3 fatty acids. Arthritis Rheum 2002; 46(6):1544–1553.

41. Jonas WB, Rapoza CP, et al. The effect of niacinamide on osteoarthritis: a pilot study. Inflamm Res 1996; 45(7):330–334.

42. McCarty MF, Russell AL. Niacinamide therapy for osteoarthritis—does it inhibit nitric oxide synthase induction by interleukin 1 in chondrocytes? Med Hypotheses 1999; 53(4):350–360.

43. Walker AF, Bundy R, et al. Bromelain reduces mild acute knee pain and improves well-being in a dose-dependent fashion in an open study of otherwise healthy adults. Phytomedicine 2002; 9(8):681–686.

44. Akhtar NM, Naseer R, et al. Oral enzyme combination versus diclofenac in the treatment of osteoarthritis of the knee—a double-blind prospective randomized study. Clin Rheumatol 2004; 23(5):410–415.

45. Bellamy N, Campbell J, et al. Viscosupplementation for the treatment of osteoarthritis of the knee. Cochrane Database Syst Rev 2005 Apr 18; (2):CD005321.

46. White P, Lewith G, et al. Acupuncture versus placebo for the treatment of chronic mechanical neck pain: a randomized, controlled trial. Ann Intern Med 2004; 141(12):911–919.

47. Vas J, Mendez C, et al. Acupuncture as a complementary therapy to the pharmacological treatment of osteoarthritis of the knee: randomised controlled trial. BMJ 2004; 329(7476):1216.

48. Segal L, Day SE, et al. Can we reduce disease burden from osteoarthritis? Med J Aust 2004; 180(5 Suppl):S11–S17.

49. van Baar ME, Assendelft WJ, et al. Effectiveness of exercise therapy in patients with osteoarthritis of the hip or knee: a systematic review of randomized clinical trials. Arthritis Rheum 1999; 42(7):1361–1369.

50. Tak E, Staats P, et al. The effects of an exercise program for older adults with osteoarthritis of the hip. J Rheumatol 2005; 32(6):1106–1113.

51. Brosseau L, MacLeay L, et al. Intensity of exercise for the treatment of osteoarthritis. Cochrane Database Syst Rev 2003; (2):CD004259.

52. Roddy E, Zhang W, Doherty M. Aerobic walking or strengthening exercise for osteoarthritis of the knee? A systematic review. Ann Rheum Dis 2005; 64(4):544–548.

53. Fransen M, McConnell S, Bell M. Exercise for osteoarthritis of the hip or knee. Cochrane Database Syst Rev 2003; (3):CD004286.

54. Huang MH, Lin YS, et al. A comparison of various therapeutic exercises on the functional status of patients with knee osteoarthritis. Semin Arthritis Rheum 2003; 32(6):398–406.

55. Brosseau L, Welch V, et al. Low level laser therapy (Classes I, II and III) for treating osteoarthritis. Cochrane Database Syst Rev 2004; (3):CD002046.

56. Arabelovic S, McAlindon TE. Considerations in the treatment of early osteoarthritis. Curr Rheumatol Rep 2005; 7(1):29–35.

57. Brouwer RW, Jakma TS, et al. Braces and orthoses for treating osteoarthritis of the knee. Cochrane Database Syst Rev 2005; (1):CD004020.

58. Manek NJ, Lane NE. Osteoarthritis: current concepts in diagnosis and management. Am Fam Physician 2000; 61(6):1795–1804.

59. Pollo FE, Jackson RW. Knee bracing for unicompartmental osteoarthritis. J Am Acad Orthop Surg 2006; 14(1):5–11.

60. Arokoski JP. Physical therapy and rehabilitation programs in the management of hip osteoarthritis. Eura Medicophys 2005; 41(2):155–161.

61. Baird CL, Sands L. A pilot study of the effectiveness of guided imagery with progressive muscle relaxation to reduce chronic pain and mobility difficulties of osteoarthritis. Pain Manag Nurs 2004; 5(3):97–104.

62. Roddy E, Zhang W, et al. Evidence-based recommendations for the role of exercise in the management of osteoarthritis of the hip or knee—the MOVE consensus. Rheumatology (Oxford) 2005; 44(1):67–73.

63. Zhang W, Doherty M, et al. EULAR evidence based recommendations for the management of hip osteoarthritis: report of a task force of the EULAR Standing Committee for International Clinical Studies Including Therapeutics (ESCISIT). Ann Rheum Dis 2005; 64(5):669–681.

64. Sarzi-Puttini P, Cimmino MA, et al. Osteoarthritis: an overview of the disease and its treatment strategies. Semin Arthritis Rheum 2005; 35(1 Suppl 1):1–10.

65. Fajardo M, Di Cesare PE. Disease-modifying therapies for osteoarthritis: current status. Drugs Aging 2005; 22(2):141–161.

PATIENT HANDOUT 13.1 – KNEE OSTEOARTHRITIS – SELF-CARE OPTIONS

Try a multipronged approach.

Triggers to avoid

- Joint malalignment → minimize distortion
  - —Strengthen quadriceps or hamstring muscles as required.
  - —Consider use of braces, foot lifts and other orthotics.
- Obesity → lose weight, refer to Patient Handouts 12.1–12.4.
  - —Exercise to increase energy consumption.
  - —Reduce dietary energy intake.

Limit further damage

- Correct triggers
- Do regular low-impact exercise
- Select appropriate footwear
- Consider nutraceuticals
  - —glucosamine sulphate 1500 mg/day; possibly for life (still to be proven).

Manage pain

Systemic intervention:

- Acetaminophen (paracetamol or Tylenol)—rapid onset, beware side effects. Beware dose >2 g/day
- Newer NSAIDs—slow onset (weeks).
- New Zealand green-lipped mussel—slow onset.

Local application:

- Capsaicin cream
- Intra-articular viscosupplementation.

Improve joint stability

- Selective muscle strengthening exercises, e.g. correct hamstring:quadriceps strength ratio
- Orthotics.

Chapter **14**

Diabetes mellitus

CHAPTER CONTENTS

A 73-year-old man presents complaining of unremitting fatigue. On examination he is found to be 2 m tall, weigh 122 kg and have a blood pressure of 165/98. His colour is good and his respiratory rate normal. He does not report a tendency to bleed or bruising. No glucose was detected in the urine. Protein was detected. He has smoked 15 cigarettes a day for the last 35 years.

- Does the absence of glucose in the urine exclude type 2 diabetes?
- Is this man at risk of type 2 diabetes?
- How could diabetes be excluded?
- Could this patient have complications resulting from diabetes in the absence of a clinical diagnosis of the disease?

INTRODUCTION

Diabetes mellitus is a metabolic disorder characterized by raised levels of blood glucose and impaired carbohydrate and lipid metabolism. Type 2 diabetes affects 150 million adults worldwide and this figure is expected to double in the next 25 years. Nearly half of all people who have diabetes are 65 years of age or older.[1] In fact, the prevalence of type 2 diabetes mellitus starts increasing from the age of 20–30 years!

Elderly people are more glucose intolerant and insulin resistant than young individuals. Whether this metabolic change is an inevitable consequence of 'biological aging' or due to environmental or lifestyle variables is, however, uncertain.[2] Certainly, physiological changes associated with aging, such as changes in body composition, decreased physical fitness, poor dietary habits and changes in hormones may aggravate any underlying insulin resistance.[3] Whereas hepatic glucose output seems to be almost unaffected, insulin resistance in elderly people appears to predominate in skeletal muscle. Biological aging is characterized by sarcopenia with increased adiposity and/or altered fat distribution.[2] Indeed, increased insulin resistance coupled with decreased insulin secretion largely explains the abnormal glucose metabolism seen in elderly people under the age of 75 years.[4] This 'long lasting diabetes', with its combination of insulin resistance and poor insulin secretion, is typical of type 2 or non-insulin dependent diabetes mellitus.

Another type of diabetes, 'senile diabetes', has also been described in persons over 75 years of age.[4] In non-obese type 2 diabetics islet beta cell secretory defects seem to dominate, with any significant degree of insulin resistance being unusual.[5] Insulin secretory defects have been consistently demonstrated in the elderly.[6] The prevailing abnormalities in insulin secretion in elderly persons may be attributed to increased amyloid deposition in pancreatic islet beta-cells, decreased amylin secretion, impaired insulin secretion pulsatility, decreased responsiveness of pancreatic beta-cells to insulinotropic gut hormones and diminished insulin response to non-glucose stimuli.[2]

PREDICTING RISK

Diabetes is an insidious condition and may remain undiagnosed for many years. Treating diabetes diagnosed through standard clinical practice reduces the risk of microvascular complications. As it is uncertain whether the additional years of treatment provided by early diagnosis through population screening would result in clinically important improvements in diabetes-related outcomes,[7] screening has been limited to those at increased risk.

Irremediable risks

Race, family history and increasing age are important non-modifiable risk factors for type 2 diabetes. Regardless of family history and race, the risk of diabetes increases with age. Fasting blood glucose increases 1–2 mg/dL for each decade of life and postprandial blood glucose increases up to

15 mg/dL over a similar period.[8,9] The mean blood glucose increase in females (2 mg/dL per decade) is double that in males (1 mg/dL). Compared to those with a diabetic parent or sibling, type 2 diabetics without a family history are older at the onset of disease, have better beta-cell function and a higher HDL cholesterol concentration.[10] Older black Americans, Australian Aboriginals, Polynesians, Indians and Maltese, with or without a family history, have particularly high rates of the disease.

Amendable risks

Obesity and sedentary lifestyle are modifiable risk factors for diabetes in younger but not necessarily in all older elderly people. Weight gained during adulthood is directly correlated with an increased risk of type 2 diabetes. The increased prevalence in diabetes parallels the increase in overweight and obesity in America and, compared to adults with a BMI < 25, the prevalence of type 2 diabetes is 3–7 times greater in obese persons (BMI > 30) and escalates to 20 times in those with a BMI > 35.[11] In addition to obesity, abdominal adiposity is an independent risk factor for type 2 diabetes. A waist circumference of at least 94 cm in men or 80 cm in women correlates with being overweight (BMI 25–30), while 102 cm or more in men and 88 cm or more in women correlates with obesity (BMI ≥ 30). A larger waist circumference reflects intra-abdominal, metabolically active fat. Both BMI and waist circumference are better predictors than waist–hip ratio.[12] BMI and physical inactivity are independent predictors of incident diabetes; however, the magnitude of the association with BMI is greater than that with physical activity in combined analyses.[13]

A sedentary lifestyle and low fitness levels are independent risk factors for all causes of mortality, including diabetes mellitus type 2. In fact the risk of developing diabetes is reduced by 40% in men of normal weight and 60% in overweight men on a regular exercise program.[14] Total physical activity time in excess of 2.5 hours a week is associated with a reduced prevalence of insulin resistance and dyslipidaemia in both sexes and a reduced prevalence of obesity and hypertension in women.[15] The risk for type 2 diabetes decreases progressively with increasing levels of physical activity[16] and even moderate levels of physical activity substantially reduce the risk of this disorder! Other lifestyle choices that increase the risk of diabetes are alcohol and smoking.[17] After controlling for known risk factors, men who smoked 25 or more cigarettes daily had a relative risk of diabetes of 1.94 compared with non-smokers. Another study found that those who currently smoked 16–25 cigarettes each day had a 3.27 times higher risk of developing type 2 diabetes compared to non-smokers. Furthermore, current smoking and starting to smoke at a younger age seem more important than the number of cigarettes smoked in determining risk. A non-linear relation between alcohol intake and diabetes has been reported. The lowest risk is recorded among moderate drinkers (16–42 units/week).[15] Other risk factors such as a low plasma vitamin E level have also been identified—a decrease of 1 μmol/L of vitamin E increases the risk of diabetes by some 22%.[18]

While population screening is not recommended, targeting those at increased risk offers a realistic alternative to population screening. In view of the prevalence and insidious nature of the disease, it has been suggested that consideration be given to screening for type 2 diabetes at 3-year intervals beginning at age 45, particularly in those with BMI ≥25.[7]

SCREENING FOR DIABETES

Screens for diabetes test for glucose in the urine or blood. In health, when plasma glucose levels do not exceed 5.5 mmol/L, glucose is absent from urine. In diabetes, blood glucose levels exceed the renal threshold, resulting in glucosuria. However, due to renal changes associated with aging, blood glucose may need to be substantially raised before it spills over into the urine. By the age of 70 years glucosuria may not be detectable until plasma glucose exceeds 15 mmol/L! In older persons, diabetes mellitus is best diagnosed using blood glucose levels. Most accurate readings are obtained after an 8 hour fast.

For screening and definitive diagnosis, plasma glucose is initially tested in fasting individuals (fasting blood glucose—FBG), followed, 2 hours after taking an oral glucose load, by the oral glucose tolerance test (OGTT). Using standard diagnostic criteria:[7]

- normoglycaemia is defined as plasma glucose levels <100 mg/dL (5.6 mmol/L) in the FBG test and <140 mg/dL (7.8 mmol/L) in the OGTT.
- impaired fasting glucose (IFG) is defined as plasma glucose levels >100 mg/dL but <126 mg/dL (5.6–7.0 mmol/L)
- impaired glucose tolerance (IGT) is defined as a level of 140 mg/dL (7.8 mmol/L) but <200 mg/dL (11.1 mmol/L) at 2 hours in the OGTT.

In view of the prevalence of altered glucose metabolism amongst elderly persons it has been suggested that the diagnosis of diabetes for persons over 65 years of age be established on the basis of repeated fasting glycaemia of ≥126 mg/dL (7 mmol/L) and 2 hour OGTT of ≥200 mg/dL (11.1 mmol/L).[4] Use of both these criteria is recommended in view of the different kinds of diabetes in the elderly resulting in a poor concordance between these two tests in elderly persons.[19] IFG (6.1–6.9 mmol/L) is characterized by basal insulin resistance and other features of the metabolic syndrome such as greater insulin responses during an OGTT, higher waist-to-hip ratios, higher triglyceride and total cholesterol concentrations with lower HDL cholesterol concentration. IGT, a glucose level of 7.8–11.0 mmol/L (140–200 mg/dL) at 2 hours on the OGTT, is characterized by waning insulin secretion in relation to glucose concentrations. The former is best suited to detect the 'long lasting diabetes' of the young old, the latter the 'senile diabetes' of the older old. Elderly patients with IFG and/or IGT are referred to as having 'prediabetes'. Motta et al feel it may be helpful to distinguish between clinically manifested diabetes (glycaemia ≥140), mild diabetes (glycaemia ≥126 and <140 mg/dL) and diabetes based on OGTT (2-h ≥200 mg/dL) in elderly persons.[4]

Using the standard diagnostic criteria for diabetes, a study based on data from the Third National Health and Nutrition Examination Survey (1988–1994) found 17.1% of overweight adults aged 45–74 years had IGT, 11.9% had IFG, 22.6% had prediabetes, and 5.6% had both IGT and IFG.[20]

Based on those data the researchers estimated that almost 12 million overweight individuals aged 45–74 years in the US may benefit from diabetes prevention intervention.

CONTROLLING BODY WEIGHT

Maintaining an ideal body weight is a major objective in prevention of 'long lasting diabetes' in elderly people. Given that the hazard ratio for diabetes is 3.7 in obese individuals with a FBG of 5.6 mmol/L or greater and a family history,[21] weight reduction would seem a logical starting point for any intervention. A systematic review of long term outcomes of weight loss studies published between 1966 and 2001 showed that diabetics who intentionally lost weight reduced their risk of dying by 25%; weight loss of 9–13 kg was most protective.[22] Metabolic handling of glucose improved in 80% of type 2 diabetics who lost weight, particularly when their abdominal adiposity decreased.

The risk of diabetes changes with alterations in body weight in all age groups. Compared to women with stable weight, i.e. those whose weight changed less than 5 kg after 18 years of age, the relative risk for diabetes mellitus amongst those who gained 5.0–7.9 kg was 1.9; for women who gained 8.0–10.9 kg, it was 2.7. In contrast, overweight women who lost more than 5.0 kg reduced their risk for diabetes mellitus by at least 50%.[23] Weight loss can be achieved by reducing energy intake and/or increasing energy expenditure. Weight loss associated with increased physical activity seems to improve insulin sensitivity and glucose tolerance, thereby preventing development of type 2 diabetes in elderly people.[2]

LIFESTYLE INTERVENTION FOR DIABETES PREVENTION AND MANAGEMENT

The relative risk of death in known diabetics may be 2 times, in just diagnosed diabetics 2.7 times and in persons with impaired glucose tolerance 1.6 times that of normoglycaemic men.[24] Furthermore, despite diabetes affecting more than 1 in 5 elderly persons, evidence-based management information specific to older adults with diabetes is surprisingly lacking.[25] As diabetes in elderly adults is metabolically distinct from diabetes in younger patient populations, the approach to therapy may need to be different in this age group.[1] Certainly it has been suggested that elderly persons whose glucose levels slightly exceed the cut off values of an FBG of ≥ 7 (126 mg/dL) or a 2 hour OGTT reading of ≥11.1 (200 mg/dL) should use diet and exercise without medication.[26]

Dietary fat

As fat is energy dense, it is not surprising that meta-analyses of intervention trials report fat reduced diets cause a 3–4 kg larger weight loss than normal fat diets.[27] A 10% reduction in dietary fat has been found to cause a 4–5 kg weight loss in individuals with initial BMI of 30,[27] and a systematic review of randomized controlled trials suggested the best long term diet for weight loss, preventing type 2 diabetes and improving cardiac risk in obese adults may be one low in fat.[28] Weight loss is, however, but an intermediate step to reach the major goal of diabetes management, which is to establish and maintain near normal blood glucose levels. The macronutrient composition of the diet is also important.

The American Diabetic Association recommends a daily energy intake from fat of less than 10% from saturated fat, 10% from polyunsaturated fat and 10–15% from monounsaturated fat.[29] Trans-fatty acids should be avoided. The more saturated the fatty acids within the membrane lipid, the greater the insulin resistance. In contrast, polyunsaturated fatty acids enhance the cell membrane's response to insulin, omega-3 fatty acids more so than omega-6 fatty acids. Fish oil has no adverse affects on glycosylated haemoglobin (HbA1c) in diabetics and it lowers triglyceride levels by almost 30%, but may be accompanied by a slight increase in LDL cholesterol concentration.[30] It is, however, diets rich in monounsaturated fat that improve lipoprotein profiles as well as glycaemic control. Better glycaemic control and lipid profiles have been reported on a diet of 33% mono-unsaturated fat and 35% carbohydrate than on the traditional 60% carbo-hydrate and 25% fat diet.[31] High monounsaturated fat diets reduce fasting plasma triacylglycerol and very low density lipoprotein (VLDL) cholesterol concentrations by 19% and 22% respectively, and cause a modest increase in HDL cholesterol concentrations without adversely affecting LDL cholesterol concentrations.[32] Good sources of monounsaturated fats include: avocados, pecans, almonds, macadamias, pistachios, hazelnuts, cashews, mustard seeds, canola oil, olives and high monounsaturated varieties of safflower and sunflower oils.

Dietary carbohydrate

Instead of a specific 'diabetic diet' that labels fats as bad and carbohydrates as good, diabetics are now encouraged to eat a healthy, well-balanced diet that provides all the essential macro- and micronutrients in appropriate amounts.[33] Although a diet with 60–70% of its daily energy derived from monounsaturated fats and carbohydrates which permits up to 10% of its total energy from sucrose is regarded as acceptable, the use of high complex carbohydrate diets is being questioned. As carbohydrate is the major secretagogue of insulin, there are those who believe some form of carbo-hydrate restriction is a prima facie candidate for dietary control of dia-betes.[34] They argue that a high carbohydrate diet raises postprandial plasma glucose and insulin secretion, thereby increasing the risk of macrovascular disease, hypertension, dyslipidaemia, obesity and diabetes. Indeed, con-trary to the traditional energy restricted low fat high carbohydrate diets, isocaloric low carbohydrate diets appear to reduce visceral fat more effec-tively, improve insulin sensitivity, increase HDL cholesterol and decrease triglyceride levels in obese type 2 diabetics.[35,36] This is relevant as a serum triglyceride concentration equal to or over 250 mg/dL (2.82 mmol/L) or HDL cholesterol concentration less than 0.90 mmol/L (35 mg/dL) carries a significant risk of diabetes.[15] Low carbohydrate diets that permit 20% rather than 50–60% of energy from carbohydrate have been associated with improved glycaemic control.[34]

While some form of carbohydrate restriction may be beneficial, targeting the type of carbohydrate eaten may further benefit glycaemic control. Although some experts maintain that the amount of carbohydrate consumed has a greater glycaemic influence than does the source,[19] selection of carbohydrates with a low glycaemic index (GI) may be advisable.[37–39] In the short term, HbA1c has been demonstrated to improve on the low compared with the high GI diet and a low GI diet may well help to improve the metabolic control in type 2 obese diabetic persons.[40] Although health authorities have yet to reach consensus about the long term benefit of using foods with low glycaemic indices,[33] foods with a GI of less than 55 appear desirable. Good choices are apples, grapefruit, beans, lentils, dense grainy bread and bran cereals. Oats and guar gum deserve particular attention. Low GI foods improve insulin sensitivity and curtail postprandial blood glucose rises thereby reducing the microvascular complications, enhance the lipid profile thereby decreasing cardiovascular risk and increase satiety thereby aiding weight loss. A low GI diet was found to improve both in vivo insulin sensitivity and in vitro adipocyte insulin sensitivity in women with a parental history of coronary artery disease.[41] On the other hand, persons consuming diets with a higher GI appear at greater risk of insulin resistance, diabetes and metabolic syndrome.

Despite strong support for a low carbohydrate diet,[34] the high carbohydrate alternative has yet to be dismissed. Contrary to the researchers' expectations, an ad libitum, low fat, high fibre diet has been found to promote weight loss in patients with type 2 diabetes without causing unfavourable alterations in plasma lipids or glycaemic control.[42] Anderson et al recommend a macronutrient diet containing carbohydrate >54%; protein 12–16%; total fat <30% with monounsaturated fat 12–15% and 25–50 g/day of dietary fibre (15–25 g/1000 kcal) for diabetics.[43] They justify their recommendations for high carbohydrate, high fibre diets, as compared to moderate carbohydrate, low fibre diets, on the grounds that these diets achieve lower total LDL and HDL cholesterol and triglycerides as well as fasting, postprandial and average plasma glucose and HbA1c levels. Furthermore, one study found that, compared to a high protein diet, it was only the high carbohydrate group that showed increased insulin sensitivity and decreased HbA1c and fasting plasma glucose.[44]

Dietary protein

The American Diabetic Association recommends that 10–20% of the energy intake of the diet should be from protein.[29] The Atkins Diet limits carbohydrate intake to 5% of energy (<30 g/day) and derives 30% of its energy from protein. Although ingested protein does not contribute to postprandial glucose concentration, in view of the increased risk of diabetic nephropathy such a high protein intake may cause concern. Nonetheless, a pilot study that compared type 2 diabetics on a hypocaloric high protein diet (40% carbohydrate, 30% protein, 30% fat) with those on a hypocaloric high carbohydrate diet (55% carbohydrate, 15% protein, 30% fat) found both diets achieved weight loss with no or minimal effects on lipid levels, or on renal or hepatic function.[44] Systolic and diastolic blood pressure decreased in the high protein group.

Dietary supplementation

For older persons the best diet for prevention of weight gain, obesity, type 2 diabetes and cardiovascular disease may well be one that is low in fat and sugar rich beverages and high in carbohydrates, fibre, grains and protein.[27] Whatever macronutrient composition may ultimately emerge as optimal, all are agreed that a BMI equal to or less than 25 is highly desirable. Furthermore, in addition to careful carbohydrate selection, dietary supplementation with psyllium or chromium may benefit glycaemic control. Psyllium (5.1 g bid), a bulk-forming laxative high in fibre and mucilage, has been shown to benefit blood indices.[45] Various studies have also shown chromium supplementation, as Brewer's yeast (23.3 μg Cr/day), CrCl3 (200 μg Cr/day) and chromium picolinate (200–1000 μg Cr/day), benefit glycaemic and lipid indices in overweight diabetics.[46,47] Diet and dietary supplements are, however, but one aspect of diabetic control; exercise is another important measure.

Exercise

Lifestyle intervention may be even more potent than drugs. A clinical trial involving non-diabetic persons with elevated fasting and postload plasma glucose concentrations compared a three way intervention trial.[48] The goals of the lifestyle program intervention arm were weight loss of at least 7% and physical activity of 150 minutes or more per week. The mean age of participants was 51 years, and mean BMI was 34.0. After the subjects had been followed for an average 2.8 years the incidence of diabetes was 11.0, 7.8, and 4.8 cases per 100 person-years in the placebo, metformin (850 mg twice daily) and lifestyle groups respectively.[48] Compared with the placebo group, lifestyle intervention reduced the incidence by 58%, metformin by 31%. The authors calculated that to prevent one case of diabetes during a period of 3 years, 6.9 persons would have to participate in the lifestyle intervention program. After an average of 3.2 years, the incidence of the metabolic syndrome in the trial groups was, compared to placebo, reduced by 41% in the lifestyle group and by 17% in the metformin group.[49]

Even in the absence of dietary control, exercise is beneficial. Daily exercise without caloric restriction was associated with substantial reductions in total, abdominal and visceral fat in women.[50] Similarly, exercise without weight loss has been associated with a substantial reduction in total and abdominal obesity.[51] In fact, it appears exercise is required for visceral fat loss in postmenopausal women with type 2 diabetes.[52] Reduction of visceral fat is relevant as abdominal obesity is perceived to play an important role in mediating insulin resistance. Exercise, through its pronounced effect on substrate utilization and insulin sensitivity, lowers blood glucose and favourably alters the dyslipidaemia associated with insulin resistance, i.e. hypertriglyceridaemia, decreased HDL cholesterol, and composition changes of low-density lipoprotein.[50,52] Moderate intensity exercise is advocated. Initially, physical activity recommendations should be largely guided by the patient's willingness to comply. Over time the duration and frequency should increase to 30–45 minutes of moderate aerobic activity on 3–5 days each week. Successful long term weight loss may, however, require greater effort; walking for at least an hour daily or jogging for half that time may be necessary. Patients with hypertension or diabetic retinopathy should avoid high intensity exercise and resistance training.

DIABETICS AT RISK

The risk of developing diabetes is directly associated with age, race, parental history of diabetes, BMI, abdominal obesity and fasting glucose. The risk of developing complications from diabetes increases with the duration of the disease (>5 years) and therapeutic compliance. The elderly are at greatest risk.

Long term complications in diabetics range from macro- to microvascular disease. The former increases the risk of a heart attack, stroke and peripheral vascular disease; the latter the probability of nephropathy, neuropathy and retinopathy. Even mild hyperglycaemia is associated with adverse health outcomes. Tight glycaemic control reduces the risk of retinopathy by 76%, of neuropathy by 60% and albuminuria by 54%. Microalbuminuria is a marker of early nephropathy and increased cardiovascular risk. Tight glycaemic control reduces microvascular complications but increases the risk of hypoglycaemia.[53]

The likelihood of complications can be predicted by monitoring glycosylated haemoglobin levels (HbA1c). An HbA1c of 6% is associated with 6.4 microvascular events per 1000 patient years and a hypoglycaemic rate of 2.8 per 1000 patient years; if HbA1c increases to 9%, microvascular events increase to 15.6 but hypoglycaemic episodes drop to 1.1. At HbA1c of 12%, 38.5 microvascular events are likely per 1000 patient years but no hypoglycaemic attacks are anticipated. Although tight glycaemic control (4–8 mmol/L) doubles or triples the risk of hypoglycaemia, it more than halves the risk of retinopathy, neuropathy and albuminuria. Glycaemic control, as exemplified by lowering glycosylated haemoglobin to less than 0.2% points (around 6.3%) above the upper limit of normal, is a central aim of therapy.[54] A combination of HbA1c and oral glucose tolerance test levels is used to predict progression to type 2 diabetes.

Diabetic complications have a major health impact. In the United States,[55,56] the following is true:

- Approximately $1 in every $7 spent on health is expended on diabetes mellitus.
- Diabetics have a 2–6 times greater risk of heart disease than non-diabetics.
- Diabetics have a 5 times greater risk of stroke than non-diabetics.

- Diabetic retinopathy is the leading cause of blindness in working age adults. Four out of five cases of blindness due to diabetes are attributable to diabetic retinopathy. Diabetics are also at increased risk of cataracts and blurred vision. The HbA1c threshold for diabetic retinopathy is 8.5%.
- Diabetic nephropathy is the leading cause of end stage renal failure. One in 10 adult onset diabetics have evidence of renal disease within 20 years of the initial diagnosis. Predictors of diabetic nephropathy are micro-albuminuria, hypertension, glucosuria and poor glycaemic control. Microalbuminuria, at a level of 30–300 mg/day, is an early sign of this complication. Albuminuria in excess of 150 mg/day in diabetics is predictive of nephropathy.[57] In type 2 diabetics, microalbuminuria is strongly linked with cardiovascular risk. Albuminuria detected on dipstick (>550 mg/24 hours) is predictive of future renal failure.

  An HbA1c level of 8.1% is a threshold above which the risk of micro-albuminaemia rises steeply. The Micral-Test can reliably assess albumin in spot urine tests in the clinic. As this test has high sensitivity and low specificity, positive findings require sending a 24 hour specimen to the laboratory for further analysis.
- Diabetes mellitus is the leading cause of non-traumatic amputations. Neuropathy affects the motor, sensory and autonomic nervous systems. Preliminary findings indicate that oral treatment with 600 mg of alpha-lipoic acid tid for 3 weeks may improve symptoms and deficits resulting from polyneuropathy in type 2 diabetic patients, without causing significant adverse reactions.[58] Two 52-week randomized placebo-controlled clinical diabetic neuropathy trials found acetyl-L-carnitine 1000 mg/day tid alleviated symptoms, particularly pain, and improved nerve fibre regeneration and vibration perception in patients with established diabetic neuropathy.[59] Carnitine and its derivative may meet energy demand by aiding regulation of fat metabolism through acetyl and acyl cellular metabolism and carbohydrate metabolism by effecting synthetic control of key glycolytic and gluconeogenic enzymes. Important risk factors for neuropathy are: poor control of blood glucose; the duration of the disease (50% have neuropathy after 25 years as a diabetic); and tall stature, longer neurons being more susceptible to biochemical damage.

PATIENT MONITORING

Red alerts suggesting unacceptable deviations of blood glucose and the need for vigorous attention to management include:

- Nocturnal polyuria, an unhelpful sign given the prevalence of nocturia in elderly persons.
- Persistent failure to meet the targets for blood sugar control. Unacceptable levels include a
  —fasting blood sugar of over 7.8 mmol/L. The target fasting blood sugar is 4.4–6.1 mmol/L
  —postprandial blood sugar level over 10 mmol/L. The target level for postprandial blood sugar is 4.4–8.0 mmol/L

—glycosylated haemoglobin of more than 7.5%. The target level is an HbA1c of less than 6.5%.

- A middle-aged well diabetic with a preprandial glucose level over 7 mmol/L and 2 hour postprandial level of 10 mmol/L or more.
- An elderly frail diabetic with a preprandial glucose of over 10 mmol/L and 2 hour postprandial level of 15 mmol/L or more.

In view of its ability to reflect longer term glycaemic control, HbA1c has emerged as a particularly valuable therapeutic aid. An HbA1c level of 7.0% or higher is considered an indication for pharmacological intervention, a level below 7.0% is generally treated with diet and exercise.[60]

In addition to being used to indicate the need to complement lifestyle intervention with drugs, HbA1c is routinely used to monitor compliance and metabolic control in individual patients. HbA1c levels increase in older obese diabetics when weight and/or energy intake from dietary saturated fat increases.[61] On the other hand, HbA1c levels can drop by up to 20% in type 2 diabetics who exercise regularly for 30–60 minutes on alternate days at 50–80% of maximum oxygen capacity.[62] Despite the efficacy of HbA1c as a monitoring tool for microvascular complications, increased fasting plasma glucose and 2-hour postchallenge plasma glucose levels with normal HbA1c levels are recognized as risk factors for macro- i.e. cardiovascular disease. Individuals with HbA1c values between 6.0% and 7.0% may have normal fasting plasma glucose levels but abnormal 2-hour postchallenge plasma glucose levels.[63] Although both fasting plasma glucose and 2-hour postchallenge plasma glucose levels increase as HbA1c increases, the 2-hour postchallenge plasma glucose level increases at a greater rate and accounts for a greater proportion of HbA1c. It has been suggested that an upper limit of normal for fasting plasma glucose at 110 mg/dL (6.11 mmol/L) is too high and that attempts to lower HbA1c in these individuals require treatment preferentially directed at lowering postprandial glucose levels.[37]

GETTING PERSPECTIVE

There are two distinct forms of diabetes mellitus in elderly people. The 'long lasting' form is similar in all respects to type 2 diabetes mellitus, the 'senile' form is characterized by an insulin secretory defect. The diverse pathogenesis underlying the development of diabetes in the elderly has implications for its early recognition rather than its management. In both instances weight control, dietary choice and exercise offer the major lifestyle options for preventing and controlling the disease.

CLINICAL CHALLENGE

A tall obese 67-year-old patient has had diabetes type 2 for 10 years. She is concerned she may develop complications. Her blood pressure is 160/95.

Questions arising

- What information would you collect in order to respond to her concerns?
- How would you advise the patient?

Clinical considerations

Step 1: Search for risk indicators

A. *Identify overt risks*

- Duration of disease >5 years
- Her height puts her at increased risk of neuropathy.

B. *Test for biochemical markers of poor metabolic control*

- Request an HbA1c. This will provide information on long term blood glucose control.
- Do a postprandial and 2-hour postprandial blood glucose test.
- Check blood lipids.

C. *Check for evidence of complications*

- Absent or decreased Achilles tendon reflexes—reflex present
- Microalbuminuria (21 µg/mL or greater)
- Paraesthesia—present.

Laboratory results were: HbA1c >7.5%; postprandial glucose 10.5 mmol/L; 2-hour postprandial glucose 15.8 mmol/L; microalbuminuria absent; total cholesterol 8.0 mmol/L; HDL 0.7 mmol/L.

Clinical assessment is that the patient has evidence of neuropathy and is at risk of the other complications of microvascular disease due to poor glycaemic control. She is at increased risk of macrovascular disease in view of her blood lipids, hypertension and smoking.

Step 2: Advise the patient as follows

Exercise for at least 30–45 minutes on alternate days of the week.

Diet recommendations include

- a low energy diet to achieve weight reduction of at least 9 kg
- a low saturated fat, moderate monounsaturated and carbohydrate diet
- favouring foods with a low glycaemic index
- limiting alcohol to one standard drink daily, with meals
- not adding salt to food when cooking or eating; avoiding highly salted items. Sodium should be restricted to less than 3 g each day.

Consider drug therapy, as her HBA1c is above 7%

- Metformin is probably the drug of choice for obese diabetics.

To reduce the likelihood of microvascular disease, the blood glucose targets are:

- HbA1c <6.5%
- fasting blood glucose 4.4–6.1 mmol/L
- postprandial blood glucose 4.4–8.0 mmol/L.

To reduce the likelihood of macrovascular disease:

- stop smoking
- blood pressure target 140/90
- blood lipid targets are
  –a total cholesterol of less than 5.5 mmol/L
  –LDL less than 3.5 mmol/L
  –triglycerides less than 2.0 mmol/L
  –HDL greater than 1.01 mmol/L for women (0.83 mmol/L for men).

The patient returns for follow-up some years later and you detect numbness and pins and needles in both legs in a stocking distribution. On examination of the lower limb there is evidence of muscle weakness and wasting. She is also experiencing calf pain when walking long distances.

Questions arising

- What is the working diagnosis?
- Should the management plan be amended?
- What other complications of diabetes should be actively excluded?

Clinical considerations

The patient has evidence of diabetic neuropathy and peripheral vascular disease.

Management should aim to:

Enhance perfusion by

- exercising to encourage the development of collateral circulation. Walking at least 3 times per week for 30 or more minutes until near maximum pain level is reached is recommended.
  - taking one or more of the following nutritional supplements
    - vitamin E 300–1600 IU/day for at least 3 months
    - niacin 100–300 mg/day (relief appears to be temporary)
    - a-tocopheryl-nicotinate 200 mg tds
    - garlic 800 mg/day.
- Avoid damage to the feet by
  - careful podiatry and avoidance of foot, ankle and leg injury or ulceration
  - good daily foot care: refer to Patient Handout 14.3
  - careful selection of footwear: refer to Patient Handout 14.3
  - knowing when to get professional care: refer to Patient Handout 14.3.
- Review metabolic control of diabetes
  - order a HbA1c, fasting and random blood glucose, blood lipid level
  - review and reiterate dietary advice
  - review weight and encourage weight loss as indicated
  - review use of pharmaceuticals—consider replacing metformin with
    - meglitinides, which stimulate insulin release, have a rapid onset and short duration of action
    - second generation sulphonylureas, but first generation sulphonylureas, e.g. chlorpropamide, tolbutamide, should be avoided in the elderly
    - determine whether the patient requires insulin. Suggestive findings are:
    - anti-glutamic acid decarboxylase (GAD) antibodies
    - an inability to achieve satisfactory HbA1c levels
    - clinically overt hyperglycaemic attacks.

Other complications that should be considered include those attributable to:

- large vessel disease, i.e. atherosclerosis, causing myocardial ischaemia
- small vessel disease, i.e.
  - neuropathy e.g. autonomic neuropathy may result in labile blood pressure, impotence
  - nephropathy—assess renal function
  - diabetic retinopathy and cataract formation.

◆ There are two kinds of diabetes mellitus in elderly people: the major defect in old elderly is impaired insulin secretion young elderly are particularly prone to increased insulin resistance.

   ◆ Chronically raised levels of blood glucose impair insulin secretion and may explain the progressive deterioration of type 2 diabetes over time.

   ◆ Age is a risk factor for type 2 diabetes and screening of overweight elderly people is advisable.

   ◆ The excess risk for diabetes with even modest and typical adult weight gain is substantial.

   ◆ Obesity increases insulin resistance and blood glucose levels and is an independent risk factor for dyslipidaemia, hypertension and cardiovascular disease.

   ◆ Moderate weight loss (5% of body weight) can improve insulin action, decrease fasting blood glucose concentrations, and reduce the need for diabetes medications.

   ◆ Regular, moderate intensity physical activity enhances long term weight maintenance and improves insulin sensitivity, glycaemic control, and major risk factors for cardiovascular disease (e.g. hypertension and dyslipidaemia).

◆ Potential developments worth watching:

   —Dairy foods, which are rich in conjugated linoleic acid, have been inversely correlated with both diabetes and metabolic syndrome in some studies—but not in others.

   —Beta-glucan may reduce the glycaemic index in diabetic patients without compromising the palatability of breakfast cereal.

   —Phytosterols may improve the lipid status of hyperlipidaemic persons. Stanol enriched margarine can be found on supermarket shelves.

   —Nicotinamide increases insulin secretion in prediabetic patients and long term use in doses up to 1 g per day has been suggested.

   —Vitamin E (900 mg/day) may enhance insulin action improving glucose utilization and non-oxidative glucose metabolism.

   —Cinnamon may promote glucose uptake and glycogen synthesis in diabetics.

   —Fasting blood sugar, glycosylated haemoglobin and serum lipid profile of type 2 diabetics may be improved by taking either ginseng (200 mg) or chromium (200 μg/day or 100 mg taken with 9 g/day Brewer's yeast).

References

1. Shorr RI, Franse LV, et al. Glycemic control of older adults with type 2 diabetes: findings from the Third National Health and Nutrition Examination Survey, 1988–1994. J Am Geriatr Soc 2000 Mar; 48(3):264–267.

2. Scheen A. Diabetes mellitus in the elderly: insulin resistance and/or impaired insulin secretion? Diabetes Metab 2005; 31 Spec No 2:5S27–5S34.

3. Moller N, Gormsen L, et al. Effects of ageing on insulin secretion and action. Horm Res 2003; 60 (Suppl 1):102–104.

4. Motta M, Bennati E, et al. Diabetes mellitus in the elderly: diagnostic features. Arch Gerontol Geriatr 2006; 42(1):101–106.

5. Hermans MP, Pepersack TM, et al. Prevalence and determinants of impaired glucose metabolism in frail elderly patients: the Belgian Elderly Diabetes Survey (BEDS). J Gerontol A Biol Sci Med Sci 2005; 60(2):241–247.

6. Chang AM, Halter JB. Aging and insulin secretion. Am J Physiol Endocrinol Metab 2003; 284(1):E7–12.

7. American Diabetes Association. Screening for type 2 diabetes. Diabetes Care 2004; 27:S11–S14.

8. Guastamacchia E, Nardelli GM, et al. The influence of aging on the normal oral glucose tolerance. Boll Soc Ital Biol Sper 1983; 59(8):1096–1101.

9. Nakano H. Clinical pathophysiology of the elderly onset diabetes mellitus. Nippon Rinsho 2006; 64(1):51–56. Abstract. (Article in Japanese).

10. Li H, Isomaa B, et al. Consequences of a family history of type 1 and type 2 diabetes on the phenotype of patients with type 2 diabetes. Diabetes Care 2000; 23(5):589–594.

11. Klein S, Sheard NF, et al. Weight management through lifestyle modification for the prevention and management of type 2 diabetes: rationale and strategies. A statement of the American Diabetes Association, the North American Association for the Study of Obesity, and the American Society for Clinical Nutrition. Am J Clin Nutr 2004; 80(2):257–263.

12. Wang Y, Rimm EB, et al. Comparison of abdominal adiposity and overall obesity in predicting risk of type 2 diabetes among men. Am J Clin Nutr 2005; 81(3):555–563.

13. Weinstein AR, Sesso HD, et al. Relationship of physical activity vs body mass index with type 2 diabetes in women. JAMA 2004; 292(10):1188–1194.

14. Keller KB, Lemberg L. Retirement is no excuse for physical inactivity or isolation. Am J Crit Care 2002; 11(3):270–272.

15. Dunstan DW, Salmon J, et al. Associations of TV viewing and physical activity with the metabolic syndrome in Australian adults. Diabetologia 2005 Oct 7; [Epub ahead of print].

16. Wannamethee SG, Shaper AG, Alberti KG. Physical activity, metabolic factors, and the incidence of coronary heart disease and type 2 diabetes. Arch Intern Med 2000; 160(14):2108–2116.

17. Rimm EB, Chan J, et al. Prospective study of cigarette smoking, alcohol use, and the risk of diabetes in men. BMJ 1995; 310(6979):555–559.

18. Salonen JT, Nyyssonen K, et al. Increased risk of non-insulin dependent diabetes mellitus at low plasma vitamin E concentrations: a four year follow up study in men. BMJ 1995; 311(7013):1124–1127.

19. Tripathy D, Carlsson M, et al. Insulin secretion and insulin sensitivity in relation to glucose tolerance: lessons from the Botnia Study. Diabetes 2000; 49(6):975–980.

20. Benjamin SM, Valdez R, et al. Estimated number of adults with prediabetes in the US in 2000: opportunities for prevention. Diabetes Care 2003; 26(3):645–649.

21. Lyssenko V, Almgren P, et al. Predictors of and longitudinal changes in insulin sensitivity and secretion preceding onset of type 2 diabetes. Diabetes 2005; 54(1):166–174.

22. Aucott L, Poobalan A, et al. Weight loss in obese diabetic and non-diabetic individuals and long-term diabetes outcomes—a systematic review. Diabetes Obes Metab 2004; 6(2):85–94.

23. Colditz GA, Willett WC, et al. Weight gain as a risk factor for clinical diabetes mellitus in women. Ann Intern Med 1995; 122(7):481–486.

24. Balkau B, Eschwege E, et al. Risk factors for early death in non-insulin dependent diabetes and men with known glucose tolerance status. BMJ 1993; 307(6899):295–299.

25. Sakharova OV, Inzucchi SE. Treatment of diabetes in the elderly. Addressing its complexities in this high-risk group. Postgrad Med 2005; 118(5):19–26, 29.

26. Kuzuya T, Nakagawa S, et al. Report of the Committee on the classification and diagnostic criteria of diabetes mellitus. Diabetes Res Clin Pract 2002; 55(1):65–85.

27. Astrup A. The role of dietary fat in obesity. Semin Vasc Med 2005; 5(1):40–47.

28. Avenell A, Brown TJ, et al. What are the long-term benefits of weight reducing diets in adults? A systematic review of randomized controlled trials. J Hum Nutr Diet 2004; 17(4):317–335.

29. American Diabetes Association. Nutritional recommendations and principles for people with diabetes mellitus. Diabetes Care 1999; 22(Suppl 1):S32–S35.

30. Friedberg CE, Janssen MJ, et al. Fish oil and glycemic control in diabetes. A meta-analysis. Diabetes Care 1998; 21(4):494–500.

31. Garg A, Bonanome A, et al. Comparison of a high carbohydrate diet with a high monounsaturated fat diet in patients with non insulin-dependent diabetes mellitus. New Eng J Med 1988; 319:829–834.

32. Garg A. High-monounsaturated-fat diets for patients with diabetes mellitus: a meta-analysis. Am J Clin Nutr 1998; 67(3 Suppl):577S–582S.

33. Choudhary P. Review of dietary recommendations for diabetes mellitus. Diabetes Res Clin Pract 2004; 65 (Suppl 1):S9–S15.

34. Arora SK, McFarlane SI. The case for low carbohydrate diets in diabetes management. Nutrition & Metabolism 2005, 2:16.

35. Miyashita Y, Koide N, et al. Beneficial effect of low carbohydrate in low calorie diets on visceral fat reduction in type 2 diabetic patients with obesity. Diabetes Res Clin Pract 2004; 65(3):235–241.

36. Yancy WSJ, Olsen MK, et al. A low-carbohydrate, ketogenic diet versus a low-fat diet to treat obesity and hyperlipidaemia: a randomized, controlled trial. Ann Intern Med 2004, 140:769–777.

37. Moran M. The evolution of the nutritional management of diabetes. Proc Nutr Soc 2004; 63(4):615–620.

38. Brand-Miller J, Hayne S, et al. Low-glycemic index diets in the management of diabetes: a meta-analysis of randomized controlled trials. Diabetes Care 2003; 26(8):2261–2267.

39. Opperman AM, Venter CS, et al. Meta-analysis of the health effects of using the glycaemic index in meal-planning. Br J Nutr 2004; 92(3):367–381.

40. Jimenez-Cruz A, Bacardi-Gascon M, et al. A flexible, low-glycemic index Mexican-style diet in overweight and obese subjects with type 2 diabetes improves metabolic parameters during a 6-week treatment period. Diabetes Care 2003; 26(7):1967–1970.

41. Frost G, Leeds A, et al. Insulin sensitivity in women at risk of coronary heart disease and the effect of a low glycemic diet. Metabolism 1998; 47(10):1245–1251.

42. Gerhard GT, Ahmann A, et al. Effects of a low-fat diet compared with those of a high-monounsaturated fat diet on body weight, plasma lipids and lipoproteins, and glycemic control in type 2 diabetes. Am J Clin Nutr 2004; 80(3):668–673.

43. Anderson JW, Randles KM, et al. Carbohydrate and fiber recommendations for individuals with diabetes: a quantitative assessment and meta-analysis of the evidence. J Am Coll Nutr 2004; 23(1):5–17.

44. Sargrad KR, Homko C, et al. Effect of high protein vs high carbohydrate intake on insulin sensitivity, body weight, hemoglobin A1c, and blood pressure in patients with type 2 diabetes mellitus. J Am Diet Assoc 2005; 105(4):573–580.

45. Ziai SA, Larijani B, et al. Psyllium decreased serum glucose and glycosylated hemoglobin significantly in diabetic outpatients. J Ethnopharmacol 2005 Nov 14; 102(2):202–207.

46. Bahijiri SM, Mira SA, et al. The effects of inorganic chromium and brewer's yeast supplementation on glucose tolerance, serum lipids and drug dosage in individuals with type 2 diabetes. Saudi Med J 2000; 21(9):831–837.

47. No authors listed. A scientific review: the role of chromium in insulin resistance. Diabetes Educ 2004; Suppl:2–14.

48. Knowler WC, Barrett-Connor E, et al. Reduction in the incidence of type 2 diabetes with lifestyle intervention or metformin. N Engl J Med 2002; 346(6):393–403.

49. Orchard TJ, Temprosa M, et al. Prevention Program Research Group. The effect of metformin and intensive lifestyle intervention on the metabolic syndrome: the Diabetes Prevention Program randomized trial. Ann Intern Med 2005; 142(8):611–619.

50. Ross R, Janssen I, et al. Exercise-induced reduction in obesity and insulin resistance in women: a randomized controlled trial. Obes Res 2004; 12(5):789–798.

51. Giannopoulou I, Ploutz-Snyder LL, et al. Exercise is required for visceral fat loss in postmenopausal women with type 2 diabetes. J Clin Endocrinol Metab 2005; 90(3):1511–1518.

52. Howard BV. Insulin resistance and lipid metabolism. Am J Cardiol 1999; 84(1A):28J–32J.

53. Holmwood C, Philips P. Insulin and type 2 diabetes. Aust Fam Phys 1999; 28:429–435.

54. Yoshinaga H, Kosaka K. High glycosylated hemoglobin levels increase the risk of progression to diabetes mellitus in subjects with glucose intolerance. Diabetes Res Clin Pract 1996; 31(1–3):71–79.

55. Edelman SV. Importance of glucose control. Medical Clinic North America 1998; 82:665–687.

56. Skyller JS. Preface. Medical Clinic North America 1998; 82:xi–xii.

57. Popplewell P. Type 2 diabetes and cardiovascular disease. Mod Med Aust 1995; 38:92–102.

58. Ruhnau KJ, Meissner HP, et al. Effects of 3-week oral treatment with the antioxidant thioctic acid (alpha-lipoic acid) in symptomatic diabetic polyneuropathy. Diabet Med 1999; 16(12):1040–1043.

59. Sima AA, Calvani M, et al; Acetyl-L-Carnitine Study Group. Acetyl-L-carnitine improves pain, nerve regeneration, and vibratory perception in patients with chronic diabetic neuropathy: an analysis of two randomized placebo-controlled trials. Diabetes Care 2005; 28(1):89–94.

60. Peters AL, Davidson MB, et al. A clinical approach for the diagnosis of diabetes mellitus: an analysis using glycosylated hemoglobin levels. JAMA 1996; 276(15):1246–1252.

61. Grylls WK, McKenzie JE, et al. Lifestyle factors associated with glycaemic control and body mass index in older adults with diabetes. Eur J Clin Nutr 2003; 57(11):1386–1393.

62. Moore H, Summerbell C, et al. Dietary advice for treatment of type 2 diabetes mellitus in adults. Cochrane Database Syst Rev 2004; (3):CD004097.

63. Woerle HJ, Pimenta WP, et al. Diagnostic and therapeutic implications of relationships between fasting, 2-hour postchallenge plasma glucose and hemoglobin A1c values. Arch Intern Med 2004; 164(15):1627–1632.

PATIENT HANDOUT 14.1 – PREVENTING DIABETES: THE LIFESTYLE CHOICES

You can reduce your risk of developing diabetes by:

- maintaining a BMI <25
- losing weight if you are overweight—losing 4.5 kg can reduce your risk by 30%
- exercising
- eating fish in preference to meat
- choosing a low fat diet rich in monounsaturated fat, e.g.
  - —olive or canola oil
  - —avocado, mustard seeds
  - —almonds, pecans, almonds, macadamias, pistachios, hazelnuts, cashews
- eating lots of fruit and vegetables
- favouring soluble fibre, e.g. legumes, oatmeal
- selecting foods with a low glycaemic index, e.g. legumes, pasta, wholegrain bread
- using less than 1.5 teaspoons of salt a day
- limiting alcohol to one standard drink daily, and only with meals
- being a non-smoker.

The complications of diabetes can be minimized by early diagnosis and effective treatment.

Diabetes is diagnosed by testing for glucose in the blood—persons at risk of diabetes should ask for a fasting and 2 hour oral glucose tolerance blood test.

You are at increased risk of developing diabetes if you:

- ☐ have a family history of diabetes
- ☐ belong to a high risk ethnic group e.g. Aboriginal, Polynesian, Indian, Maltese
- ☐ are over 65 years of age
- ☐ had a low foetal birth weight
- ☐ are overweight (BMI 28 or greater)
- ☐ gained over 5 kg since the age of 18 years
- ☐ have an abdominal girth >80 cm female/ 94 cm male
- ☐ have a waist–hip ratio >1.0 in males; >0.9 in females
- ☐ lead a sedentary lifestyle, especially if you are over 45 years of age
- ☐ eat a high fat diet
- ☐ are a smoker
- ☐ are a woman, especially if you gave birth to babies of 4.5 kg or more.

The more boxes you ticked the greater your risk.

To avoid having undiagnosed diabetes, ask your doctor to check your blood sugar if you:

- are over 45 years of age, especially if you are overweight
- are always thirsty and wanting a drink
- frequently pass urine
- have unexplained weight loss
- have recurrent blurred vision
- are extremely tired
- have recurrent infections.

PATIENT HANDOUT 14.2 – AVOIDING COMPLICATIONS: SELF-CARE FOR DIABETICS

Your risk of developing complications from diabetes is increased if you/your:

- blood glucose level is poorly controlled
- have protein in your urine—microalbuminuria 21 μg/mL or greater)
- are depressed
- are over 50 years of age
- have had diabetes for 5 years or longer
- have hyperlipidaemia
- have hypertension: blood pressure exceeds 140/90 mmHg
- have lost or decreased Achilles tendon reflexes
- drink more than 60 g of alcohol daily
- are pregnant
- are obese (BMI 30 or more)
- are tall.

Complications may already be present if you have:

- numbness in the hands and feet
- pins and needles (sensory neuropathy)
- muscle cramps, weakness or wasting
- foot drop
- cranial nerve palsy
- dizziness, diarrhoea/constipation, impotence (autonomic neuropathy).

Better blood sugar control is necessary. Consult your doctor.

PATIENT HANDOUT 14.3 – FOOT CARE FOR DIABETICS

Aim to improve circulation by:

- exercising to encourage the development of collateral circulation. Walking at least three times per week for 30 or more minutes until near maximum pain level is reached is recommended.
- taking nutritional supplements such as one or more of the following:
  - vitamin E 300–1600 IU/day for at least 3 months
  - niacin 100–300 mg/day (relief appears to be temporary)
  - a-tocopheryl-nicotinate 200 mg tds
  - garlic 800 mg/day.

Avoid damage to the feet by:
- Using the services of a careful podiatrist.
- Good daily foot care, including
  - □ washing feet in lukewarm water using a mild soap
  - □ blotting feet dry with a soft towel; remember to dry between the toes
  - □ applying lotions/creams to keep feet soft
  - □ cutting toenails straight
  - □ keeping sweaty feet dry by dusting with powder
  - □ keeping bedclothes loose around your feet at night
  - □ washing foot injuries carefully before applying antibiotic ointment
  - □ leaving blisters intact
  - □ switching socks and shoes more than once a day
  - □ don't soak your feet.

- Selecting footwear with care
  - □ wear socks with shoes
  - □ select well-padded seamless socks 2.5 cm longer than your foot
  - □ buy new shoes late in the day when your feet are at their largest
  - □ only wear comfortable shoes and break in new shoes an hour at a time
  - □ wear good shoes when walking
  - □ choose shoes with
    - a well-cushioned heel, firm heel counter and padded Achilles tendon collar
    - a comfortable well fitted insole with an arch support
    - a flexible curved sole
    - a wide toe box
    - leather uppers or other breathable materials
    - a padded tongue and ankle collar
  - □ avoid going barefoot or wearing sandals or shoes with open toes.
- Checking for and getting professional care if you notice
  - □ redness, swelling
  - □ prolonged pain or tingling
  - □ wounds that don't heal
  - □ calluses or corns
  - □ any foot, ankle and leg ulcers, especially if they won't heal.

Internet resources

http://www.niapublications.org/engagepages/ footcare.asp

PATIENT HANDOUT 14.4 – TRAVEL TIPS FOR DIABETICS

When undertaking long haul travel:
- carry a personal identification kit with details of your condition
- be prepared to cope with blood sugar fluctuations
  - —carry sweets or glucose tablets to treat low blood glucose
  - —take snack pack foods such as cheese, biscuits, peanut butter
  - —carry insulin, syringes, needles and blood testing equipment for self-care
  - —include an extra battery or glucose meter on overseas trips
- stay hydrated: drink a lot of water or non-alcoholic decaffeinated low energy beverages on long air flights.

Internet resources

For general information on diabetes and resource addresses refer to:
http://www.niapublications.org/engagepages/diabetes.asp

Chapter 15

Hypertension

CHAPTER CONTENTS

An asymptomatic 55-year-old woman is found to have a blood pressure of 139/89 mmHg. Her general practitioner concluded she was at increased risk of cardiovascular disease and advised her to lose at least 4 kg to reduce her BMI below 25, to increase her fruit and vegetable intake, to avoid salt and to limit her alcohol intake to no more than nine standard drinks a week. He also suggested she walk for 1 hour on alternate days.

- Is this woman at risk of hypertension as she ages?
- Is lifestyle intervention justified at this stage?
- How may exercise influence her risk of hypertension?

INTRODUCTION

Persons who are normotensive at 55 years of age have a 90% lifetime risk of developing hypertension. Reduced cardiac, renal and hepatic reserves all contribute to the development and maintenance of hypertension in the elderly. Factors contributing to the prevalence of hypertension in elderly persons include:

- reduced cardiac output and myocardial reserve
- reduced aortic elasticity and baroreceptor sensitivity
- increased susceptibility to orthostatic hypotension
- increased peripheral resistance
- increased salt sensitivity
- increased plasma catecholamine levels with decreased B-adrenergic responsiveness.

MAKING A DIAGNOSIS

Blood pressure (BP) increases with age. Depending on the criteria used, 3 in 4 persons over 60 years of age may be deemed hypertensive. While a blood pressure of under 145/95 mmHg was previously considered 'normotensive' in the elderly, younger adults only fell into this category when their blood pressure was under 140/90 mmHg. The age-related rise in blood pressure is particularly steep for women. As the risk of cardiovascular disease starts to increase at 115/75 mmHg and doubles with each increment of 20/10 mmHg, a new definition of 'normotensive' is required.

The Seventh Report of the Joint National Committee on Prevention, Detection, Evaluation, and Treatment of High Blood Pressure[1] has redefined normal blood pressure as less than 120/80 mmHg and estimated that in the United States:[2]

- 41.9 million men and 27.8 million women over 20 years of age have prehypertension (120–139/80–89 mmHg)
- 12.8 million men and 12.2 million women over 20 years of age have stage 1 hypertension (140–159/90–99 mmHg)
- 4.1 million men and 6.9 million women over 20 years of age have stage 2 hypertension (≥160/100 mmHg).

Specific blood pressure levels determine the need for antihypertensive medications; however, lifestyle modifications are advisable for all, particularly those with 'prehypertension'.[3]

ISOLATED SYSTOLIC HYPERTENSION

Although diastolic BP reaches a plateau around the age of 40, systolic BP increases until 70 or 80 years of age and has emerged as a major independent risk factor in the elderly. The age-related rise in systolic blood pressure is primarily responsible for an increase in both incidence and prevalence of hypertension with increasing age.[1] A number of structural and functional changes contribute to the development of isolated systolic hypertension in elderly persons.[4] Intimal thickening, migration of small muscle cells to the intima, medial fibrosis and elastic fibre degeneration result in increased arterial stiffness. These structural changes are associated with overactivity of the sympathetic nervous system, reduced neuronal plasma norepinephrine uptake and baroreceptor dysfunction. An age-related increase of sodium sensitivity coupled with endothelial dysfunction leading to changes in aortic smooth muscle cells and collagen accumulation results in increased arterial stiffness and early wave reflections.[5] Elevated pulse pressure, a consequence of stiffening of the arterial wall, is a strong predictor of cardiovascular morbidity and mortality. In persons 60 years and older elevated pulse pressure is also associated with an impaired glomerular filtration rate.[6] Altered aortic properties associated with augmented wave reflection of arterial pressure are also related to orthostatic hypertension in the elderly.[7]

Isolated systolic hypertension is associated with impaired renal function, coronary and cerebrovascular morbidity and mortality. Blood pressure variability, common in hypertensive patients 60 years and older, is suspected to further aggravate this cardiovascular risk.[8] Fortunately, there is good evidence that lifestyle modifications such as weight reduction, increased physical activity, moderation of dietary sodium and decreased alcohol intake, in combination with pharmacological therapy can effectively reduce blood pressure in elderly individuals with isolated systolic hypertension.[4] Unfortunately, management of hypertension, and particularly its control among treated hypertensive patients, needs to be improved in elderly people.[9] Even blood pressure targets in the elderly remain controversial.[10]

Among patients who have not had a previous stroke or significant cardiovascular or renal disease, the benefits of reducing systolic blood pressure below 159 mmHg are well documented. However, if doing so either increases the day–night difference in blood pressure by more than 20% or leads to decline in diastolic blood pressure below 65 mmHg, then the benefits of treatment may be attenuated or lost. In addition, there is some suggestion that reducing systolic blood pressure consistently below 135 mmHg may accelerate cognitive decline. Midlife hypertension enhances cognitive impairment later in life, but at old age, mild hypertension may increase cognitive performance.[11] Perhaps, like osteoporosis prevention, blood pressure management should routinely be addressed in younger people. Maybe lifestyle intervention should be enthusiastically initiated in prehypertensive individuals who give systolic readings of 120–139 mmHg or diastolic pressures between 80 and 89 mmHg.[1]

Although control of established hypertension is less successful in the elderly, treatment dramatically reduces hypertension-related cardiovascular complications in this age group.[12] Clinical trials strongly support drug treatment of older persons with systolic pressure of 160 mmHg or greater.[13] The risks of cardiovascular, cerebrovascular, peripheral artery and end-stage renal disease are linearly related to systolic blood pressure, whereas successful lowering of systolic blood pressure effectively modulates these risks.[3]

MANAGEMENT

Management of hypertension initially relies on lifestyle measures. These may need to be complemented by drug therapy, depending on the blood pressure lowering response and the presence of target organ damage.

Lifestyle management

The major lifestyle modifications to reduce and manage blood pressure include weight management, dietary sodium reduction, physical activity and moderation of alcohol consumption.[1,10] The potential population impact of lifestyle measures should not be underestimated given that around 122 million Americans are overweight or obese, their mean sodium intake is approximately 4100 mg per day (men) and 2750 mg per day (women), less than 20% engage in regular physical activity and fewer than 1 in 4 consume five or more servings of fruits and vegetables daily.[1]

Implementation of self-management measures to correct unhealthy lifestyles has been shown to decrease systolic blood pressure by 5 mmHg and diastolic blood pressure by 4.3 mmHg.[14] Combinations of two or more lifestyle modifications achieve even better results. For overall cardiovascular risk reduction, patients should also be strongly counselled to quit smoking.

Body mass index (BMI)

BMI is positively associated with systolic, diastolic and mean arterial pressure. Although BMI has little effect on persons with a BMI of less than 19, systolic blood pressure increases with increasing BMI, even in persons falling within a 'normal' BMI range of 20–25.[15] The impact of BMI on blood pressure is greater in males than females, especially in those over 45 years of age. Other measures of adiposity also correlate with increases in blood pressure. One study found a 1 mmHg rise in systolic BP resulted if men increased their BMI by 1.7 kg/m^2, their waist circumference by 4.5 cm or their waist–hip ratio by 3.4%.[16] For women, corresponding figures were 1.25 kg/m^2, 2.5 cm and 1.8% respectively. Another study concluded that average blood pressure and the prevalence of hypertension stopped increasing when waist–hip ratio equalled or exceeded 0.76.[17] The authors suggested a waist–hip ratio equal to or greater than 0.80 could be used as a cut-off value for the prediction of hypertension risk. A third study concluded that compared to those with a waist circumference of less than 94 cm, males with a waist circumference equal to or greater than 102 cm were 3–5 times more likely to present with hypertension.[18] Compared to those with a waist circumference of less than 80 cm, females whose waist measured 88 cm or more had twice the risk for hypertension. In this study, age shows a significant relationship to hypertensive risk only in males aged 55 and females aged 50 years and over. Age, BMI and increments in BMI appear strong predictors for hypertension and increased systolic and diastolic BP in older women.[19] BMI and age appear to act synergistically in creating a strong association with hypertension.[15] Short term weight gain is associated with a predictable rise in arterial pressure and is a strong risk factor for developing hypertension in obese individuals.[20] However, even small weight losses are associated with improvement in blood pressure control—loss of as little as 4 or 5 kg may normalize blood pressure.[1] Currently the recommendation is to maintain a healthy body weight, i.e. a BMI of 18.5–24.9, and waist circumference under 102 cm if male or less than 88 cm if female.[21]

A plant rich diet

An Australian trial of overweight men found that for a comparable 5 kg weight loss, a diet high in low-fat dairy products, vegetables and fruit results in a greater decrease in BP than a low fat diet.[22] Energy is not the only dietary factor that influences blood pressure. In fact, a diet rich in fruits, vegetables and low-fat dairy foods with a low cholesterol, total and saturated fat content reduces systolic hypertension without associated weight loss.[23] The beneficial aspect of the Dietary Approaches to Stop Hypertension (DASH) diet may be its low saturated fat content (< 7%) or its relatively high potassium–sodium ratio. The current recommendation is to follow a reduced fat, low cholesterol diet with an adequate intake of potassium, magnesium and calcium and to restrict salt intake.[21]

Sodium restriction

Dietary guidelines for sodium are far in excess of any physiological need; furthermore, it is likely that harmful effects of sodium are expressed above a threshold of approximately 2300 mg sodium daily (about 100 mmol), roughly 1 teaspoon or 6 g of salt each day.[24] While a randomized controlled trial found that persons on 8.5 servings of fruit and vegetables each day had greater reduction in blood pressure than those on 3.6 serves a day,[25] sodium restriction has been shown to be more effective than increasing fruit and vegetable content.[26] A decrease of 6.3 mmHg in systolic and 2.2 mmHg in diastolic BP per 100 mmol decrease in daily sodium intake was observed in hypertensive people over 44 years of age. Sodium restriction is more effective in older persons![21]

Salt-sensitive persons demonstrate an increase in blood pressure and in body weight when switched from a low to a high sodium intake. Salt-sensitive hypertensive subjects exhibit alterations of autonomic cardiovascular control,[27] and appear to have an endothelial dysfunction characterized by defective endothelium dependent vasodilation due to impairment of the L-arginine-nitric oxide pathway.[28] Nitric oxide production is a homeostatic mechanism that may regulate BP during salt loading. The vascular endothelium plays a key role in the local regulation of vascular tone by the release of vasodilator substances such as nitric oxide and prostacyclin, and vasoconstrictor substances including thromboxane A2, free radicals or endothelin. Endothelial dysfunction is associated with impaired tissue perfusion, particularly during stress, and paradoxical vasoconstriction of large conduit vessels including the coronary arteries.[29] Endothelial dysfunction, especially of the nitric oxide system, is implicated in both experimental and clinical hypertension.[30]

Animal studies show endogenous nitric oxide plays an important role in renal haemodynamics and sodium homeostasis, inducing renal vasodilation and natriuresis. Endothelial nitric oxide, in addition to producing endothelium dependent vasodilation, has potent antiatherogenic properties, including inhibition of platelet aggregation and adhesion molecule expression.[31] Oxidative stress reduces the bioavailability of nitric oxide in the cardiovascular system, causing vasoconstriction and increasing BP.[32] Endothelial dysfunction appears to be reversible by administering L-arginine, the precursor of nitric oxide, lowering cholesterol levels, undertaking physical training and taking angiotensin converting enzyme (ACE) inhibitors or antioxidants such as vitamin C.[29]

Exercise

The shear stress of blood flow acting on the endothelium is responsible for flow-induced nitric oxide release. Regular exercise appears to enhance nitric oxide bioavailability as a result of both enhanced synthesis and reduced oxidative stress-mediated destruction. Exercise training is thought to target endothelial nitric oxide synthase and the antioxidant enzyme, superoxide dismutase.[33]

The extent of the improvement in humans depends upon the muscle mass subjected to training; forearm exercise produces local vasodilation but lower body training induces generalized benefit.[34] Short term training increases nitric oxide bioactivity which acts to homeostatically regulate the shear stress associated with exercise; prolonged training leads to nitric oxide dependent structural changes with arterial remodelling and structural normalization of shear.[34]

The current recommendation is to perform 30–60 minutes of aerobic exercise on 4–7 days of the week.[21] Furthermore, moderate intensity physical activity involving rhythmic movements of the lower limbs, as in brisk walking, appears to be more effective than vigorous exercise.

Alcohol limitation

While all agree exercise is beneficial, there is some disagreement regarding alcohol.[35,36] Nonetheless, observational studies and clinical experiments strongly suggest an empiric relationship between heavy drinking, i.e. 3 or more standard drinks (30 g) per day, and higher blood pressure.[36] Moreover, drinking outside meals appears to increase the risk of hypertension independent of the amount of alcohol consumed.[37] A reduction in alcohol consumption to no more than two standard drinks per day reduces the blood pressure of both hypertensive and normotensive people. A standard drink is 12 oz of beer, 5 oz of wine, or 1.5 oz of 80 proof liquor. In randomized clinical trials systolic and diastolic BP fell by approximately 1 mmHg for each daily drink not consumed.[38] Healthy adults who choose to drink should limit alcohol consumption to 2 or fewer standard drinks per day, with consumption not exceeding 14 standard drinks per week for men and 9 standard drinks per week for women.

Stress management

Although lacking the strong validation of the previously mentioned lifestyle measures, stress reduction may be helpful. Psychosocial stress is believed to contribute to high blood pressure. Data pooled from two randomized controlled trials suggest specific stress-decreasing approaches such as transcendental meditation may contribute to decreased mortality from all causes and from cardiovascular disease in older hypertensive subjects.[39]

DRUG THERAPY

Drug therapy should always be combined with lifestyle modification. Most patients with hypertension require two or more antihypertensive medications to reach a satisfactory blood pressure goal. For patients with uncomplicated hypertension a reputable BP target is less than 140/90 mmHg. In patients with diabetes or chronic kidney disease, the goal may be lower—below 130/80 mmHg.

Thiazide diuretics are the mainstay of treatment. Agents appropriate for first line therapy of diastolic hypertension include, amongst others, thiazide diuretics, beta-blockers, ACE inhibitors, long-acting calcium channel blockers and angiotensin receptor antagonists.[1,21] Globally, the efficacy of the major classes of antihypertensive drugs appears roughly equivalent.[40] Consequently, therapeutic choice is largely governed by the type of hypertension, systolic or systolic–diastolic, the rapidity of the desired effect, drug tolerance and the presence of comorbid conditions, particularly coronary or renal disease.[40] In systolic hypertension, thiazide diuretics and long-acting calcium channel blockers are considered first line therapy.[13]

It is worth noting that population mortality trends for stroke paralleled those for hypertension control.[41]

LOOKING AHEAD

An ideal body weight, a diet rich in plant foods and low in salt and alcohol, along with exercise, are proven lifestyle measures for preventing and controlling blood pressure. Introduction of these measures in normotensive adults may reduce the need for drug therapy at a later date. Furthermore, increased understanding of the role of endothelial dysfunction in raising BP may offer novel nutraceutical approaches to blood pressure management. Any combination of these measures, with the assistance of pharmaceuticals, may be used to prevent, delay the onset of, reduce severity and more effectively control hypertension.[42]

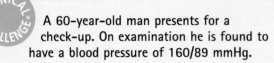

A 60-year-old man presents for a check-up. On examination he is found to have a blood pressure of 160/89 mmHg.

Questions arising

■ Does this patient require treatment for hypertension?
■ How could this patient be counselled?
■ Are any special investigations warranted?

Clinical considerations

The patient has systolic hypertension and, in the absence of active intervention, the condition is likely to worsen as he ages:

■ Lifestyle intervention is recommended, see Patient Handout15.1.
■ Thiazide diuretics and/or long-acting calcium channel blockers should be considered.
■ As peripheral, cardio- and cerebrovascular disease and renal failure are linearly related to systolic blood pressure, this patient should be investigated for evidence of renal disease e.g. albuminuria, cardiac ischaemia (ECG), and risk of atherosclerosis including LDL and HDL cholesterol levels.

A 72-year-old female presents for her annual check-up. You notice that she seems unusually clumsy when getting onto the treatment table. On examination you find she has elevated blood pressure and you detect some weakness of the left leg.

She reports she has recently had episodes of clumsiness, dizziness and weakness previously. She says it doesn't last long.

Questions arising

■ What working diagnosis comes to mind?
■ What clinical findings would you particularly wish to explore/exclude in this patient?

Clinical considerations

Transient ischaemic attack needs to be considered.

Other symptoms suggestive of the problem include:

■ slurred speech
■ an unsteady gait
■ difficulty swallowing
■ an altered or loss of sensation or weakness of a single limb on one side of the body or face or bilaterally
■ a loss of vision in one eye or half or the whole of the visual field in both eyes
■ dizziness
■ difficulty with the expression or understanding of verbal or written language.

◆ All elderly persons are at increased risk of hypertension.
◆ Aortic stiffness is an independent predictor of progression to hypertension in non-hypertensive subjects.
◆ Systolic BP over 140 mmHg presents a greater risk of cardiovascular disease than raised diastolic BP in persons over 50 years of age.
◆ Lifestyle intervention to prevent cardiovascular disease is recommended for persons with a systolic pressure between 120 and 139 mmHg or a diastolic blood pressure of 80–89 mmHg.

◆ Lifestyle modification combined with drug therapy should be considered once BP exceeds 140/90 mmHg.
◆ Thiazide-type diuretics are the drug treatment of choice in most cases of uncomplicated hypertension.
◆ A thiazide-type diuretic plus another drug is usually required to control BP that exceeds the recommended goal by 20/10 mmHg or more.
◆ Endothelial dysfunction, a risk factor for hypertension, may be improved by reducing oxidative stress and promoting nitric oxide synthesis.

References

1. Chobanian AV, Bakris GL, et al. The Seventh Report of the Joint National Committee on Prevention, Detection, Evaluation, and Treatment of High Blood Pressure: the JNC 7 report. JAMA 2003; 289(19):2560–2572.

2. Qureshi AI, Suri MF, et al. Prevalence and trends of prehypertension and hypertension in United States: National Health and Nutrition Examination Surveys 1976 to 2000. Med Sci Monit 2005; 11(9):CR403–409.

3. Lackland DT. Population strategies to treat hypertension. Curr Treat Options Cardiovasc Med 2005; 7(4):253–258.

4. Wong J, Wong S. Evidence-based care for the elderly with isolated systolic hypertension. Nurs Health Sci 2005; 7(1):67–75.

5. Safar ME. Systolic hypertension in the elderly: arterial wall mechanical properties and the renin-angiotensin-aldosterone system. J Hypertens 2005; 23(4):673–681.

6. Verhave JC, Fesler P, et al. Elevated pulse pressure is associated with low renal function in elderly patients with isolated systolic hypertension. Hypertension 2005; 45(4):586–591.

7. Hoshide S, Kario K, et al. Altered aortic properties in elderly orthostatic hypertension. Hypertens Res 2005; 28(1):15–19.

8. Eto M, Toba K, et al. Impact of blood pressure variability on cardiovascular events in elderly patients with hypertension. Hypertens Res 2005; 28(1):1–7.

9. Brindel P, Hanon O, et al; 3C Study Investigators. Prevalence, awareness, treatment, and control of hypertension in the elderly: the Three City study. J Hypertens 2006; 24(1):51–58.

10. Maddens M, Imam K, Ashkar A. Hypertension in the elderly. Prim Care 2005; 32(3):723–753.

11. Anson O, Paran E. Hypertension and cognitive functioning among the elderly: an overview. Am J Ther 2005; 12(4):359–365.

12. Lackland DT, Egan BM. The dominant role of systolic hypertension as a vascular risk factor: evidence from the southeastern United States. Am J Med Sci 1999; 318(6):365–368.

13. Chaudhry SI, Krumholz HM, Foody JM. Systolic hypertension in older persons. JAMA 2004; 292(9):1074–1080.

14. Chodosh J, Morton SC, et al. Meta-analysis: chronic disease self-management programs for older adults. Ann Intern Med 2005; 143(6):427–438.

15. Mufunda J, Mebrahtu G, et al. The prevalence of hypertension and its relationship with obesity: results from a national blood pressure survey in Eritrea. J Hum Hypertens 2006; 20(1):59–65.

16. Doll S, Paccaud F, et al. Body mass index, abdominal adiposity and blood pressure: consistency of their association across developing and developed countries. Int J Obes Relat Metab Disord 2002; 26(1):48–57.

17. Zhao WH, Xu HQ, et al. The association of BMI and WHR on blood pressure levels and prevalence of hypertension in middle-aged and elderly people in rural China. Biomed Environ Sci 2000; 13(3):189–197.

18. Guagnano MT, Ballone E, et al. Large waist circumference and risk of hypertension. Int J Obes Relat Metab Disord 2001; 25(9):1360–1364.

19. Kristjansson K, Sigurdsson JA, et al. Blood pressure and pulse pressure development in a population sample of women with special reference to basal body mass and distribution of body fat and their changes during 24 years. Int J Obes Relat Metab Disord 2003; 27(1):128–133.

20. Schulz M, Liese AD, et al. Associations of short-term weight changes and weight cycling with incidence of essential hypertension in the EPIC-Potsdam Study. J Hum Hypertens 2005; 19(1):61–67.

21. Khan NA, McAlister FA, et al. The 2005 Canadian Hypertension Education Program recommendations for the management of hypertension: part II—therapy. Can J Cardiol 2005; 21(8):657–672.

22. Nowson CA, Worsley A, et al. Blood pressure change with weight loss is affected by diet type in men. Am J Clin Nutr 2005; 81(5):983–989.

23. Svetkey LP, Simons-Morton D, et al. Effects of dietary patterns on blood pressure: subgroup analysis of the Dietary Approaches to Stop Hypertension (DASH) randomized clinical trial. Arch Intern Med 1999; 159(3):285–293.

24. Kaplan NM. The dietary guideline for sodium: should we shake it up? No. Am J Clin Nutr 2000; 71(5):1020–1026.

25. Appel LJ, Moore TJ, et al. A clinical trial of the effects of dietary patterns on blood pressure. DASH Collaborative Research Group. N Engl J Med 1997; 336(16):1117–1124.

26. Delichatsios HK, Welty FK. Influence of the DASH Diet and other low-fat, high-carbohydrate diets on blood pressure. Curr Atheroscler Rep 2005; 7(6):446–454.

27. Coruzzi P, Parati G, et al. Effects of salt sensitivity on neural cardiovascular regulation in essential

hypertension. Hypertension 2005 Oct 24; [Epub ahead of print].

28. Bragulat E, de la Sierra A, et al. Endothelial dysfunction in salt-sensitive essential hypertension. Hypertension 2001; 37(2 Part 2):444–448.

29. Drexler H, Hornig B. Endothelial dysfunction in human disease. J Mol Cell Cardiol 1999; 31(1):51–60.

30. Bragulat E, de la Sierra A. Salt intake, endothelial dysfunction, and salt-sensitive hypertension. J Clin Hypertens (Greenwich) 2002; 4(1):41–46.

31. Landmesser U, Harrison DG, Drexler H. Oxidant stress-a major cause of reduced endothelial nitric oxide availability in cardiovascular disease. Eur J Clin Pharmacol 2005 Oct 12;1–7 [Epub ahead of print].

32. Malinski T. Understanding nitric oxide physiology in the heart: a nanomedical approach. Am J Cardiol 2005; 96(7B):13–24.

33. Rush JW, Denniss SG, et al. Vascular nitric oxide and oxidative stress: determinants of endothelial adaptations to cardiovascular disease and to physical activity. Can J Appl Physiol 2005; 30(4):442–474.

34. Green DJ, Maiorana A, et al. Effect of exercise training on endothelium-derived nitric oxide function in humans. J Physiol 2004; 561(Pt 1):1–25.

35. Lip GY, Beevers DG. Alcohol and cardiovascular disease—more than one paradox to consider. Alcohol and hypertension—does it matter? (no!). J Cardiovasc Risk 2003; 10(1):11–14.

36. Klatsky AL. Alcohol and cardiovascular disease—more than one paradox to consider. Alcohol and hypertension: does it matter? Yes. J Cardiovasc Risk 2003; 10(1):21–24.

37. Stranges S, Wu T, et al. Relationship of alcohol drinking pattern to risk of hypertension: a population-based study. Hypertension 2004; 44(6):813–819.

38. Cushman WC. Alcohol consumption and hypertension. J Clin Hypertens (Greenwich) 2001; 3(3):166–170.

39. Schneider RH, Alexander CN, et al. Long-term effects of stress reduction on mortality in persons > or = 55 years of age with systemic hypertension. Am J Cardiol 2005; 95(9):1060–1064.

40. Blickle J. Management of hypertension in elderly diabetic patients. Diabetes Metab 2005; 31 Spec No 2:82–91.

41. Luepker RV, Arnett DK, et al. Trends in blood pressure, hypertension control, and stroke mortality: the Minnesota Heart Survey. Am J Med 2006; 119(1):42–49.

42. Houston MC. Nutraceuticals, vitamins, antioxidants, and minerals in the prevention and treatment of hypertension. Prog Cardiovasc Dis 2005; 47(6):396–449.

PATIENT HANDOUT 15.1 – PREVENTING HYPERTENSION: THE LIFESTYLE CHOICES

The older you are the greater your risk of hypertension. Hypertension is a risk factor for coronary heart disease, stroke, congestive heart failure and renal disease.
Lowering blood pressure levels reduces this risk.

The risk of cardiovascular disease starts to increase once blood pressure exceeds 115/75 mmHg and doubles with each increment of 20/10 mmHg. If your blood pressure exceeds 120/80 mmHg you are likely to benefit from adopting protective lifestyle measures.

Protective lifestyle measures are to:

- Maintain an ideal body weight
- Restrict salt intake
- Limit alcohol consumption
- Take regular exercise
- Not smoke.

Maintain an ideal body weight

Aim for:

- BMI = 18.5–24.9. The lower the better!
- Waist circumference < 102 cm in males; < 88 cm in females.

See Patient Handouts 12.1–12.4.

Note: A diet rich in fruit and vegetables (>8 serves per day!) and low in saturated fat and cholesterol is best!

Restrict salt intake

Limit sodium intake to 1 teaspoon or 6 g of salt each day.
To achieve this you need to:

- Avoid processed foods and restrict processed foods to lower sodium varieties. Always read the Nutrition Facts Label and choose foods lower in sodium. Consume milk and yogurt (less sodium and more potassium) in preference to cheese.
- Never add salt in cooking or at the table. Use spices, herbs and lemon juice to enhance flavour. Avoid condiments e.g. soy, sauces, pickles, olives, excess ketchup, mustard.
- Choose fresh foods.

Limit alcohol consumption

- More than 20 g of alcohol per day increases blood pressure.
- Men should have 2 or fewer standard drinks per day and not more than 14 standard drinks per week.
- Women should have 2 or fewer standard drinks per day and not more than 9 standard drinks per week.

Take regular exercise

Do moderate intensity aerobic exercise e.g. brisk walking or swimming, for 30 minutes daily or 60 minutes on alternate days.

Doing rhythmic activity that involves the lower limbs benefits the whole body—arm exercises only benefit the arms!

Internet resources

http://www.niapublications.org/engagepages/hiblood.asp
hypertension

http://www.niapublications.org/engagepages/stroke.asp
stroke

http://www.agingwell.state.ny.us/selfcare/articles/high_hp.htm
tips for controlling blood pressure

Chapter 16

Coronary heart disease

CHAPTER CONTENTS

A 59-year-old man presents for a check-up. You note he is overweight, has slightly raised blood pressure and has high total cholesterol and low HDL-cholesterol. He smokes 15 cigarettes a day.

- Is the man at increased risk of a heart attack?
- What other information would be helpful in determining his risk?
- What measures could be taken to reduce his risk of a heart attack?

INTRODUCTION

In 1995, Americans 65 years of age and older comprised 13% of the population but accounted for 35% of total personal health care dollars spent—heart disease was responsible for most deaths in this age group.[1] A review of the scientific literature to assess the importance of cardiovascular preventive measures concluded smoking cessation, regular physical activity and healthy diet were appropriate and effective measures and urged active implementation of these measures in persons 65 years of age and older.[2] A UK study found that mortality rates for coronary heart disease (CHD) fell by 54% between 1981 and 2000.[3] During this time overall smoking prevalence declined by 35%, total cholesterol concentrations fell by 4.2% and mean population blood pressure fell by 7.7%. Approximately 45 370 fewer deaths were attributable to reductions in these major risk factors, some 81% occurring in people without recognized heart disease and 19% in patients with coronary artery disease. Compared with secondary prevention, primary prevention achieved a fourfold larger reduction in deaths.[3]

RECOGNIZING RISK

In addition to increasing age and family history, traditionally the major risk factors for ischaemic heart disease are smoking, hypertension and hypercholesterolaemia.

Smoking

Nicotine adversely affects lipids, blood coagulation and vascular stability. Males who are current smokers are 2.9 times more likely than non-smokers to have a first myocardial infarct or fatal heart attack; women are 3.5 times more likely. Current male smokers with hypertension are 4.5 times more likely, and current female smokers are 7.9 times more likely, to have a heart attack than non-smokers.[4] Giving up smoking can halve the risk of dying in 5–10 years. Women who stop smoking reduce their excess risk of coronary heart disease by one quarter to one third within 2 years and approximate the risk of those who have never smoked in 10–14 years.[5] Smoking cessation translates into a reduction in overall mortality and morbidity rates at least equal to that of other preventive measures such as aspirin or beta-blocker therapy.[6]

Hyperlipidaemia

Clinical trials of lipid modification by diet and different drugs have also provided convincing evidence that the risk of CHD associated with rising cholesterol can be substantially reduced.[7] While it remains controversial whether the correlation between lipid abnormality and CHD becomes weaker in the elderly, it has been shown that high total and LDL cholesterol levels correlate with a high risk of cardiac ischaemia even in people over 80 years of age.[8] Recent studies have confirmed that lowering LDL cholesterol levels to below 100 mg/dL substantially reduces CHD mortality and non-fatal myocardial infarction rates even in older patients over 75 years of age.[6] Minimal intervention targets are a total cholesterol consistently below 5 mmol/L (190 mg/dL) and an LDL cholesterol below 3 mmol/L (115 mg/dL). For high risk individuals the intervention goal is even lower levels. Concentrations of HDL cholesterol <1.0 mmol/L (40 mg/dL) in men and <1.2 mmol/l (46mg/dL) in women are considered markers of increased CHD risk, as are fasting triglycerides >1.7 mmol/L (150 mg/dL).

Hypertension

Hypertension is the second most prevalent chronic condition in persons over 65 years of age. Hypertension, which manifests mostly as isolated systolic blood pressure elevation in the elderly, should be treated aggressively. In both cohort studies and clinical trials, coronary artery disease risk differences associated with a given blood pressure increase with age. For those 60–69 years of age, a 10 mmHg lower systolic blood pressure is associated with about one fifth lower risk of a CHD event.[9] Conventional medical therapies for hypertension (e.g. diuretics, beta blockers) and newer agents (e.g. calcium channel blockers, angiotensin-converting enzyme inhibitors), together with sodium restriction, have had a positive effect on cardiovascular mortality and morbidity rates in older patients.[6] In some cases lifestyle measures alone may achieve the minimal therapeutic goal of a blood pressure level consistently less than 140/90 mmHg.[7] In fact, 30 minutes of dynamic exercise 3–4 times a week lowers raised BP as effectively as increasing the dietary intake of potassium.[10] In other cases of sustained systolic BP >180 mmHg and/or a diastolic BP >100 mmHg, drug intervention is required. Furthermore, as the strong association between blood pressure and a heart attack is continuous down to levels of at least 115 mmHg systolic, considerable benefit is likely with lowering blood pressure below traditional hypertension thresholds.[9] The presence of multiple risk factors also lowers the blood pressure threshold at which lifestyle intervention needs to be complemented with drug intervention.

The metabolic syndrome

The metabolic syndrome is recognized as a risk factor for CHD. Sarcopenia increases the predilection of elderly persons to the metabolic syndrome.[11] Detectable as early as the fourth decade, loss of muscle mass coupled with decreased physical activity reduces the resting metabolic rate and increases the prevalence of the metabolic syndrome in the elderly. The metabolic syndrome predicts future CHD in hypercholesterolaemic men and in any person with essential hypertension without a history of cardiovascular disease. Diagnosed when at least three of abdominal obesity (or BMI >30), hypertension, high fasting glucose, high triglycerides or reduced levels of HDL cholesterol are present, the metabolic syndrome has emerged as an independent predictor of both cardiac and cerebrovascular events.[12] A combination of hypertension and the metabolic syndrome appears to amplify cardiovascular risk.

Other risks

In addition to the more traditional risk factors for coronary artery disease, low vitamin E, high fibrinogen and plasma S-adenosylhomocysteine have all been recognized as important predictors of CHD. Another risk factor that has been observed to be associated with an increased risk for coronary heart disease incident, mortality and a poor prognosis is sympathovagal imbalance.[13] Autonomic dysfunction, as indicated by a reduced heart rate variability, increases with age. Adverse psychosocial factors such as anxiety and hostility also appear associated with a reduced heart rate variability.[14]

PRIMARY PREVENTION

Lifestyle modification, focusing on diet, exercise, maintaining a healthy body weight and avoiding smoking, constitutes the first step in risk reduction for old and young alike.

Dietary options

Recent American Heart Association guidelines place greater emphasis on recommendations about food and food groups and less on advice about nutrients and the percentage of energy that they provide.[15] A significant inverse association between fruit and vegetable intake and the risk of cardiovascular disease, including myocardial infarction has been detected.[16,17] The risk of CHD is about 15% lower in persons eating four times more fruit and double the amount of vegetables. Similarly, subjects consuming relatively large amounts of whole grain cereals have significantly lower rates of CHD.[18] Three generally effective dietary strategies for preventing CHD have emerged. These are to substitute non-hydrogenated unsaturated fats for saturated and trans fats, to increase consumption of omega-3 fatty acids from fish, fish oil supplements or plant sources, and to consume a diet low in refined grain products and high in fruits, vegetables, nuts and whole grains.[19]

Dietary patterns

The major dietary patterns derived from the food frequency questionnaires appear to predict the risk of heart disease, independent of other lifestyle variables.[20] A 12-year follow-up study found a 'prudent' diet, characterized by higher consumption of vegetables, fruit, fish, poultry and whole grains, reduced the risk of CHD compared to the 'Western' diet, characterized by higher consumption of red meat, processed meat, French fries, high fat dairy products, refined grains, sweets and desserts.[20] Coincidentally, the prudent diet is rich in n-3 fatty acids, antioxidant vitamins (especially vitamins E and C), folic acid and L-arginine—all dietary factors emerging as important modulators of endothelial function.[21]

Consideration has also been given to the five food groups. An epidemiological study found the relative risk of mortality in men and women consuming two or fewer food groups was 1.5 and 1.4 respectively.[22] In addition to eating from all five food groups, one food group deserves particular mention.

Selecting fats

Restricting fat to 30% of total energy intake has long been advocated; however, simply lowering the percentage of energy from fat does not suffice. The quantity and quality of fat is relevant. Particular attention needs to be paid to limiting the intake of saturated and trans unsaturated fatty acids to less than 8% of total energy and permitting greater flexibility in eating more appropriate fat sources, namely polyunsaturated and cis-monounsaturated fatty acids.[7]

Increasing energy consumed as saturated fats by 1% elevates serum cholesterol levels by around 2.7 mg/dL. Trans fatty acids, which increase LDL and lower HDL cholesterol levels, appear to carry an even greater risk. The effect of trans fatty acids on total cholesterols is double that of saturated fatty acids![23] The intake of trans fats increases the risk of heart disease by over 1.3-fold comparing those with highest and lowest intakes.[24] Trans fats may also have other adverse effects on thrombogenesis and Lp(a) lipoprotein levels, high blood levels of which have been independently linked with an increased risk of CHD.[24]

Because processing increases saturation and the concentration of trans fats, cold pressed vegetable oils are a better source of fats than processed spreadable fats. Because fish is a richer source of polyunsaturated fat, it is considered a healthier option than meat. Fish is rich in long chain omega-3 fatty acids. However, it appears uncertain whether omega-3 fats, whether from fish, plant or supplemental sources, do indeed alter total mortality, combined cardiovascular events or cancers in people whether or not at high risk of cardiovascular disease.[25] This stance is not supported by another review which suggested omega-3 polyunsaturated fatty acids from seafood or plant sources may reduce the risk and recurrence of CHD events, possibly by influencing platelet function, inflammation, endothelial cell function, arterial compliance, and arrhythmia.[26] Daily dietary consumption of 2–3 g of alpha-linolenic acid is recommended as an alternative to fish for primary and secondary prevention of CHD. Alpha-linolenic acid is the omega-3 polyunsaturated fatty acid found mainly in plants, including flaxseed oil, canola oil, and walnuts.

Monounsaturated fats, plentiful in olive oil and avocados, provide another acceptable fat source. An inverse association between intake of monounsaturated fatty acids and death from CHD has been noted.[27] Oleic acid exerts significant protection against atherosclerosis and thrombosis.

Exercise

Exercise provides another lifestyle measure that influences cardiovascular risk. Compared with active persons, sedentary men almost quadruple their risk of dying from cardiovascular disease.[28] A decade of regular exercise training by older adults has been shown to reduce the likelihood of developing metabolic risk factors for cardiovascular disease.[29]

Whether the exercise-induced reduction in cardiovascular risk is attributable to increased fitness or associated weight loss is unclear.[30,31] Central fat mass is associated with atherogenic tendencies while peripheral fat seems to exhibit an independent dominant antiatherogenic effect.[32] A change in body composition, attributable to moderate intensity aerobic exercise training reducing abdominal fat in middle aged and older men, provides a plausible explanation for the cardiovascular benefits detected.[33] Certainly, localization of fat mass in elderly women is apparently more important for atherosclerosis than obesity per se.

Exercise also affects other risk factors. Thirty minutes of dynamic exercise 3–4 times a week lowers raised blood pressure as effectively as increasing the dietary intake of potassium.[34] A study of obese, sedentary, hypertensive middle aged men found 6 months of aerobic exercise training plus weight loss substantially lowered blood pressure and improved glucose and lipid metabolism.[35] Another study found total physical activity of at least 2.5 hours weekly reduced the prevalence of both insulin resistance and dyslipidaemia in both sexes, and reduced the prevalence of both obesity and hypertension in women.[36]

A word of caution. It does appear that while physical activity during leisure is beneficial, workplace activity may not be protective.[37] Regardless of the mechanism or mechanisms involved, exercise has undisputedly been shown to enhance cardiovascular health in older persons.

TARGETING SPECIFIC RISKS

The pathogenesis of a heart attack may involve two discrete processes.[5] Risk factors strongly related to the arterial wall inflammation that underlies atheromatous plaque formation include vessel shear associated with hypertension and vessel wall infiltration by denatured cholesterol. Risk factors strongly related to the critical event precipitated by vascular occlusion are smoking causing vasospasm and thrombosis associated with a hypercoagulable state.

Targeting cholesterol

Both the concentration and the redox state of cholesterol are relevant.

Much emphasis has been placed on the adverse impact of saturated fats and the potential benefits of mono- and polyunsaturated dietary fats on blood cholesterol levels, yet the concentration of dietary cholesterol also influences risk. While shellfish are a rich source of cholesterol and their intake should be limited, eggs provide more of a conundrum. Despite health authorities having traditionally recommended that eggs be limited, the relationship between heart disease and egg intake remains obscure. The yolk of a single egg contains about 210 mg of cholesterol, i.e. 70% of the daily cholesterol permitted. Nevertheless, people eating 4 or more eggs each week had significantly lower mean serum cholesterol concentration than those who reported eating no more than one egg weekly![38] Furthermore, in addition to dietary cholesterol only increasing plasma cholesterol in around

3 in 10 people, egg intake may be protective in that it increases the concentration of HDL cholesterol and, although increasing LDL circulating levels, shifts individuals from the LDL pattern B to the less atherogenic pattern A.[39]

HDL cholesterol is protective, improving endothelial function, inhibiting endothelium induced cytokines and enhancing vasodilation. Taking 900 mg/day garlic over 12 weeks reduced total cholesterol by over 11%— and it did this without reducing HDL.[40] Supplementation with n-3 fatty acids and isoflavones has also been shown to raise HDL cholesterol.[41,42] Fruit is rich in pectin and pectin enhances faecal excretion of bile acids and cholesterol. Eating 400 g of apples a day lower blood cholesterol by up to 11%; eating 200 g of fresh carrots daily achieves an 11% drop, 0.5–1 kg of guava a day an 8% drop and 100 g/day of prunes a 5% decline.[43] Whole fruits rather than juices are recommended. Indeed, care must be exercised in choosing a diet rich in carbohydrate.

For every 15 unit increase in the glycaemic index , the HDL concentration drops by 0.06 mmol/L.[44] Dietary choices rich in simple sugars, e.g. bread, pasta, cornflakes, potato, bananas, honey and fruit juice, create a high glycaemic load and should be limited. Dietary choices with a low glycaemic index, e.g. apples, peaches, legumes, barley, oat bran cereals, milk and yogurt are preferable options. Four weeks of consuming 35–50 g daily of oat bran, plus a fat modified diet with caloric restriction, reduced total cholesterol and LDL cholesterol levels in overweight hypercholesterolaemic men.[45]

In addition to the amount of dietary cholesterol consumed, consideration needs to be given to the nature of the cholesterol eaten. Eating hard boiled eggs with denatured cholesterol may be hazardous, but drinking an eggnog may be beneficial. Oxidized, but not native, LDL inhibits macrophage migration, attracts circulating monocytes, appears to be cytotoxic to endothelial cells and may enhance arterial vasoconstriction. Several dietary choices can reduce oxidation of LDL cholesterol. These include drinking red wine, eating garlic and increasing fruits and vegetables rich in Beta-carotene and vitamins E and C. Not only does a dietary change that increases plant foods increase plasma antioxidants, it also reduces both systolic and diastolic blood pressure.[46]

A successful cholesterol modulating regime provides 1 g EPA/DHA taken four times daily accompanied by a daily dose of 3 g garlic, 2 tablespoons psyllium, 2 tablespoons lecithin and 4 teaspoons of plant sterol margarine and includes a general antioxidant.[47] However, despite the belief that antioxidant supplements can prevent heart disease, the most prudent current recommendation for the general public is to obtain antioxidants from fruits, vegetables and whole grains.[48]

Targeting hypertension

BMI correlates strongly with systolic blood pressure. Compared to those with a BMI of 19, a BMI of 29 increases the risk of hypertension 3.9 times. Weight loss reduces blood pressure.

Salt intake also has a direct vascular effect and as its effects on blood pressure are not diminished by weight loss, weight loss and sodium restriction appear independently beneficial.[49] The reduction of daily sodium intake to 1.5 g rather than the currently recommended 2.4 g (100 mmol) combined with a diet which emphasizes fruit, vegetables and low fat dairy foods (DASH) substantially lowered blood pressure in both normotensive (systolic dropped 7.1 mmHg) and hypertensive (systolic decreased 11.5 mmHg) participants.[50] The high potassium and calcium content of the DASH diet also confers benefit. For a comparable 5 kg weight loss, a diet high in low fat dairy products, vegetables and fruit produces a greater decrease in blood pressure than does a diet that merely emphasizes a low fat intake.[51]

Another dietary consideration is alcohol. Women consuming 1–14 units weekly had a reduction in CHD, but there was an increased prevalence of hypertension among those consuming 15 or more units/week.[52] It would seem prudent for women to restrict their alcohol consumption to 14 units/week or less.

Avoiding the critical event

The risk of vascular occlusion can be reduced by smokers quitting, and also by modifying platelet function. The tendency to clot formation may be reduced by taking fish, garlic, ginger, red wine, vitamin E and aspirin. Persons contemplating surgery are sometimes advised to moderate their consumption of ginger and garlic.

Deep sea cold water fish such as leather jacket, yellowfin, blue grenadier, tuna, mackerel and herring are all good options. A serving of 150 g of any of the following types of fish will provide at least 500 mg of omega-3 fatty acids: Atlantic salmon, bonito, gem fish, mackerel, mullet, oreo dory, sardines, swordfish and trevally. Omega-3 fatty acids increase bleeding time—even to the extent that the fish rich diet of Eskimos results in a bleeding tendency. Supplementation with fish oil, in addition to having an anticoagulant effect, decreases blood pressure (1.2 g/day) and reduces death following a heart attack (3 g/day).

Platelet aggregation has been shown to be profoundly and reversibly inhibited by vitamin E in a dose dependent fashion.[53] The dose of vitamin E appears critical to its physiological impact: a-tocopherol in daily doses of 400 IU and above reduces oxidation of LDL, doses in excess of 800 IU impair platelet function and enhance immunity, while at 1200 IU the function of vitamin K and the immune response are compromised.[54]

The impact of aspirin is also dose dependent. A dose as low as 75 mg/day may reduce the risk of coronary occlusion. The US Preventive Services Task Force recommends aspirin therapy be offered to adults at increased risk for heart disease.[55] Meta-analysis of pooled data showed aspirin therapy reduced the risk for coronary heart disease by 28%; no significant effects on total mortality and stroke were noted.[55]

MONITORING PROGRESS

A number of non-intrusive measures are available for monitoring progress ranging from blood cholesterol readings through blood pressure measurements. More recently increasing waist–hip ratio has been associated with increasing risk of myocardial infarction.[56] This relationship remains significant after adjustment of various risk factors including BMI. In fact, the association of waist–hip ratio to the risk of myocardial infarction has been found to apply to those of normal weight and across different countries![56] Men should aim to have a waist circumference of no more than 94 cm, women should aim for 80 cm or less.

LIFESTYLE CONTROL

Diet and exercise elicit complementary effects on lipid profiles.[57] More specifically, diet therapies, with some exceptions, lower total triglyceride and LDL cholesterol concentrations, whereas exercise interventions increase HDL cholesterol while decreasing triglyceride levels. Furthermore, the health benefits of physical activity are at least as great as treating hypertension or successful cholesterol reduction.[58] A useful lifestyle approach would seem to include at least the following:[59]

- weight reduction of around 7–10% over 6–12 months for overweight persons
- a reduced calorie intake with a low dietary intake of saturated fats, trans fats and cholesterol, and a low glycaemic index
- a practical, regular and moderate exercise regime, with a daily minimum of 30–60 minutes and an equal balance between aerobic exercise and strength training
- consideration of nutritional supplements as required.

Lifestyle control should always be included. When this does not achieve the desired effect, drug therapy should be added. Different trials in elderly individuals have shown that use of statins, antithrombotic agents, beta-adrenoceptor antagonists and ACE inhibitors plays an important role both in primary and in secondary cardiovascular prevention.[2]

CLINICAL CHALLENGE

A 78-year-old woman presents with chest tightness. She says the discomfort only lasts a couple of minutes. It tends to comes on if she tries to run for the bus. She smokes 25 cigarettes a day. Her BMI is 21 and her blood pressure 140/90. You detect a bruit over her carotid artery.

She is afraid of needles and refuses to have any examinations that involve 'skin piercing' such as blood taken for laboratory investigations. Her ECG is normal.

Questions arising

- What is a working diagnosis?
- How could this patient be managed?

Clinical considerations

It is reasonable to assume the patient has atherosclerosis given her age, the carotid bruit and her current presenting complaint. She is consequently not only at risk of a heart attack but also a stroke.

Angina pectoris is a reasonable working diagnosis. Treat her angina: provide sublingual nitroglycerine.

Select interventions to target risk factors for atherosclerosis. The major modifiable risk factor definitely present is her cigarette smoking. Refer to *www.jamisonhealth.com* Handouts 14.4–14.11.

Ask her to complete a dietary diary. Consider advising her to adopt a diet consistent with that advocated at *www.jamisonhealth.com* in Handout 20.5.

In order to reduce her risk of thrombosis and vascular occlusion, particular consideration should be given to her taking aspirin and/or Vitamin E and including garlic and ginger in her diet.

PRACTICE GEMS

- Age is a major risk factor for CHD.
- Modifiable risk factors include cigarette smoking, hypercholesterolaemia (high LDL and low HDL cholesterol) and hypertension.
- There is a graded dose–response relationship between activity and all-cause mortality and coronary heart disease deaths—aerobic or vigorous activities are not essential for these cardiovascular benefits.
- Low intensity physical activity results in a slight increase in breathing and is achieved by walking at 3 km/h on flat hard surfaces, tidying the house, social lawn bowls or leisurely stationary cycling at <50 watts.
- Moderate intensity physical activity results in a modest but noticeable increase in the depth and rate of breathing but still allows for comfortable talking while walking and can be achieved by walking at 3–6 km/h on a flat firm surface, cleaning the house, cycling for pleasure at less than 16 km/h or doing water aerobics.
- Low vitamin E levels, raised fibrinogen, the metabolic syndrome and raised plasma S-adenosylhomocysteine are important predictors of a heart attack.
- Quitting smoking reduces the risk of atherosclerosis and coronary artery spasm.
- Dietary modification can reduce LDL cholesterol and increase HDL cholesterol.
- A plant based diet supplemented with cold deep water fish and low fat dairy products that includes garlic and ginger is cardioprotective.
- Weight loss improves cholesterol and corrects hypertriglyceridaemia.
- Exercise is beneficial and should be included in any management regime.
- Soy protein is more beneficial than animal protein both for correcting dyslipidaemia and in weight reduction.
- Nutritional supplements such as fish oil, oat bran or plant sterol are particularly advantageous.

References

1. Desai MM, Zhang P, Hennessy CH. Surveillance for morbidity and mortality among older adults— United States, 1995–1996. MMWR CDC Surveill Summ 1999; 48(8):7–25.

2. Andrawes WF, Bussy C, Belmin J. Prevention of cardiovascular events in elderly people. Drugs Aging 2005; 22(10):859–876.

3. Unal B, Critchley JA, Capewell S. Modelling the decline in coronary heart disease deaths in England and Wales, 1981–2000: comparing contributions from primary prevention and secondary prevention. BMJ 2005; 331(7517):614.

4. Chun BY, Dobson AJ, Heller RF. Smoking and the increase of coronary heart disease in an Australian population. Med J Aust 1993; 159:508–512.

5. Kawachi I, Colditz GA, et al. Smoking cessation and time course of decreased risks of coronary heart disease in middle-aged women. Arch Intern Med 1994; 154(2):169–175.

6. Hanna IR, Wenger NK. Secondary prevention of coronary heart disease in elderly patients. Am Fam Physician 2005; 71(12):2289–2296.

7. Third Joint Task Force of European and Other Societies on Cardiovascular Disease Prevention in Clinical Practice. European guidelines on cardiovascular disease prevention in clinical practice. Eur Heart J 2003; 24(17):1601–1610.

8. Li JZ, Chen ML, et al. A long-term follow-up study of serum lipid levels and coronary heart disease in the elderly. Chin Med J (Engl) 2004; 117(2):163–167.

9. Lawes CM, Bennett DA, et al. Blood pressure and coronary heart disease: a review of the evidence. Semin Vasc Med 2002; 2(4):355–368.

10. Morgan TO. Hypertension. Medicine Today 2000; 1(1):51–55.

11. Karakelides H, Sreekumaran Nair K. Sarcopenia of aging and its metabolic impact. Curr Top Dev Biol 2005; 68:123–148.

12. Schillaci G, Pirro M, et al. Prognostic value of the metabolic syndrome in essential hypertension. J Am Coll Cardiol 2004; 43(10):1817–1822.

13. Greiser KH, Kluttig A, et al. Cardiovascular disease, risk factors and heart rate variability in the elderly general population: design and objectives of the CARdiovascular disease, Living and Ageing in Halle (CARLA) Study. BMC Cardiovasc Disord 2005; 5:33.

14. Virtanen R, Jula A, et al. Anxiety and hostility are associated with reduced baroreflex sensitivity and increased beat-to-beat blood pressure variability. Psychosom Med 2003; 65:751–756.

15. Mann J. Importance of dietary management and practical patient counseling, the European/Australasian perspective. Atheroscler Suppl 2002; 3(3):23–29.

16. Liu S, Manson JE, et al. Fruit and vegetable intake and risk of cardiovascular disease: the Women's health study. Am J Clin Nutr 2000; 72(4):922–928.

17. Law MR, Morris JK. By how much does fruit and vegetable consumption reduce the risk of ischaemic heart disease? Eur J Clin Nutr 1998; 52(8):549–556.

18. Truswell AS. Cereal grains and coronary heart disease. Eur J Clin Nutr 2002; 56(1):1–14.

19. Hu FB, Willett WC. Optimal diets for prevention of coronary heart disease. JAMA 2002; 288(20):2569–2578.

20. Hu FB, Rimm EB, et al. Prospective study of major dietary patterns and risk of coronary heart disease in men. Am J Clin Nutr 2000; 72(4):912–921.

21. Brown AA, Hu FB. Dietary modulation of endothelial function: implications for cardiovascular disease. Am J Clin Nutr 2001; 73(4):673–686.

22. Kant AK, Schatzkin A, et al. Dietary diversity and subsequent mortality in the First National Health and Nutrition Examination Survey Epidemiologic Follow-up Study. Am J Clin Nutr 1993; 57(3):434–440.

23. Mensink RPM, Katan MB. Effect of dietary trans fatty acids on high-density and low-density lipoprotein cholesterol levels in healthy subjects. N Engl J Med 1990; 323:439–445.

24. Murray S, Flegel K. Chewing the fat on trans fats. CMAJ November 8, 2005; 173(10):1158–1159.

25. Hooper L, Thompson RL, et al. Omega 3 fatty acids for prevention and treatment of cardiovascular disease. Cochrane Database Syst Rev 2004 Oct 18; (4):CD003177.

26. Mozaffarian D. Does alpha-linolenic acid intake reduce the risk of coronary heart disease? A review of the evidence. Altern Ther Health Med 2005; 11(3):24–30.

27. Khor GL. Dietary fat quality: a nutritional epidemiologist's view. Asia Pac J Clin Nutr 2004; 13(Suppl):S22.

28. Haapanen N, Miilunpalo S, et al. Characteristics of leisure time physical activity associated with decreased risk of premature all-cause and cardiovascular disease mortality in middle-aged men. Am J Epidemiol 1996; 143(9):870–880.

29. Petrella RJ, Lattanzio CN, et al. Can adoption of regular exercise later in life prevent metabolic risk for cardiovascular disease? Diabetes Care 2005; 28(3):694–701.

30. Stewart KJ, Bacher AC, et al. Exercise and risk factors associated with metabolic syndrome in older adults. Am J Prev Med 2005; 28(1):9–18.

31. Watkins LL, Sherwood A, et al. Effects of exercise and weight loss on cardiac risk factors associated with syndrome X. Arch Intern Med 2003; 163(16):1889–1895.

32. Tanko LB, Bagger YZ, et al. Peripheral adiposity exhibits an independent dominant antiatherogenic effect in elderly women. Circulation 2003; 107(12):1626–1631.

33. Pratley RE, Hagberg JM, et al. Aerobic exercise training-induced reductions in abdominal fat and glucose-stimulated insulin responses in middle-aged and older men. J Am Geriatr Soc 2000; 48(9):1055–1061.

34. Morgan TO. Hypertension. Medicine Today 2000; 1(1):51–55A.

35. Dengel DR, Hagberg JM, et al. Improvements in blood pressure, glucose metabolism, and lipoprotein lipids after aerobic exercise plus weight loss in obese, hypertensive middle-aged men. Metabolism 1998; 47(9):1075–1082.

36. Dunstan DW, Salmon J, et al. Associations of TV viewing and physical activity with the metabolic syndrome in Australian adults. Diabetologia 2005 Oct 7; [Epub ahead of print].

37. Nordstrom CK, Dwyer KM, et al. Leisure time physical activity and early atherosclerosis: the Los Angeles Atherosclerosis Study. Am J Med 2003; 115(1):19–25.

38. Dawber TR, Nickerson RJ, et al. Eggs, serum cholesterol, and coronary heart disease. Am J Clin Nutr 1982; 36(4):617–625.

39. Fernandez ML. Dietary cholesterol provided by eggs and plasma lipoproteins in healthy populations. Curr Opin Clin Nutr Metab Care 2006; 9(1):8–12.

40. Ford ES, Liu S. Glycemic index and serum high-density lipoprotein cholesterol concentration among US adults. Arch Intern Med 2001; 161(4):572–576.

41. Goodman-Gruen D, Kritz-Silverstein D. Usual dietary isoflavone intake is associated with cardiovascular disease risk factors in postmenopausal women. J Nutr 2001; 131(4):1202–1206.

42. Nilsen DW, Albrektsen G, et al. Effects of a high-dose concentrate of n-3 fatty acids or corn oil introduced early after an acute myocardial infarction on serum triacylglycerol and HDL cholesterol. Am J Clin Nutr 2001; 74(1):50–56.

43. Robertson J, Brydon WG, et al. The effect of raw carrot on serum lipids and colon function. Am J Clin Nutr 1979; 32(9):1889–1892.

44. Adler AJ, Holub BJ. Effect of garlic and fish-oil supplementation on serum lipid and lipoprotein concentrations in hypercholesterolemic men. Am J Clin Nutr 1997; 65(2):445–450.

45. Berg A, Konig D, et al. Effect of an oat bran enriched diet on the atherogenic lipid profile in patients with an increased coronary heart disease risk. Ann Nutr Metab 2003; 47(6):306–311.

46. Oxford Fruit and Vegetable Study Group. Effects of fruit and vegetable consumption on plasma antioxidant concentrations and blood pressure: a randomised controlled trial. Lancet 2002; 359(9322):1969–1974.

47. Tomas L. Hypercholesterolaemia. J Comp Med 2003; 2(6):14–22.

48. Tran TL. Antioxidant supplements to prevent heart disease. Postgraduate Medicine 2001; 109:109–114.

49. Keogh JB, Torpy DJ, et al. Salt and blood pressure: relationship with obesity, weight loss and direct effects on vascular function. Asia Pac J Clin Nutr 2005; 14 Suppl:S59.

50. Sacks FM, Svetkey LP, et al. Effects on blood pressure of reduced dietary sodium and the Dietary Approaches to Stop Hypertension (DASH) diet. DASH-Sodium Collaborative Research Group. N Engl J Med 2001; 344(1):3–10.

51. Nowson CA, Worsley A, et al. Blood pressure change with weight loss is affected by diet type in men. Am J Clin Nutr 2005; 81(5):983–989.

52. Nanchahal K, Ashton WD, et al. Alcohol consumption, metabolic cardiovascular risk factors and hypertension in women. Int J Epidemiol 2000; 29(1):57–64.

53. Bakaltcheva I, Gyimah D, Wood DA. Effects of alpha-tocopherol on platelets and the coagulation system. Platelets 2001; 12(7):389–394.

54. Jamison JR. Clinical guide to nutrition and dietary supplements in disease management. Edinburgh: Churchill Livingstone; 2003:733–741.

55. US Preventive Services Task Force. Guide to clinical preventive services. 2nd edn. Washington DC: Office of Disease Prevention and Health Promotion, US Government Printing Office; 1996.

56. Murray S. Is waist-to-hip ratio a better marker of cardiovascular risk than body mass index? CMAJ 2006 January 31; 174 (3):308.

57. Varady KA, Jones PJ. Combination diet and

exercise interventions for the treatment of dyslipidemia: an effective preliminary strategy to lower cholesterol levels? J Nutr 2005; 135(8):1829–1835.

58. Briffa TG, Maiorana A, et al. Physical activity for people with cardiovascular disease: recommendations of the National Heart Foundation of Australia. Med J Aust 2006; 184(2):71–75.

59. Deedwania PC, Volkova N. Current treatment options for the metabolic syndrome. Curr Treat Options Cardiovasc Med 2005; 7(1):61–74.

PATIENT HANDOUT 16.1 – HEART ATTACK: REDUCING THE RISK

Heart attacks are the major cause of death in industrialized countries. You can reduce your personal risk of a heart attack. *Keep your waist circumference under 94 cm (men) or 80 cm (women).*

See *www.jamisonhealth.com* Handout 20.7 which provides a more comprehensive approach that:

- Helps you to recognize your personal risk of heart disease.
- Suggests how to approach reducing your risk.
- Makes you aware of the early signs of a heart attack.

Lifestyle choices

The lifestyle of our ancestors was more conducive to cardiovascular health than that of our peers. Our ancestors were leaner, had more exercise, and ate less sodium and more vitamin C and calcium. Their diet had less energy from fat and relatively more unsaturated than saturated fatty acids. It also had more of the type of unsaturated fatty acids found in fish than in vegetable oils. The diet and lifestyle of our ancestors was cardioprotective. We need to protect our hearts by:

- maintaining an ideal body weight
- not smoking
- eating five or more fruit and vegetables each day. Favour a plant based diet.
- spending 30 minutes of our leisure time exercising on five or more occasions each week.

See *www.jamisonhealth.com* Handout 20.1 for more detailed lifestyle guidelines on how to reduce your risk of a heart attack.

Modifying the major risk factors

Three of the major risk factors for a heart attack can be changed by lifestyle choices!

1. The high blood cholesterol problem

Health authorities recommend a diet that gets less than 30% of its energy from fat. They also advise that less than one third of energy from fat should come from saturated fat, up to one third from polyunsaturated fats and more than one third from monounsaturated fats.

Dietary cholesterol should be less than 300 mg a day. For those at greater risk even more stringent guidelines are suggested.

Refer to *www.jamisonhealth.com* Handout 20.5 to help you select and prepare food that is more likely to conform to this advice. In general avoid:

- animal fat except for fish.
- spreadable vegetable fats – use vegetable oils.

Refer to *www.jamisonhealth.com* Handout 20.6 for advice on how to:

- improve your lipid profile.
  −increase HDL cholesterol
  −decrease LDL cholesterol
  −decrease triglycerides by losing weight
- avoid the dangerous form of cholesterol−reduce oxidation of LDL cholesterol
- prevent thrombosis.

2. Smoking
Refer to *www.jamisonhealth.com*:

- Handout 14.11 for a stepwise approach to quitting
- Handouts 14.4 and 14.5 for a cost–benefit analysis of quitting
- Handout 14.6 for a diary template to make you aware of your smoking behaviour
- Handout 14.7 for the various approaches used to quit
- Handouts 14.8–14.10 for increasing self-awareness and suggestions as to which approach is most successful for your type of smoking.

3. High blood pressure
A plant based diet that includes low fat dairy products benefits blood pressure. Blood pressure is increased by being overweight, having a high salt intake and drinking too much alcohol. Blood pressure is reduced by weight loss, a low salt diet and limiting alcohol intake.

Refer to *www.jamisonhealth.com* Handout 23.6 for 7 steps to an ideal body weight. Also refer to Handouts 23.3 and 23.4 for dietary advice on food selection.

Refer to *www.jamisonhealth.com* Handout 19.2 for help in avoiding excess sodium/salt.

Refer to *www.jamisonhealth.com* Handout 15.5 for tips on how to control social drinking.

For information on how lifestyle can reduce your risk of a heart attack see:

Ornish D, Brown SE, et al. Can lifestyle changes reverse coronary disease? Lancet 1990; 336:129–33.

Internet resources

http://www.americanheart.org/
http://www.healthstatus.com/

Chapter 17

Leg ulcers

CHAPTER CONTENTS

A 70-year-old woman presents with a shallow ulcer over her medial malleolus. Her ankle is thickened and pigmented. She complains of persistent itching.

- What type of ulcer presents in this fashion?
- What predisposes to this problem?
- How may the condition be treated?

INTRODUCTION

Elderly persons are at increased risk of compromised blood supply and drainage to the lower limb. Chronic lower limb ischaemia results in a cool pale limb and chronic venous congestion in a thickened dusky ankle. In both conditions the microcirculation is impaired and skin may break down to cause ulcers which resist healing.

VARICOSE ULCERS

Most leg ulcers are of venous origin. The risk of developing leg ulcers increases dramatically with age; those aged 60 years and over are particularly at risk.[1] A prospective survey confirmed rates of ulceration are highly dependent on age, increasing to 8.29 (men) and 8.06/1000 (women) in those aged over 85 years.[2]

Pathogenesis

Venous ulcers are the result of disturbed venous flow patterns and chronic inflammation. In persons with chronic venous insufficiency, distortion of hydrostatic and centrifugal pressures disrupts shear stress along the vessel wall and around valves.[3] Shear stress acts as a mechanical physical force activating receptors and transducers in the vessel wall. At the level of microcirculation, reduced shear stress induces hypoxia, accumulation of white cells and haemorrheological disorders in microvenulae.[3] In the case of varicose veins, transmission of high venous pressures to the dermal microcirculation stimulates inflammation. The release of cytokines and growth factor in response to leukocyte migration into the interstitium initiates further inflammatory events, leading to the intense dermal fibrosis and tissue remodelling characteristic of chronic venous insufficiency.[4] Inappropriate leukocyte activation and interaction with the endothelium contribute to venous ulceration.

Venous ulcers heal slowly. A Portuguese study found the median duration of ulceration was 18 months, with 66% of ulcers present for longer than 1 year, and 17% for longer than 5 years.[5] Along with old age and a high body mass index, local factors predicting poor ulcer healing include arterial lower limb disease, ulcer duration of more than 3 months and an initial ulcer length of 10 cm or more.[6]

Management

Standard care for venous leg ulcers, based on local wound care and application of compression therapy, reports up to 83% success within 6 months. Local treatment includes mechanical cleaning, normal saline perfusion and covering with moist pads. Use of hydrocolloid dressings, silver nitrate solution, silver sulfadiazine and paraffin are all popular options. Compression using stockings or bandages to exert pressure of at least of 30 mmHg at the ankle is appropriate. More invasive options include surgical treatments such as ulcer excision by 'shave therapy' and mesh grafting.

Those ulcers that are larger than 5 cm^2 or have been present for over 6 months may require more specialized intervention. Oral treatment with micronized purified flavonoid fraction (MPFF) 2×500 mg daily appears beneficial for ulcers of 5–10 cm^2 in size and/or present for 6–12 months.[7]

However, MPFF appears only to achieve a better outcome than conventional therapy in patients whose ulcers meet these parameters. MPFF appears to protect the microcirculation both from damage secondary to raised ambulatory venous pressure by improved venous tone and lymphatic drainage, and from inflammatory processes by reducing capillary hyperpermeability.[8] MPFF is usually most appropriate when the venous ulcer disease has been present for less than 5 years. Another novel option is prostaglandin E-1 (PGE-1). A randomized, placebo-controlled, single blind study reported that venous leg ulcers treated for 20 days with an infusion of PGE-1 showed enhanced healing.[9]

ARTERIAL ULCERS

Arterial ulcers result from impaired limb perfusion and present as deep, painful ulcers in a cool pale limb. Patients may have a long history of cold feet and report slow growing toenails. Intermittent claudication, the most common symptom of peripheral arterial disease, increases sharply in late middle age.

Pathogenesis

Persons with peripheral arterial disease due to atherosclerosis are not only at increased risk of arterial leg ulcers, they are also at risk of coronary heart disease and stroke. Risk factors for peripheral arterial disease are the same as those for atherosclerosis. They include cigarette smoking, diabetes or impaired glucose tolerance, hypertension, low levels of high density lipoprotein cholesterol, and high levels of triglycerides, apolipoprotein B, lipoprotein(a), homocysteine, fibrinogen and increased blood viscosity.[10,11] The mortality rate of persons with claudication due to peripheral arterial disease increases with the duration of the problem, rising from 30% for those who have had the condition for 5 years, to 50% for 10 years, to 70% in those in whom the condition has persisted for 15 years.[12]

The most common presenting complaint of persons with peripheral arterial disease is intermittent claudication. Muscle ischaemia or intermittent claudication presents as pain in the calf, buttocks, thigh or feet. The pain is worsened by exercise. The distance a patient can walk without needing to stop and rest is used as an indication of the severity of the disease. The prevalence of exercise induced ischaemic pain in persons under 60 years of age is 2.5%, it rises to 8.3% in persons aged 60–69 years and to 18.8% in those over 70.[10] While 2–3% of men and 1–2% of women aged 60 years experience intermittent claudication,[13] non-invasive testing suggests the true prevalence of peripheral arterial disease is at least five times higher than would be expected from such prevalence reports.[10]

Walking distance is a useful clinical measure of severity. In mild ischaemia pain is experienced after walking 500 or more metres, in moderate ischaemia the patient requires a rest after 250 metres, in severe ischaemia pain halts the patient trying to walk more than 125 metres. In more severe cases, rest pain presents as a persistent gnawing ache which is often worst at night when the cardiac output drops. While an absent pulse is a useful indicator, a more precise correlate of severity, progress and prognosis is the ankle–brachial index.[14] The ankle–brachial index is the ratio of the systolic pressure in the ankle to that in the arm. A 5–7 MHz Doppler is used to measure pressure in the brachial artery and the ankle, either the posterior tibial or dorsalis pedis artery of that side. An ankle–brachial index of over 0.90 is normal, 0.71–0.90 indicates mild obstruction, 0.41–0.70 moderate obstruction and 0.00–0.4 severe obstruction. An exercise ankle–brachial index can provide additional functional information.

Persons most at risk of arterial ulcers are those with rest pain or an ankle–brachial index of less than 0.4.

Management

Management of arterial ulcers focuses on treating the underlying vascular disease as well as the ulcer itself. Intervention for peripheral arterial disease focuses both on minimizing risk factors and on enhancing perfusion.

Risk factors

Hypertension doubles the risk of claudication.[5] Refer to Chapter 15 for information on controlling hypertension. Some 80% of persons with claudication smoked at some stage and 30–40% are current smokers.[14] Refer to Patient Handout 16.1 for information on quitting. Management of hypercholesterolaemia, (see Chapter 16) can also reduce risk. Statins have been demonstrated to decrease the incidence of intermittent claudication and delay the onset of intermittent claudication during treadmill exercise in hypercholesterolaemic persons with peripheral arterial disease.[15]

Increasing perfusion

Enhancing perfusion improves symptoms and decreases the risk of future or recurrent ulceration. Claudication symptoms limit functional capacity and decrease the quality of life.

Leg pain is often effectively relieved through exercise. The greatest improvement is achieved by walking at least 30 minutes for 3 or more sessions every week over a period of 6 or more months.[14] Exercise should lead to moderately severe claudication with training beginning at 50–85% of the patient's functional capacity as determined by treadmill walking. Exercise effectively increases functional independence in both smoking and non-smoking patients,[16] and may even improve functioning for individuals with peripheral arterial disease who do not have classical symptoms of intermittent claudication.[17] In fact, exercise therapy can significantly improve maximal walking time and achieve an overall improvement in walking ability of approximately 150% (range 74–230%), a result comparable to surgical intervention and better than that provided by angioplasty at 6 months and antiplatelet therapy.[18]

Drugs to reduce the risk of thrombotic occlusion such as antiplatelet drugs, e.g. aspirin or clopidogrel, are also routinely given to patients with peripheral vascular disease.[15] Another option is cilostazol (100 mg or 50 mg bd), a phosphodiesterase III inhibitor, which in addition to having a mild antiplatelet effect is a vasodilator.[14] Drug induced vasodilation and training combine to improve exercise capacity.[15]

Lower extremity angioplasty provides another option. In future, therapeutic angiogenesis using angiogenic growth factors such as hepatocyte growth factor or vascular endothelial growth factor may be possible.[19,20] Introduction of the relevant naked plasmid encoding for the appropriate gene appears to be a safe and feasible strategy for improving ischaemic limbs. In the meantime, lower extremity angioplasty is a surgical option. Stenting or bypass surgery are considered only when claudication is incapacitating, rest pain is present, ulcers are non-healing and infection or gangrene suggest limb salvage is needed and feasible.[15]

The best treatment for arterial ulcers is improved perfusion. Modern wound dressing may accelerate healing; however, there is insufficient evidence to recommend any specific dressing type.[21]

LOOKING AHEAD

Researchers are identifying interventions that promise to improve the healing rates of vascular ulcers in the elderly. Prevention is, however, better than cure and exercise remains an important intervention both for preventing blood stasis in venous disease and for enhancing tissue perfusion in arterial disorders.

CLINICAL CHALLENGE

A 60-year-old man presents with a painful ulcer at the tip of his right big toe. The ulcer has clearly demarcated edges, is punched out and has a necrotic base. The leg is cool, pale and hairless.

The man has severe emphysema and leads a highly sedentary life. He was a heavy smoker but has not smoked for the last 5 years.

Questions arising

- What is the working diagnosis?
- What additional information would confirm the diagnosis?
- How should the patient be counselled?
- What is his prognosis?

Clinical considerations

A reasonable working diagnosis is an arterial ulcer due to peripheral arterial disease. The diagnosis can be confirmed by data collection demonstrating impaired perfusion.

Inquire about symptoms of hypoxia
- Intermittent claudication
- Slow growing toenails
- Cold feet/ankles/legs
- Shooting pains, paraesthesia.

Search for signs of chronic ischaemia
- Cool pale hairless leg with thin shiny skin
- Calf muscle atrophy and weakness
- Absent pedal pulses and a zone of temperature change
- Check for pedal colour change
  - pallor developing in the leg when it is slightly raised
  - pallor developing rapidly on high elevation of the leg/foot

  - dependency rubor (beefy redness) when the foot is returned to a dependent position
  - a flushing time which exceeds 20 seconds. Elevate the lower limb for 2 minutes. Return the limb to the dependent position and note the time taken for the leg to flush.
- Check venous filling. In patients with an intact saphenous system, the time taken for venous filling after elevating the leg for 2 minutes provides information about limb perfusion. Normal venous filling time is 7 seconds. Venous filling of 30 seconds indicates poor perfusion.

Do special investigations:
- Determination of the ankle–brachial index.

Results: The flushing time exceeded 20 seconds and the venous filling time exceeded 30 seconds. The posterior tibial pulse is absent and the ankle–brachial index is 0.03.

Definitive diagnosis: arterial ulcer due to severe peripheral arterial disease. There is a risk of dry gangrene.

The ultimate prognosis is influenced, in view of the patient's compromised respiratory system, by the potential to enhance limb perfusion without surgery.

Other determinants of this patient's outcome are influenced by the likelihood of widespread atherosclerosis and the risk of a heart attack or stroke. Associated risk factors such as hypertension, diabetes and dyslipidaemia should be investigated.

◆ The clinical presentation of occlusive arterial disease is determined by the extent of occlusion, the collateral circulation and the functional demands of the area.

◆ The ankle–brachial index correlates with severity and prognosis.

◆ To determine impaired limb perfusion check the pulses and look for pedal colour changes—impaired perfusion is present in a limb that rapidly develops pallor on elevation and becomes beefy red when lowered.

◆ Think chronic hypoxia in a patient with a pale, cool, pulseless, shiny hairless limb, atrophied cramping muscles and deformed, slow growing nails.

◆ Think peripheral arterial disease in patients with ulcers on the dorsum of the foot and/or anterior aspect of the leg that fail to heal.

◆ Think an arterial ulcer when a painful punched out ulcer with a dry base is found between or on the toes.

◆ Think venous disease in patients with thickened, warm, cyanotic ankles with persistent or recurrent skin ulceration and venous eczema.

◆ Think a venous ulcer when a moist, superficial ulcer with a ragged edge and granulating base is found in the lower third of the leg.

◆ Leg pain precipitated by exercise and relieved by rest suggests peripheral arterial disease, heavy aching legs relieved by leg elevation suggests venous disease.

References

1. Walker N, Rodgers A, et al. The occurrence of leg ulcers in Auckland: results of a population-based study. N Z Med J 2002; 115(1151):159-162.

2. Moffatt CJ, Franks PJ, et al. Prevalence of leg ulceration in a London population. QJM 2004; 97(7):431–437.

3. Boisseau MR. Roles of mechanical blood forces in vascular diseases. A clinical overview. Clin Hemorheol Microcirc 2005; 33(3):201–207.

4. Nicolaides AN. Chronic venous disease and the leukocyte–endothelium interaction: from symptoms to ulceration. Angiology 2005; 56 (Suppl 1):S11–19.

5. Pina E, Furtado K, et al. Leg ulceration in Portugal: prevalence and clinical history. Eur J Vasc Endovasc Surg 2005; 29(5):549–553.

6. Meaume S, Couilliet D, Vin F. Prognostic factors for venous ulcer healing in a non-selected population of ambulatory patients. J Wound Care 2005; 14(1):31–34.

7. Coleridge-Smith P, Lok C, Ramelet AA. Venous leg ulcer: a meta-analysis of adjunctive therapy with micronized purified flavonoid fraction. Eur J Vasc Endovasc Surg 2005; 30(2):198–208.

8. Lyseng-Williamson KA, Perry CM. Micronised purified flavonoid fraction: a review of its use in chronic venous insufficiency, venous ulcers and haemorrhoids. Drugs 2003; 63(1):71–100.

9. Milio G, Mina C, et al. Efficacy of the treatment with prostaglandin E-1 in venous ulcers of the lower limbs. J Vasc Surg 2005; 42(2):304–308.

10. Criqui MH, Denenberg JO, et al. The epidemiology of peripheral arterial disease: importance of identifying the population at risk. Vasc Med 1997; 2(3):221–226.

11. Ness J, Aronow WS, et al. Prevalence of symptomatic peripheral arterial disease, modifiable risk factors, and appropriate use of drugs in the treatment of peripheral arterial disease in older persons seen in a university general medicine clinic. J Gerontol A Biol Sci Med Sci 2005; 60(2):255–257.

12. Dormandy JA, Rutherford RB. Management of peripheral arterial disease (PAD). TASC Working Group. TransAtlantic Inter-Society Consensus (TASC). J Vasc Surg 2000; 31(1 Pt 2):S1–S296.

13. Bradberry JC. Peripheral arterial disease: pathophysiology, risk factors, and role of antithrombotic therapy. J Am Pharm Assoc (Wash DC) 2004; 44(2 Suppl 1):S37–44.

14. Treat-Jacobson D, Walsh ME. Treating patients with peripheral arterial disease and claudication. J Vasc Nurs 2003; 21(1):5–14.

15. Aronow WS. Management of peripheral arterial disease. Cardiol Rev 2005; 13(2):61–68.

16. Gardner AW, Killewich LA, et al. Response to

exercise rehabilitation in smoking and non-smoking patients with intermittent claudication. J Vasc Surg 2004; 39(3):531–538.

17. McDermott MM, Tiukinhoy S, et al. A pilot exercise intervention to improve lower extremity functioning in peripheral arterial disease unaccompanied by intermittent claudication. J Cardiopulm Rehabil 2004; 24(3):187–196.

18. Leng GC, Fowler B, Ernst E. Exercise for intermittent claudication. Cochrane Database Syst Rev 2000; (2):CD000990.

19. Morishita R, Aoki M, et al. Safety evaluation of clinical gene therapy using hepatocyte growth factor to treat peripheral arterial disease. Hypertension 2004 Aug; 44(2):203–209.

20. Kim HJ, Jang SY, et al. Vascular endothelial growth factor-induced angiogenic gene therapy in patients with peripheral artery disease. Exp Mol Med 2004; 36(4):336–344.

21. Bouza C, Munoz A, Amate JM. Efficacy of modern dressings in the treatment of leg ulcers: a systematic review. Wound Repair Regen 2005; 13(3):218–229.

PATIENT HANDOUT 17.1 – LEG ULCERS

The risk of ankle and foot ulcers due to vascular disease increases with age. Leg ulcers in the elderly take a long time to heal.

Venous ulcers

Persons at greatest risk of ulcers due to venous disease usually have leaky valves in their veins resulting in increased pressure in veins around the region of the ankle. Damage to the vein's valves is often the result of a deep vein thrombosis.

Is this a venous ulcer?

- ☐ Thickened ankle
- ☐ Reddish-brown discoloured ankle
- ☐ Shallow weeping ulcer
- ☐ Itchy surrounding skin
- ☐ Leg discomfort eased by raising the leg (reducing congestion)

The more boxes you tick the greater the likelihood this is a venous ulcer.

Tips to heal a venous ulcer:

- ■ Wear a compression bandage or stocking.
- ■ Local ulcer treatment: mechanical cleaning and dressing by a health professional.

Arterial ulcers

The risk factors for peripheral vascular disease and lower limb ulcers are the same as those for a heart attack. In addition to age, major risk factors are smoking, diabetes, hypertension and abnormal cholesterol levels.

Peripheral vascular disease results when perfusion of the lower limb is impaired.

Is this an arterial ulcer?

- ☐ A cool, pale leg
- ☐ Cold feet
- ☐ Thin hairless shiny skin
- ☐ Deformed slow growing toenail
- ☐ Calf/leg pain on exercise. The pain is relieved by rest
- ☐ Deep painful ulcer (often found on the toes or foot)

The more boxes you tick, the greater the likelihood this is an arterial ulcer.

Tips to manage peripheral vascular disease:

- ■ Stop smoking.
- ■ Exercise regularly. Walk at least 30 minutes on alternate days. If walking causes pain, exercise until pain becomes moderately severe. After resting to relieve the pain, continue exercising.
- ■ Take half an aspirin each day.

Professional monitoring of the condition and intervention as necessary may prevent limb amputation.

Chapter 18

Depression

CHAPTER CONTENTS

A 75-year-old man witnessed his cat of 10 years being mauled by a dog 10 days ago. He has been down ever since his cat died. He has lacked energy and been off his food but has still regularly provided assistance at his favourite charities on three days of the week. In view of his age he has been unable to decide whether it would be 'fair' to get a new kitten. His friends are concerned about how he is coping with his recent loss.

- Is the patient depressed?
- Is this patient's depression physiological or clinical?
- Is there a risk of suicide?
- Does the patient require professional intervention?

INTRODUCTION

The prevalence of depression increases with age, escalating from 5.6% at the age of 70 to 13.0% by the age of 85.[1] The incidence of depression is higher in women, being 30 per 1000 person-years, and only 12 per 1000 person-years in men between the ages of 70 and 85. Moreover the incidence of depression between 79 and 85 years of age is some 2.5 times that between the ages of 70 and 79.[1] The impact of depression on wellness is not limited to depressed mood.

Depression, like age, gender, functional disability and medical disorders, based on use of prescription drugs, is a strong and consistent independent predictor of mortality in older adults. Depression alone predicts mortality in the short term, and when combined with a self-rating of poor health, it strongly predicts mortality at all end points.[2] Furthermore, although subjective views of wellbeing may be more important predictors of mortality in older adults than the classic symptoms of depression,[3] depressed older people may be at increased risk of physical disability. One longitudinal epidemiological study with a follow-up of 5 years concluded that depression was associated with an increased risk of impaired function;[4] another concluded that depressive symptoms did not consistently contribute to greater decline.[5]

Causal relationships are difficult to define as depression in the elderly may be linked to overall immunoendocrine dysregulation.[6] Animal studies have clearly demonstrated that cytokine mediated illnesses are associated with behavioural changes and high levels of cytokines have been shown to induce systemic symptoms, such as fatigue, anorexia, weight loss, sleep disturbances, anhedonia and decreased psychomotor activity–all sentinel indicators of depressive disorder.[7] Inflammatory markers have been linked to depression and cytokines may themselves both cause and be a consequence of depression.[6–8] Certainly depression may be the result of medical problems. Viral infections, connective tissue disorders, endocrine diseases, vitamin deficiencies (B12, B3), pancreatic cancer and drugs including alcohol, sedative-hypnotics, certain antihypertensive agents and oral contraceptives may trigger depression.

Late life depression is strongly associated with poor health.[9] Late life depressive symptoms have been shown to increase the risk for subsequent cardiovascular disease, mortality, disability, and physical function decline; similarly, increased levels of inflammatory cytokines in old age have been shown to lead to cardiovascular disease, loss of skeletal muscle mass, and a subsequent increased risk of disability and mortality.[7] Furthermore, although older adults appear to be at greater risk for major depression attributable to biological changes, e.g. depression resulting from vascular changes,[10] the depressogenic effect of stress dominates even in the presence of significant vascular risk.[11] A biopsychosocial approach to depression is therefore desirable.[12]

DIAGNOSING DEPRESSION

Regardless of age, depressed persons lack motivation and experience a mood change. Depression has emotional, physical and social repercussions. The major features of depression are:

- Mood changes. Pervasive feelings of sadness or depressed mood accompanied by a loss of interest or pleasure that persist for 2 or more weeks is typical. Elderly patients with depression are prone to present with unexplained somatic complaints and a sense of hopelessness rather than sadness. Sadness in elderly patients with depression is often masked by other symptoms.

- Three or more of the following are present:
  —significant loss or gain of appetite or weight.
  —a sleep disturbance. This ranges from early morning waking, through difficulty falling asleep to excessive sleep.
  —psychomotor retardation or agitation, particularly when anxiety is marked. Lack of personal care may be evident
  —feelings of worthlessness or guilt. A loss of self-esteem is a characteristic of clinical depression.
  —impaired thinking or concentration and indecisiveness. Cognitive impairment is often marked in elderly depressed patients.
- Autonomic nervous system problems such as constipation, palpitations, dry mouth or menstrual disorders.
- Psychosomatic problems such as arthralgia, chest pain, weakness, nausea or psychogenic vomiting. Elderly depressed patients often express concern about their physical wellbeing.
- Normal laboratory investigations.

Several useful screening questionnaires providing a quick method for detecting major depression are available,[13,14] such as the Mini-International Neuropsychiatric Interview (MINI) and the DSM-IV screening questions.

THE VARIOUS PRESENTATIONS OF DEPRESSION

Depression can take various forms. It may be physiological or clinical. Before depression is considered a clinical problem it must have been present for at least 14 days and be associated with a significant mood disturbance, poor self-esteem and social impairment. In contrast, physiological depression lasts less than 14 days, is not associated with loss of self-esteem, has no diurnal mood variation and no or mild mood disturbance. The patient may express feelings of despair or rejection but continues to function at a satisfactory level socially.

Depression may be overt or masked. Masked depression may be present when the patient displays:

- flatness of mood
- lack of interest in work and hobbies
- loss of self-worth
- avoidance of people
- loss of physical energy, lethargy
- an inability to cope with stress
- a disturbed sleep pattern
- an all-pervading anxiety
- suicidal thoughts.

Depression may present as an acute event or a chronic mildly incapacitating mood disturbance. Dysthymia is a mood disorder and refers to low grade affective pathology with an intermittent course that persists for at least 2 years.[15] Gloominess, anhedonia, low drive and energy, low self-confidence and pessimism dominate. Unlike patients with a major depressive disorder, dysthymic patients are no slower than controls in performing the fine motor tasks, with neither initiation nor movement time being prolonged.[16] Psychomotor retardation is consequently helpful for differentiating between dysthymia and a major depressive disorder.[16] Persons with medical problems may experience either a major depressive episode or dysthymia.

Depression must not be confused with dementia. In contrast to patients with dementia who have a long history of progressive gradual memory loss most marked for recent events, depressed patients have a short history of fluctuating memory loss that started abruptly and was accompanied by a sleep, appetite and mood disturbance. Furthermore, depressed persons emphasize their cognitive disability while demented patients are usually unaware and unconcerned.

SUICIDE

Depression carries a risk of suicide. Those at highest risk are white males, over 45 years of age, who live alone and have a history of drug or alcohol abuse. Depressed anxious patients are at increased risk.[17] Ominous warning signs include talking about suicide and a personal or family history of a previous suicide attempt. It is of some concern that one study found health providers largely failed to explore the risk of suicide amongst very old depressed patients.[18] In fact, health professionals were less likely to inquire about depression or to refer elderly patients for specialist care of this condition.

MANAGEMENT

Active treatment of depression is important and effective. Lifestyle management is an important component of any treatment plan. This includes self-monitoring and exercise. Self-monitoring of mood and other symptoms provides evidence of progress and encouragement while increasing feelings of control. Moderate intensity exercise for 20 minutes at least three times a week significantly reduces symptoms of depression. While physiological depression resolves over time and may be assisted with exercise, clinical depression requires more vigorous intervention on the part of both patients and health care providers.

Professional intervention options include referral to specialists. Psychologists offer cognitive behaviour therapy and may reduce relapse rates without any risk of suicide due to drug overdose. Psychiatrists can provide drug therapy and electroconvulsive therapy (ECT) as well as counselling and these additional interventions may be required for a successful outcome.

Herbs and nutraceuticals offer another viable option. Herbal therapy has been shown to be effective for mild to moderate depression. St John's wort in doses of 300 mg of extract standardized to 0.3% hypericin given tds is effective and has fewer side effects than other antidepressants.[19,20] It may, however, take 8 weeks before any benefit is felt. Photosensitivity may be a problem and the herb should be discontinued 14–21 days prior to surgery. Similarly, parenteral or oral S-adenosyl-methionine(SAMe) in doses of 200–1600 mg daily has been shown to be superior to placebo and as effective as tricyclic antidepressants in alleviating depression.[21] One clinical trial found a daily 400 mg intramuscular dose of SAMe comparable to 150 mg/day of oral imipramine in terms of antidepressive efficacy.[22] SAMe was significantly better tolerated with only mild and transient side effects. SAMe acts quickly, detectably improving depression within 7 days at a dosage of 400 mg.[23]

A number of pharmaceuticals are effective. As a general rule, it has been suggested that initial treatment of depression should be continued at full drug dosage for 6–12 weeks to achieve complete remission of symptoms. Full dosage may be continued for a further 4–5 months as maintenance to stabilize the patient at a fully functional level. On discontinuation of the drug the dose should be tapered off—reducing the dose by 25% each week over a 1–5 month period.[14] Imipramine, a popular option for treating depression, is prescribed in doses of 75 mg/day increasing to 150 mg/day if necessary. The patient should respond in 10–14 days. Fluoxetine (Prozac) is another well-liked alternative. It is taken as a single morning dose of 20 mg. The dose may be increased after several weeks if necessary. The maintenance dose ranges from 20 to 80 mg/day. Patients usually respond in 10–14 days. Venlafaxine (Effexor), another alternative, carries a risk of sustained hypertension, abnormal ejaculation and impotence. None of these pharmaceuticals may be used with monoamine inhibitors. As overdosing and suicide can be a problem with pharmaceuticals, weekly prescriptions should be provided.

IN PERSPECTIVE

The elderly should be screened for depression and when it is present, active intervention is indicated.

CLINICAL CHALLENGE

You notice that a 75-year-old man who attends your clinic for monitoring and drug management of his hypertension is becoming increasingly withdrawn and is losing weight. He says he has no appetite, is constipated and feels generally tired and weak, especially in the morning. He says he is sleeping badly and wakes early in the morning. He lost his wife 6 months ago.

On examination his temperature and pulse are normal. His chest is clear, and his abdomen is soft and no masses were palpated. His reflexes are normal. He has no dependency oedema and his liver is within normal limits. His faecal occult blood test is negative as is his rectal examination. Five years ago his sigmoidoscopy was normal. He does not have a history of alcoholism. His blood pressure is being well controlled.

Questions arising

- Is depression a plausible working diagnosis?
- Are there any underlying conditions that require investigation/intervention?

Clinical considerations

Depression is plausible given the following:

- age—depression is a common problem in the elderly
- apathy/withdrawal
- anorexia and weight loss
- diurnal psychomotor variations and early waking
- propranolol is associated with depression in some patients
- his quality of life is likely to have declined since the death of his wife.

Depression is more likely to present with somatic complaints than guilt and worthlessness in the elderly. While his 'bowel blockage' may represent a somatic delusion, common in the depressed elderly, bowel cancer should be excluded.

A 56-year-old woman presents complaining of tiredness. She has been unable to find work since being made redundant 6 months ago. She finds it difficult to make ends meet and now she says she has lost her 'get up and go'. Everything is just too much trouble.

She complains of neck stiffness, headaches, backache. She has previously been diagnosed with osteoarthritis in the right hip and left knee.

On further questioning she acknowledges she has been:

- consistently depressed or down, most of the day, nearly every day, for the past 2 weeks
- less interested in most things and less able to enjoy the things she used to enjoy most of the time over the past 2 weeks.

Clarifying her presenting complaint reveals:

- her appetite had been decreased nearly every day over the last 2 week
- she has felt tired almost every day over the last 2 weeks
- she had trouble sleeping, both with getting to sleep and then waking up during the night, nearly every night over the last 2 weeks.

Questions arising

- What is the diagnosis?
- How should she be managed?

Clinical considerations

She fulfils the criteria for diagnosing a major depressive episode. However, recent life events e.g. being made redundant, financial difficult and the persistent pain of osteoarthritis would justify reactive depression. In either case, counselling and 20 minutes of moderate intensity exercise on alternate days, are indicated. Furthermore, attention to her underlying health problem is required—glucosamine sulphate, pain management and consideration of surgery for her osteoarthritis require investigation.

Making a definitive diagnosis

Refer to Ballenger JC et al to make a definitive diagnosis.

In the case of a major depressive episode consider the following management strategy:

- If the depression is judged to be moderate: St John's wort is effective although it may take up to 8 weeks before improvement is noted. SAMe provides a safe alternative which should achieve improvement in around 7 days.
- Refer to a psychiatrist if depression is severe and warrants drug therapy and/or ECT.

In the case of reactive depression referral to a psychologist for cognitive behaviour therapy could reduce the risk of a relapse.

References

1. Ballenger JC, Davidson JR, et al. A proposed algorithm for improved recognition and treatment of the depression/anxiety spectrum in primary care. Prim Care Companion J Clin Psychiatry 2001 Apr; 3(2):44–52.

- ◆ Depression is often overlooked and not treated in elderly persons.
- ◆ Minor depression in the elderly is most typically an episodic phenomenon.
- ◆ Clinical depression requires active treatment.
- ◆ Clinically depressed persons are as frail as persons who have survived a stroke.
- ◆ For a diagnosis of clinical depression, a depressed mood that shows a diurnal variation, an impaired self-image and psychomotor retardation must have persisted for more than 14 days.
- ◆ Dysthymia is characterized by a depressed mood that persists for more than 2 years and is not associated with detectable psychomotor retardation.
- ◆ Dysthymic and clinically depressed patients are at increased risk of suicide.

- ◆ Exercise elevates mood.
- ◆ St John's wort is an effective treatment for mild to moderate depression but 2 months may lapse before benefit is felt.
- ◆ SAMe produces mild, transient side effects and starts lifting depression within 1 week.
- ◆ Pharmaceuticals used for the treatment of depression, such as the tricyclic antidepressants and monoamine oxidase inhibitors, raise the concentration of the amines e.g. serotonin, in the brain.
- ◆ A concern with drug therapy of depressed patients is the use of pharmaceuticals to overdose in suicide attempts—an avoidance strategy is to limit the quantity prescribed at any one time to the weekly requirement.

References

1. Palsson SP, Ostling S, Skoog I. The incidence of first-onset depression in a population followed from the age of 70 to 85. Psychol Med 2001; 31(7):1159–1168.

2. Ganguli M, Dodge HH, Mulsant BH. Rates and predictors of mortality in an aging, rural, community-based cohort: the role of depression. Arch Gen Psychiatry 2002; 59(11):1046–1052.

3. Blazer DG, Hybels CF. What symptoms of depression predict mortality in community-dwelling elders? J Am Geriatr Soc 2004; 52(12):2052–2056.

4. Kivela SL, Pahkala K. Depressive disorder as a predictor of physical disability in old age. J Am Geriatr Soc 2001; 49(3):290–296.

5. Everson-Rose SA, Skarupski KA, et al. Do depressive symptoms predict declines in physical performance in an elderly, biracial population? Psychosom Med 2005; 67(4):609–615.

6. Dentino AN, Pieper CF, et al. Association of interleukin-6 and other biologic variables with depression in older people living in the community. J Am Geriatr Soc 1999; 47(1):6–11.

7. Penninx BW, Kritchevsky SB, et al. Inflammatory markers and depressed mood in older persons: results from the Health, Aging and Body Composition study. Biol Psychiatry 2003; 54(5):566–572.

8. Reichenberg A, Yirmiya R, et al. Cytokine-associated emotional and cognitive disturbances in humans. Arch Gen Psychiatry 2001; 58(5):445–452.

9. Tiemeier H, Breteler MM, et al. Multivariate score objectively assessed health of depressed elderly. J Clin Epidemiol 2005; 58(11):1134–1141.

10. Blazer DG 2nd, Hybels CF. Origins of depression in later life. Psychol Med 2005; 35(9):1241–1252.

11. Holley C, Murrell SA, Mast BT. Psychosocial and vascular risk factors for depression in the elderly. Am J Geriatr Psychiatry 2006; 14(1):84–90.

12. Blazer DG 2nd, Hybels CF. Origins of depression in later life. Psychol Med. 2005; 35(9):1241–1252.

13. Whooley MA, Avins AL, et al. Case-finding instruments for depression. J Gen Intern Med 1997; 12: 439–445.

14. Ballenger JC, Davidson JR, et al. A proposed algorithm for improved recognition and treatment of the depression/anxiety spectrum in primary care. Prim Care Companion J Clin Psychiatry 2001; 3(2):44–52.

15. Akiskal HS. Dysthymia and cyclothymia in psychiatric practice a century after Kraepelin. J Affect Disord 2001; 62:17–31.

16. Pier MP, Hulstijn W, Sabbe BG. No psychomotor slowing in fine motor tasks in dysthymia. J Affect Disord 2004; 83(2–3):109–120.

17. Jeste ND, Hays JC, Steffens DC. Clinical correlates of anxious depression among elderly patients with depression. J Affect Disord 2006; 90(1):37–41.

18. Fischer LR, Wei F, et al. Treatment of elderly and other adult patients for depression in primary care. J Am Geriatr Soc 2003; 51(11):1554–1562.

19. Miller AL. St. John's Wort (Hypericum perforatum): clinical effects on depression and other conditions. Alt Med Rev 1998; 3(1):18–26.

20. Monograph. Hypericum perforatum. Altern Med Rev 2004; 9(3):318–325.

21. Mischoulon D, Fava M. Role of S-adenosyl-L-methionine in the treatment of depression: a review of the evidence. Am J Clin Nutr 2002; 76(5):1158S–1161S.

22. Pancheri P, Scapicchio P, Chiaic RD. A double-blind, randomized parallel-group, efficacy and safety study of intramuscular S-adenosyl-L-methionine 1,4-butanedisulphonate (SAMe) versus imipramine in patients with major depressive disorder. Int J Neuropsychopharmacol 2002; 5(4):287–294.

23. Fava M, Giannelli A, et al. Rapidity of onset of the antidepressant effect of parenteral S-adenosyl-L-methionine. Psychiatry Res 1995; 56(3):295–297.

PATIENT HANDOUT 18.1 – DEPRESSION

Depression is a common problem. 1 in 4 women and 1 in 10 men have a major episode of depression during their lifetime. The chances of suffering depression rise with increasing age. Depression is a real disease that requires and responds to treatment.

Depression is a normal reaction to loss. It only becomes a health problem when it persists for longer than 2 weeks and is associated with an impaired self-image. A major depressive episode interferes with one's social and physical functioning. Clinical depression requires active treatment.

Am I depressed?

If you have consistently experienced four or more of the following for the last 2 weeks or longer you may be suffering from depression. Tick the box if you have:

- [ ] been worried
- [ ] felt sad or depressed
- [ ] felt life is not worth living
- [ ] enjoyed activities less than you did a year ago
- [ ] enjoyed yourself less than you used to because you feel depressed or nervous
- [ ] felt pessimistic or empty and seen the future as bleak
- [ ] wished you were dead
- [ ] felt unhappy.

Depression can be successfully treated! Depressed persons benefit from professional help.

Depressed persons are at increased risk of suicide.

You do *not* increase the risk of suicide by asking a depressed friend:

- Are you thinking of suicide/ending it all?
- Are you repeatedly thinking of hurting yourself?
- Do you wish you were dead?

Professional help is urgently required if a depressed individual acknowledges they have:

- recently developed a suicide plan, i.e. within the last month
- previously attempted suicide
- been depressed for over 2 years.

Internet resources

http://www.niapublications.org/engagepages/depression.asp

Chapter **19**

Dementia

CHAPTER CONTENTS

Ben is 76 years old. He says he seems to be having memory problems. He forgets appointments, where he put his keys and when to pay his bills. He often finds himself looking for words and finds it difficult to read a novel.

His daughter says he has become very rigid and doesn't pay attention. He has also become tactless and becomes quite abusive when asked to deviate from his routine. He has been getting gradually worse.

- Does Ben have dementia?
- Should Ben's condition be discussed with him, his daughter or both parties?
- What non-medical considerations are involved in caring for patients with dementia?

INTRODUCTION

As many as 1 in 10 people over 65 years have cognitive and functional difficulties; this number escalates to 4 in 10 for those over 85 years of age.[1]

A North American study estimated that the risk of dementia doubles every 5 years after the age of 65 years;[2] a UK study estimated that the prevalence of dementia almost doubled every 5 years after the age of 35 years![3] It has been suggested that in European countries 1 year of life with dementia can be expected for every person over the age of 65.[4] One study found the rate of Alzheimer's disease rose from 2.8 per 1000 person-years in the 65–69 year age group to 56.1 per 1000 person-years in those over 90 years—in fact, rates nearly tripled from the 75–79 year to the 80–84 year age group.[5] The risk of dementia increases with age.

IDENTIFYING RISK

A genotype has been linked with dementia. A single apolipoprotein E4 (Apo-E4) on chromosome 19 increases the risk of Alzheimer-type dementia 2.2–4.4 times; the presence of two Apo-E4 genotypes (E4/E4) raises the risk by a factor of 5.1–17.9.[1,2] Nonetheless, a systematic search for this genotype is not recommended as its absence does not protect against dementia. Other factors intervene.

Modifiable medical risk factors include anaemia,[6] diabetes,[7] oral hypoglycaemic therapy[8] and midlife hypertension.[9] Although mild hypertension in the very old may be protective,[9] the risk of dementia nonetheless increases with cerebral injury whether this results from vascular insult or physical trauma.

Lifestyle choices influence risk. Even behavioural choices at a young age can have a long term impact. Persons with only an elementary education run four times the risk of dementia compared to those with at least 10 years of education![1,2] Midlife choices may also affect long term cognition. Fish consumption may be associated with slower cognitive decline with age; however, whether this is linked to omega-3 fatty acid intake remains uncertain.[10] Some studies suggest hormone replacement increases the risk for dementia and fails to prevent mild cognitive impairment in postmenopausal women aged 65 years or older,[11,12] others are less certain.[13] Soy products which are rich in phyto-oestrogens may actually be protective.[14] Current behaviours also have an impact. Current smoking increases risk, but only in persons over 75 years of age.[15] On the other hand, increased leisure activity, physical activity or a modest alcohol intake appear to lower the risk of dementia.[16] Gardening, which appears to provide both mental and physical stimulation, seems to be particularly protective.

DIAGNOSIS

Dementia may result from: a degenerative process, e.g. senile and pre-senile (Alzheimer-type); multiple cerebral infarcts as in atherosclerotic dementia; infection e.g. acute onset dementia; or may be attributable to a local brain tumour or result from harmful behaviours, e.g. alcoholism. Typically,

Alzheimer-type dementia, the most common variety in old age, progresses slowly and becomes worse over several years, on average 6–8 years after diagnosis. In contrast, vascular dementia progresses in stages with fluctuations in cognitive and functional performance, sometimes from one day to the next.

Diagnosis of dementia requires a full physical examination plus mini-mental status examination. Dementia is characterized by demonstrably impaired memory. Memory problems are characterized by impaired concentration and poor short term memory. Recent events are readily forgotten; however, long term memory is retained. Familiar tasks are well performed, learning new tasks presents difficulty.

In addition to memory changes, dementia is associated with intellectual dysfunction and/or a personality change. After 30 years of age personality tends to be stable.[17,18] Sudden changes suggest disease. Blunting of affect, tactlessness, increasing coarseness, apathy and loss of initiative develop over time.

A clinical diagnosis of dementia requires impaired memory plus four or more of the following:[2]

- Aphasia i.e. difficulty with language either in terms of comprehension and/or expression
- Apraxia i.e. an inability to accomplish skilled tasks despite the absence of sensory or motor deficit
- Agnosia i.e. an inability to recognize objects, people, parts of the body despite normal sensory and motor function
- Impaired ability to plan ahead, organize, judge or think abstractly
- Persistent cognitive deficits sufficient to impair daily functioning
- A marked decline from previous levels of functioning.

To diagnose dementia these impairments must be sufficient to interfere with work, and with usual social activities and/or relationships with others.[4] Laboratory investigations are normal.

Conditions which may be confused with dementia are depression, thyroid disease and drug responses. Depression is not unusual in the early stages of dementia when sufferers are aware they are unable to cope. However, demented patients are more likely to be unsociable, hostile, confused and disoriented than depressed patients. Thyroid function tests can discriminate between dementia and thyroid disease while drugs particularly prone to cause confusion include sedatives, anticholinergics, centrally acting antihypertensive agents, digoxin and some beta-blockers.

MANAGEMENT

Both care for patients and support for caregivers are important considerations in management.

Clinicians should inform patients and their families of the diagnosis so that anticipatory counselling can be provided to enable families to prepare for the long term responsibility of caring for someone with dementia.[2]

Anticipatory counselling creates awareness of various resources that are available and provides information about:

- Legal aspects. Matters such as power of attorney, finances and making a will are best resolved when the patient is still able to make meaningful decisions.
- The hazards of polypharmacy. Patients and their families must be cautious about modifying prescribed and/or taking over-the-counter medications. New medication should be carefully monitored, started using a low dose and only gradually increased.
- The need to monitor driving. While a diagnosis of dementia does not automatically revoke a driver's licence, vigilance is required to identify when driving does become a hazard. While only a road test can ultimately assess a driver's ability, screening for problems with vision and reaction time, intellectual impairment, a poor safety record, alcohol abuse, use of certain medications, poor attention, impaired executive functions, and a family report of driving problems can all provide useful information. Despite the absence of standardized guidelines, practical screening approaches are available.[19]

The main expectations family caregivers have of doctors are that they will provide regular follow up, communicate information on various subjects and acknowledge the important role played by families.[2] Psychological support for caregivers is imperative as more than 50% of family members develop serious mental problems including anxiety or depression during their time as caregivers. Behavioural disturbances are encountered in 9 out of 10 persons with dementia and early intervention and treatment can reduce the burden on caregivers.[20] A point worth emphasizing for both sufferers and caregivers is that physical activity appears to protect against all forms of cognitive decline, particularly for women.[21] Regular exercise should be encouraged in any daily schedule!

One aspect of care that may be of some concern is underestimation by caregivers of the personhood of individuals with dementia. Although dementia has been identified with the loss of 'self', the majority of patients change, rather than completely lose, their identity. Of four roles, professional, family role, hobbies/leisure activities, and personal attributes, the family role identity is most likely to be maintained and carer awareness of this may be used to enhance wellbeing in patients.[22]

In addition to lifestyle and psychosocial intervention, drug therapy for dementia is available for elderly patients. Although there is no solid evidence for efficacy of drug therapy in severe dementia, elderly patients with mild to moderate Alzheimer's disease should be offered drug therapy.[23]

IN PERSPECTIVE

Although one study suggests the prevalence of dementia in the US, particularly of vascular and mixed dementias may be declining due to improved medical therapy,[24] in view of an expanding aging population dementia remains a major problem.

Two years ago Mr Jones reported having 'senior moments'. Now at 70 years of age, both he and his wife are concerned because he has become very forgetful and sometimes feels confused. His wife reports that he becomes quite agitated when asked to change his routine. He says he often has difficulty finding the right word, hasn't done the crossword for at least 6 months and no longer feels able to take care of their financial affairs. He has become apathetic, doesn't want to mix with people and mopes around the house. His wife has noticed he seems to be dwelling on the past. She sometimes feels she doesn't know him anymore.

On questioning, it appears he is sleeping badly and seems to be more down since his last visit to the surgery 8 weeks ago when his blood pressure treatment was changed to a beta-blocker.

Aside from slightly raised blood pressure, physical and laboratory findings are normal. A mini mental status examination confirms memory problems and cognitive difficulties.

Questions arising

- What is the working diagnosis?
- How should the patient be managed?

Clinical considerations

Step 1: Make a diagnosis

The patient's age, short term memory loss, difficulty with intellectual functions and changed personality all suggest dementia. The problem started well before his changed medication. In view of the gradual worsening of his condition, the suggestive results of his mini mental status examination and normal physical/laboratory evaluation, a diagnosis of Alzheimer's disease is made.

Step 2: Management

The needs of both the patient and his wife require attention. Anticipatory counselling helps the patient and family. It encompasses:

- Addressing everyday lifestyle. Patients in the early stages of dementia, aware they are failing to cope, suffer stress. Refer to Patient Handout 2.2 for simple coping strategies.
- Heightening awareness of the legal implications of failing cognition.
- Preliminary screening of competence to handle a motor vehicle.
- Careful monitoring of medication. Caution against use of over-the-counter medications and alcohol abuse.
- Monitoring disease progression. A simple and useful strategy is the clock method. Sufferers are asked to draw a clock and show different time settings. Early problems may be detected when difficulty is encountered drawing 20 after 8; more advanced cases have difficulty drawing 3 o'clock.
- Provide information on resources available for sufferers and their carers. See Patient Handout 19.1.

◆ Alteration in mental status is an important sign in the elderly and may indicate disease or medication problems.

◆ Dementia is a problem that becomes increasingly common with advancing age.

◆ Confused behaviour due to dementia is slowly progressive while that due to delirium is sudden in onset.

◆ Demented patients are more likely than depressed patients to be unsociable, hostile, confused and disoriented.

◆ Dementia is characterized by grossly impaired short term memory, reduced intellectual functioning and/or a personality change.

◆ Dementia in people with Alzheimer's disease is gradually progressive over years; dementia due to vascular causes tends to be associated with fluctuating levels of confusion.

◆ The cause of Alzheimer's disease is uncertain and there is no cure for the condition.

◆ Both the patient and the caregivers require support.

◆ Anticipatory counselling includes consideration of everyday lifestyle, legal matters and the use of pharmaceuticals.

◆ Facilitating access to resources is an important aspect of management.

◆ People who have a diet rich in fish (omega-3 fatty acids) appear to reduce their risk of dementia.

◆ Although alcohol abuse is a risk factor for cognitive dysfunction among older subjects, a daily alcohol consumption of less than 40 g for women or 80 g for men might be protective.

◆ Malnourished elderly patients, especially those with deficiency of antioxidants, folic acid and vitamins B6 and B12, may be at increased risk of dementia.

References

1. Lechky O. Diagnosing dementia. Canadian Medical Association Leadership Series: Elder Care 2005; 4:25–28.

2. Frenette G, Beauchemin JP. Sad but true: your father has dementia. An approach to announcing the diagnosis. Can Fam Physician 2003; 49:1296–1301.

3. Harvey RJ, Skelton-Robinson M, Rossor MN. The prevalence and causes of dementia in people under the age of 65 years. J Neurol Neurosurg Psychiatry 2003; 74:1206–1209.

4. Berr C, Wancata J, Ritchie K. Prevalence of dementia in the elderly in Europe. Eur Neuropsychopharmacol 2005; 15(4):463–471.

5. Kukull WA, Higdon R, et al. Dementia and Alzheimer disease incidence: a prospective cohort study. Arch Neurol 2002; 59(11):1737–1746.

6. Atti AR, Palmer K, et al. Anaemia increases the risk of dementia in cognitively intact elderly. Neurobiol Aging 2006; 27(2):278–284.

7. Arvanitakis Z, Wilson RS, et al. Diabetes mellitus and risk of Alzheimer disease and decline in cognitive function. Arch Neurol 2004; 61(5):661–666.

8. Logroscino G, Kang JH, Grodstein F. Prospective study of type 2 diabetes and cognitive decline in women aged 70–81 years. BMJ 2004; 328(7439):548.

9. Anson O, Paran E. Hypertension and cognitive functioning among the elderly: an overview. Am J Ther. 2005; 12(4):359–365.

10. Morris MC, Evans DA, et al. Fish consumption and cognitive decline with age in a large community study. Arch Neurol 2005; 62(12):1849–1853.

11. Shumaker SA, Legault C, et al. Estrogen plus progestin and the incidence of dementia and mild cognitive impairment in postmenopausal women. The Women's Health Initiative Memory Study: a randomized controlled trial. JAMA 2003; 289:2651–2662.

12. Rapp SR, Espeland MA, et al. Effect of estrogen plus progestin on global cognitive function in postmenopausal women. The Women's Health Initiative Memory Study: a randomized controlled trial. JAMA 2003; 289(20):2663–2672.

13. LeBlanc ES, Janowsky J, et al. Hormone replacement therapy and cognition: systematic review and meta-analysis. JAMA 2001; 285:1489–1499.

14. Duffy R, Wiseman H, File SE. Improved cognitive function in postmenopausal women after 12 weeks of consumption of a soya extract containing isoflavones. Pharmacol Biochem Behav 2003; 75(3):721–729.
15. Reitz C, Luchsinger J, et al. Effect of smoking and time on cognitive function in the elderly without dementia. Neurology 2005; 65(6):870–875.
16. Simons LA, Simons J, et al. Lifestyle factors and risk of dementia: Dubbo Study of the elderly. Med J Aust 2006; 184(2):68–70.
17. US Department of Health and Human Services. With the passage of time: the Baltimore Longitudional Study of Aging. Washington DC: Public Health Service, NIH Pub No 93–3685; 1993:1–52.
18. US Department of Health and Human Services. In search of the secrets of aging. Washington DC: Public Health Service, NIH Pub No 93–2756; 1993:1–46.
19. Molnar FJ, Byszewski AM, et al. In-office evaluation of medical fitness to drive: practical approaches for assessing older people. Can Fam Physician 2005 Mar; 51: 372–379.
20. Desai AK, Grossberg GT. Recognition and management of behavioral disturbances in dementia. Prim Care Companion J Clin Psychiatry 2001; 3(3):93–109.
21. Lindsay J, Sykes E, et al. More than the epidemiology of Alzheimer's disease: contributions of the Canadian Study of Health and Aging. Can J Psychiatry 2004; 49(2):83–91.
22. Cohen-Mansfield J, Parpura-Gill A, Golander H. Salience of self-identity roles in persons with dementia: differences in perceptions among elderly persons, family members and caregivers. Soc Sci Med 2006; 62(3):745–757.
23. Olsen CE, Poulsen HD, Lublin HK. Drug therapy of dementia in elderly patients. A review. Nord J Psychiatry 2005; 59(2):71–77.
24. Manton KC, Gu XL, Ukraintseva SV. Declining prevalence of dementia in the US elderly population. Adv Gerontol 2005; 16:30–37.

PATIENT HANDOUT 19.1 – DEMENTIA

Dementia is the result of impaired brain function severely compromising the ability to carry out the normal functions of daily living. It can result from brain degeneration in the elderly but may also result from brain trauma due to vascular disease or physical injury.

Dementia should be suspected if there is evidence of:

- Memory failure. Although sufferers may have good recall of the past, they have difficulty remembering recent events.
- Declining cognitive function. Sufferers are incapable of learning new tasks. They have difficulty understanding, analysing and planning for the future.
- A personality change. Sufferers become indifferent and tactless.

The above changes progress gradually over a number of years in persons with senile and pre-senile dementia. The cause is unknown and there is currently no cure for Alzheimer's disease. Age is a major risk factor for this condition. In contrast to senile dementia, the course of dementia in persons with vascular causes fluctuates.

In the early stages of dementia, the patient has insight into his/her failing intellect. Awareness that they are not coping is stressful and it may be helpful to introduce simple measures to allay anxiety.

Useful tips are:

- Create memory pegs. Prepare lists of things to do.
- Create routines. Establish habits to impose structure on the environment.
- Employ simple stress management strategies:
  - Take a walk
  - Jog on the spot for 3 minutes
  - Yawn or sigh to release tension
  - Loosen tight muscles by rotating shoulders and rolling the head

- Do a windmill stretch (sweep your arms up in a wide arc from waist to above head level)
- Try a helicopter stretch (hold arms horizontal and gently swing arms in a semi-circle).

Be wary of problems with medication:

- Reduce the risk of incorrect dosage by using a medication dispenser. Weekly dispensers, providing separate compartments into which daily medication requirements can be inserted, offer a useful strategy for monitoring medications.
- Interactions between prescribed and over-the-counter drugs can have adverse effects.
- Changes in prescribed medication can have untoward effects—start with low doses and increase slowly, monitoring any changes in patient behaviour.

Internet resources

There are a number of resources to help sufferers and their families:

http://www.alzheimers.org/pr04-05/Progress_Report_on_Alzheimers_Disease_ 2004-2005-small.pdf
for recent in formation on Alzheimer's disease

http://www.alzheimers.org/pubs/homesafety.htm
home safety for dementia sufferers

http://www.niapublications.org/engagepages/home.asp
tips for helping elderly people stay at home

http://www.alzheimers.org/careguide.htm
a guide for care givers

http://www.niapublications.org/engagepages/carelist.asp
resources for caregivers

Chapter 20

Prostate disease

A 55-year-old man says he is having trouble with his 'waterworks'. He has heard that prostate cancer is a common malignancy in men. He asks if he has prostate cancer and what he can do to avoid dying from this disease.

- What distinguishes prostatic hyperplasia from prostate cancer?
- Can lifestyle choices influence the risk of prostate disease?
- What measures can be taken to ensure early diagnosis of prostate cancer?
- Can prostate cancer be treated?

INTRODUCTION

Prostate disease is a prevalent problem in older males. Prostate cancer is the commonest male cancer in developed countries and benign prostatic hyperplasia is so common many consider it a natural concomitant of aging.

BENIGN PROSTATIC HYPERPLASIA(BPH)

BPH is a chronic progressive condition, the prevalence of which increases with age. This androgen dependent metabolic disorder begins around 40 years of age and continues slowly until death. Moderate to severe lower urinary tract symptoms, depressed peak urinary flow rates and enlarged prostate volume have all been shown to increase across successively older age groups.[1] Patients with a presentation suggestive of prostate disease require a history, physical examination and urinalysis. In some cases a symptom inventory is also recommended.[2]

Diagnosis

A validated symptom index for clinically diagnosing benign prostatic hyperplasia includes seven questions covering frequency, nocturia, weak urinary stream, hesitancy, intermittence, incomplete emptying and urgency.[3] See Patient Handout 20.1. Digital palpation followed by transrectal sonographic imaging of the prostate is used to detect prostate enlargement.[3] In addition to prostate volume, clinical progression is most effectively monitored and predicted using prostate specific antigen (PSA).[4] PSA, a serine protease produced by the epithelium of the prostate gland, is elevated in men with an enlarged prostate, regardless of whether the increase in size is attributable to a benign or malignant condition.

The type and level of PSA detected can be used to discriminate between hyperplasia and cancer. PSA can be measured in the peripheral circulation in two forms: a free, non-complexed form and a form complexed to α_1-antichymotrypsin. Total serum PSA and serum-free PSA provide measures of prostate growth; however, the concentration of serum-free PSA is relatively higher in men with BPH than in men with prostate cancer.[3] A PSA in excess of 10 ng/mL suggests prostate disease while an increase in excess of 30 ng/mL excludes benign prostatic hypertrophy.[5] To complicate matters, PSA increases with age. High normal PSA levels are 2.5 ng/mL for 49-year-olds, 3.5 ng/mL for 59-year-olds, 4.5 ng/mL for 69-year-olds and 6.5 ng/mL for 79-year-olds.[5]

Management

Although three out of four elderly men have an enlarged prostate, only every second male with an enlarged prostate requires therapy. Moreover, although it is suspected that increased conversion of testosterone to dihydrotestosterone may result from an increase in 5-alpha-reductase due to drugs or pesticides, prevention of the condition has proved difficult. Nonetheless, a pilot study found a diet with less than 20% of energy from fat supplemented with 30 g daily of flaxseeds statistically significantly reduced PSA levels and the proliferation rate of benign prostatic epithelium.[6] No changes were noted in total testosterone.

A systematic review of the efficacy and safety of phytotherapeutic compounds used to treat men with symptomatic benign prostatic hyperplasia concluded saw palmetto, extracted from the berries of Serenoa, is the most widely used and most effective phytotherapeutic agent.[7] Although Hypoxis rooperi and Pygeum africanum show promise, Urtica dioica or Curcubita pepo lack any convincing evidence supporting their individual use. In contrast, clinical trials have shown Serenoa repens (160 mg bd between meals) improves urinary tract symptoms and flow measures, decreasing nocturia and improving peak urine flow, apparently with minimal side effects. The active ingredients in Serenoa repens appear to inhibit 5-alpha-reductase and block dihydrotestosterone from binding to the androgen receptors in the prostate gland. Improvement in symptoms on Serenoa repens is comparable to men receiving finasteride, a synthetic 5-alpha-reductase inhibitor. Clinical studies suggest most patients experience improvement in BPH-related lower urinary tract symptoms with alpha-adrenergic blockade or 5-alpha-reductase inhibition.[8,9] These drugs may even slow the progression of lower urinary tract symptoms, reducing both the need for surgery and the risk of complications, such as acute urinary retention. Unfortunately, finasteride is associated with sexual side effects, including decreased libido, ejaculatory dysfunction, and erectile dysfunction. Third-generation alpha-blockers, e.g. alfuzosin and tamsulosin are only infrequently associated with cardiovascular side effects.[8]

PROSTATE CANCER

Prostate cancer is around 22 times more frequent among elderly than younger men.[10]

Diagnosis

Like BPH, prostate cancer has a high incidence and a long term natural history. Early diagnosis is best achieved by screening. PSA screening is considered reasonable for men up to the age of 75 years. Case-finding based on screening serum for PSA has resulted in detection of prostate cancer 5–10 years before the disease becomes symptomatic and some 17 years before causing death of the patient.[11] Furthermore, the rate of increase in serum PSA reflects tumour growth rate and prognosis; however, reliable estimation of the rate of PSA increase requires follow-up for at least 2 years. Meta-analysis has shown the sensitivity, specificity, and positive predictive value for PSA are around 72%, 93% and 25% respectively; this compares favourably to digital rectal examination where the respective values are 53%, 83% and 18%.[12] The chance of cancer is over 20% in a patient with abnormal findings on either of these measures; conversely, the chance of missing a cancer is about 10% when these tests are within normal limits.[12]

In more advanced disease, rectal examination detects a hard irregular prostate gland in which the median sulcus has been obliterated. Further confirmation can be obtained by transrectal ultrasound guided biopsy which remains the gold standard for making a definitive diagnosis.

Prevention

Lifestyle may influence prostate cancer risk.

Epidemiological evidence suggests sun exposure may be relevant given regional variation in prostate cancer mortality rates. In fact, men with the lowest sun exposure have a three times greater incidence of prostate cancer than do men with a high lifetime exposure, and sunburn in childhood has been found to be particularly protective of prostate cancer![13]

Choosing a fitness lifestyle may also be protective. Men with the highest cardiorespiratory fitness level appear less likely to develop prostate cancer than men with a low fitness level.[14] This protective effect is limited to men under 60 years of age. Physically active men with energy expenditure >1000 kcal/week reduce their risk of developing prostate cancer. The researchers note that physical activity and cardiorespiratory fitness tend to lower testosterone levels, and androgenic stimulation over a period of time has been suggested as a cause of prostate cancer.[14]

Dietary modification may also be helpful.[15,16] A small number of studies have suggested that flaxseed-supplemented, fat-restricted diets may thwart prostate cancer growth in both animals and man.[6] Data from descriptive studies support the hypothesis that a dietary fat intake around 40% of energy consumption promotes the progression of focal prostatic cancer to clinical disease.[17] Furthermore, epidemiological evidence suggests a positive relationship between prostate cancer and land animal, but not vegetable, fat.[18] In addition, men who never eat fish were found to run at least double the risk of prostate cancer of those who eat moderate to high amounts of fatty fish such as salmon, herring and mackerel, i.e. fish rich in omega-3 fatty acids.[19] A prospective study over 12 years confirmed eating fish more than three times per week was associated with a reduced risk of prostate cancer.[20] Furthermore, in those participants who did develop prostate cancer, daily ingestion of an additional 0.5 g of marine fatty acid as fish decreased the risk of metastatic disease by 24%. A clear correlation between the blood level of long chain omega-3 fatty acids and prostate cancer has been established and researchers speculate that fish oils may prevent the progression of prostate cancer by inhibiting the biosynthesis of eicosanoids from arachidonic acid.[21]

Vegetables, but not fruit, have also been linked to a protective effect. Men who consumed 28 or more servings of vegetables each week were found to have a 35% lower risk than those who consumed fewer than 14 servings each week.[22] Men who ate three or more servings of cruciferous vegetables (broccoli, cauliflower, brussels sprouts, cabbage) each week had a 41% lower risk of developing prostate cancer than did men who ate less than one serving a week. A population-based, case control study also found that men who ate more than 10.0 g a day of allium vegetables, including garlic, scallions, onions, chives and leeks, had a statistically significantly lower risk of prostate cancer.[23] The reduced risk of prostate cancer associated with allium vegetables was more pronounced for men with localized than with advanced prostate cancer. Tomatoes are another vegetable that deserve special mention. Men who consumed 10 or more servings of tomato products per week reduced their risk of prostate cancer by 35%.[24] Moreover, the protective effect of tomato sauce (ripe tomatoes cooked in oil) was substantial compared to that of tomato juice. Oil or fat is thought necessary for proper absorption of the lycopene from the tomatoes. Lycopene is highly concentrated in the prostate. Supplementation with an oil-based tomato extract significantly lowers the level of PSA in patients with prostate cancer. Men who consumed tomato sauce two to four times per week had a 35% lower risk of developing prostate cancer than did men who never ate tomato sauce.[25] Lycopene is a powerful antioxidant with a singlet oxygen quenching capacity 10 times greater than that of vitamin E.

Epidemiological and laboratory evidence suggest a diet low in fat, with good sources of soy proteins, vitamin E and selenium, may have a protective effect against prostate cancer.[25] A case control study found higher consumption of tofu, soy foods and daidzein was associated with a reduced risk of prostate cancer.[26] It appears genistein-enriched isoflavonoids may dampen growth signalling pathways.[27]

It should, however, be noted that not all dietary measures reduce risk. Higher dietary calcium intake (2000 versus <700 mg/day) was associated with an increased risk of prostate cancer.[28] On the other hand, dairy intake is not associated with prostate cancer risk—this may be linked to vitamin D having an anti-proliferative effect. Similarly, a high intake of supplemental zinc (>100 mg/d) was associated with an increased risk of prostate cancer.[29] A low intake is not protective.

Disease management

Given the trend towards an increasing population, it has been estimated that by the year 2020, the number of people 80 years and over will soar by 135%. As the major risk factor for prostate cancer is increasing age, the notion of preventive drug therapy for elderly persons deserves consideration. As disease progression is influenced by androgenic stimulation, androgen deprivation therapy should theoretically prevent prostate cancer. Possible intervention ranges from the use of oestrogens to drugs such as finasteride which decrease prostatic androgenic stimulation by inhibiting 5-alpha-reductase. Finasteride successfully decreases prostate size but, although promising, has yet to be convincingly shown to halt the transition of normal prostatic epithelium through precancer to invasive cancer and clinically active systemic disease.[26]

Early diagnosis, in stages T1 and T2 of the disease, commonly leads to cure with current treatment modalities which include radical prostatectomy, external beam radiotherapy and brachytherapy.[30] Although radical prostatectomy reduces prostate cancer-related mortality for individuals aged 65–75, it does not seem to reduce the overall mortality of this age group.[31] Yet, high-dose conformal radiation therapy for prostate cancer is well tolerated in patients aged 75 years or older and radiation therapy with curative intent has been recommended for otherwise fit elderly patients with intermediate or locally advanced prostate cancer, taking into account concomitant disease and life expectancy.[32] Age alone is deemed not to constitute a barrier to curative intervention.

Metastatic prostate cancer is incurable and treatment is based on hormonal therapy.[30] Radioisotopes and bisphosphonates may alleviate bone pain and prevent osteoporosis and pathological fractures in such cases. Cytotoxic chemotherapy has only a limited role in hormone-independent prostate cancer. Promising treatments under development include cryotherapy and high-intensity focused ultrasound. Treatment decisions should be based on clinical status and comorbidities.[33]

An 85-year-old man presents with persistent backache. The pain is not relieved by rest. He has no previous history of backache. He worked for many years as a bus driver. He is a vegetarian and has lactose intolerance. He has a long history of difficulty passing urine and reports hesitancy, a poor stream and nocturia.

Questions arising

- Which medical conditions come to mind?
- How should a definitive diagnosis be made?
- What is the prognosis?

Clinical considerations

The patient may have developed backache due to an osteoporotic vertebral collapse or he may have prostate cancer with spinal secondaries.

In view of his history of prostatism and the prevalence of prostate cancer in this age group, rectal examination, blood for a prostate specific antigen and a spinal X-ray are indicated.

Results: On rectal examination the prostate gland is hard and irregular. You are unable to detect the median sulcus. The blood result reports a PSA 32 ng/mL.

The working diagnosis is prostate cancer with spinal secondaries. Prognosis is poor given the presence of metastasis. Pain management and bisphosphonates to reduce the risk of further osteoporosis and spinal fractures should be prescribed.

- ◆ Prostate problems are highly likely in elderly persons.
- ◆ Diagnosis of prostate disease is based on digital rectal examination and prostate specific antigen assessment.
  - ◆ Prostate specific antigen increases with age, prostatic hyperplasia and malignancy. The level of PSA influences the diagnostic decision.
  - ◆ An enlarged prostate that is firm with smooth convex lateral lobes suggests benign

hyperplasia; a hard irregular gland in which the median sulcus has been obliterated is likely to be malignant.
- ◆ Age is the greatest risk factor for prostate cancer.
- ◆ It is an ominous sign when a man with prostate cancer develops chronic low backache.
- ◆ Eight ounces of pomegranate juice daily may benefit men with prostate cancer.

References

1. Jacobsen SJ, Girman CJ, Lieber MM. Natural history of benign prostatic hyperplasia. Urology 2001; 58(6 Suppl 1): 5–16.

2. Nickel JC, Herschorn S, et al. Canadian guidelines for the management of benign prostatic hyperplasia. Can J Urol 2005; 12(3):2677–2683.

3. Barry MJ, Fowler FJ Jr, et al. The American Urological Association symptom index for benign prostatic hyperplasia. The Measurement Committee of the American Urological Association. J Urol 1992; 148(5):1549–1557.

4. Fong YK, Milani S, Djavan B. Natural history and clinical predictors of clinical progression in benign prostatic hyperplasia. Curr Opin Urol 2005; 15(1):35–38.

5. Hostetler RM, Mandel IG, Marshburn J. Prostate cancer screening. Medical Clinics of North America 1996; 80:83–98.

6. Demark-Wahnefried W, Robertson CN, et al. Pilot study to explore effects of low-fat, flaxseed-supplemented diet on proliferation of benign prostatic epithelium and prostate-specific antigen. Urology 2004; 63(5):900–904.

7. Wilt TJ, Ishani A, et al. Phytotherapy for benign prostatic hyperplasia. Public Health Nutr 2000; 3(4A):459–472.

8. Kuritzky L. Noninvasive management of lower urinary tract symptoms and sexual dysfunction associated with benign prostatic hyperplasia in the primary care setting. Compr Ther 2005; 31(3):194–208.

9. Logan YT, Belgeri MT. Monotherapy versus combination drug therapy for the treatment of benign prostatic hyperplasia. Am J Geriatr Pharmacother 2005; 3(2):103–114.

10. Hansen J. Common cancers in the elderly. Drugs Aging 1998; 13(6):467–478.

11. Stenman UH, Abrahamsson PA, et al. Prognostic value of serum markers for prostate cancer. Scand J Urol Nephrol Suppl 2005; (216):64–81.

12. Mistry K, Cable G. Meta-analysis of prostate-specific antigen and digital rectal examination as screening tests for prostate carcinoma. J Am Board Fam Pract. 2003; 16(2):95–101.

13. Luscombe CJ, Fryer AA, et al. Exposure to ultraviolet radiation: association with susceptibility and age at presentation with prostate cancer. The Lancet 2001; 358; 641–642.

14. Oliveria SA, Kohl HW, et al. The association between cardiorespiratory fitness and prostate cancer. Medicine and Science in Sports and Exercise 1996; 28:97–104.

15. Brawley OW, Barnes S, Parnes H. The future of prostate cancer prevention. Ann N Y Acad Sci 2001; 952:145–152.

16. Fujimoto N, Chang C, et al. Can we prevent prostate cancer? Rationale and current status of prostate cancer chemoprevention. Urol Int 2005; 74(4):289–297.

17. Zhou J, Blackburn GL. Bridging animal and human studies: what are the missing segments in dietary fat and prostate cancer? Am J Clin Nutr 1997; 66:1572S–1580S.

18. Willett WC. Specific fatty acids and risks of breast and prostate cancer: dietary intake. Am J Clin Nutr 1997; 66:1557S–1563S.

19. Terry P, Lichtenstein P, et al. Fatty fish consumption and risk of prostate cancer. The Lancet 2001; 357:1764–1766.

20. Augustsson K, Michaud DS, et al. A prospective study of intake of fish and marine fatty acids and prostate cancer. Cancer Epidemiol Biomarkers Prev 2003; 12:64–67.

21. Norrish AE, et al. Prostate cancer risk and consumption of fish oils: a dietary biomarker-based case-control study. British Journal of Cancer 1999; 81:1238–1242.

22. Cohen J, et al. Fruit and vegetable intakes and prostate cancer risk. Journal of the National Cancer Institute 2000; 92:61–68.

23. Hsing AW, Chokkalingam AP, et al. Allium vegetables and risk of prostate cancer: a population-based study. J Natl Cancer Inst 2002; 94(21):1648–1651.

24. Giovannucci E, Ascherio O, et al. Intake of carotenoids and retinol in relation to risk of prostate cancer. Journal of the National Cancer Institute 1995; 87: 1767–1776

25. Fair WR, Fleshner NE, Heston W. Cancer of the prostate: a nutritional disease? Urology 1997; 50(6):840–848.

26. Lee MM, Gomez SL, et al. Soy and isoflavone consumption in relation to prostate cancer risk in China. Cancer Epidemiol Biomarkers Prev 2003; 12(7):665–668.

27. Lieberman R, Nelson WG, et al. Executive Summary of the National Cancer Institute Workshop: Highlights and recommendations. Urology 2001; 57(4 Suppl 1):4–27.

28. Rodriguez C, McCullough ML, et al. Calcium, dairy products, and risk of prostate cancer in a

prospective cohort of United States men. Cancer Epidemiol Biomarkers Prev 2003; 12(7):597–603.

29. Leitzmann MF, Stampfer MJ, et al. Zinc supplement use and risk of prostate cancer. J Natl Cancer Inst 2003; 95(13):1004–1007.

30. Konstantinos H. Prostate cancer in the elderly. Int Urol Nephrol 2005; 37(4):797–806.

31. Carreca I, Balducci L, Extermann M. Cancer in the older person. Cancer Treat Rev 2005; 31(5):380–402.

32. Geinitz H, Zimmermann FB, et al. 3D conformal radiation therapy for prostate cancer in elderly patients. Radiother Oncol 2005; 76(1):27–34.

33. Syrigos KN, Karapanagiotou E, Harrington KJ. Prostate cancer in the elderly. Anticancer Res 2005; 25(6C):4527–4533.

PATIENT HANDOUT 20.1 – BENIGN PROSTATIC HYPERPLASIA

As men age, their prostate enlarges. The enlarged prostate may compress the urethra, obstructing urine flow.

Recognizing the presence of prostate enlargement

Men with an enlarged prostate may:

- Experience delay before being able to start passing urine.
- Produce a weak, intermittent urine stream. It is easier to pass urine sitting than standing.
- Find it takes a long time to empty the bladder. The rate of urine flow is often reduced to half that of their younger years.
- Find straining does not improve the urine stream.
- Dribble urine after they have finished urinating.

As obstruction to urine flow worsens, it becomes difficult to completely empty the bladder and urine may be retained in the bladder.

An incompletely emptied bladder is prone to infection.

Useful tips for self-care

Tips for managing the problem:

- Void frequently and allow sufficient time to void completely.
- Avoid drinks before going to bed; cut down on fluids after 5.00 p.m.
- Avoid decongestants, coffee, alcohol and nicotine.
- Eat foods rich in phytosterols. Soybeans and soy products are particularly good choices.

Other foods to consider include apples, onion, flaxseeds, cereals and whole grains.

Recognizing bladder infection

Infection causes irritation of the urinary tract. This requires treatment. Suspect urinary infection if urine is passed:

- frequently during the day
- at night, resulting in disturbed sleep
- with urgency—when you gotta go you gotta go—incontinence may result
- in small volumes
- causing discomfort—burning is common.

Treatment is available

Treatment options include:

- Drugs. Saw palmetto (Serenoa repens) is a recognized herbal treatment for benign prostatic hyperplasia and may be as effective as finasteride, a pharmaceutical prescribed for the condition.
- Surgery. Surgical resection of the prostate may be necessary if symptoms are distressing and cannot be satisfactorily controlled, if there is a risk of kidney damage, or if bladder stones form. Complications of prostatectomy include sexual dysfunction, urinary infection, incontinence and bleeding.

Internet resources

http://www.niapublications.org/engagepages/prostate.asp
prostate problems

PATIENT HANDOUT 20.2 – PROSTATE CANCER

Early diagnosis reduces the risk of dying from prostate cancer.

A man with prostate cancer may have no symptoms and appear healthy. On the other hand he may have complaints indistinguishable from those suggesting benign prostatic hypertrophy. Screening is therefore recommended for all men over the age of 50 years.

Early diagnosis

- Digital rectal examination
- A blood test for prostate specific antigen (PSA).

A combination of digital rectal examination and PSA results is almost as effective in diagnosing this disease as using routine transurethral ultrasound.

Tips for preventing prostate cancer

Good lifestyle choices may reduce the risk of prostate cancer:

- Limit fat intake. Good sources of fat are fish such as salmon, herring, sardines and mackerel; olive oil and avocados. Limit or avoid processed meats, bacon, beef, pork or lamb, and dairy products.
- Eat lots of fruit and vegetables especially tomatoes and cruciferous vegetables i.e. cabbage, cauliflower, broccoli. Tomato sauce offers better protection than fresh tomatoes!
- Eat soy products.
- Take regular exercise.
- Consider taking nutritional supplements e.g. zinc (30 mg/day), vitamin E (55–100IU/day).
- Avoid excess calcium. However, 29-33 kcal of tomatoes may fully counter the effects of calcium contained in 1 cup of non-fat milk, with 86 kcal and 300 mg calcium.

Although these lifestyle measure may reduce risk, convincing evidence has yet to be produced. It is therefore important that older men are regularly screened for prostate cancer.

Internet resources

http://www.niapublications.org/engagepages/prostate.asp
prostate problems

Chapter 21

Gastrointestinal problems

An elderly patient presents complaining of the recent onset of constipation. He says his stool looks dark. He has a long history of heartburn and regurgitation. His wife recently put him on an iron supplement because he was complaining of tiredness and she felt he looked 'pale'.

- What may explain the sudden onset of this man's constipation?
- Could gastro-oesophageal reflux explain this patient's pallor i.e. possible anaemia?
- Once serious pathology has been excluded, how could this patient's reflux and constipation be managed?

INTRODUCTION

A number of gastrointestinal problems, present in all age groups, become more pronounced with aging. Two complaints prevalent amongst elderly patients are constipation and gastro-oesophageal reflux.

CONSTIPATION

It has been suggested that constipation affects some 4.5 million Americans and accounts for over 2.5 million physician visits annually.[1] The elderly and women are most at risk. Some 26% of women and 16% of men 65 years of age and older suffer from constipation.[2] While the prevalence of constipation ranges from 15–20% in the community-dwelling elderly population, it increases and may reach 50% in nursing home residents. The latter are at increased risk of a reduced fibre and fluid intake, decreased physical activity and multiple medications.[3] Drugs commonly causing constipation include calcium and iron supplements, opioid analgesics such as codeine, antacids such as aluminium hydroxide, calcium channel antagonists, drugs with anticholinergic side effects and laxatives, when abused. Laxatives are the third or fourth most commonly used over-the-counter drug purchases and over $350 million is spent in this manner in the US each year.[1,2] Furthermore, while a decline in bowel movement frequency is not an invariable concomitant of aging, laxative use has been found to increase substantially with aging.[4]

Diagnosing constipation

Constipation is defined as a change in the frequency, volume, weight, consistency and ease of the passage of stool. It may present as infrequent defecation, an excessively hard stool or an inability to evacuate without prolonged straining. Constipation may be attributed to poor dietary and bowel habits, bowel motility disorders or organic disease. While it is particularly important to exclude constipation secondary to organic disease such as colorectal cancer, hypothyroidism or depression in the elderly, primary constipation remains the prevalent problem.

Anal fissure and haemorrhoids are complications of chronic constipation. Despite popular belief, there is as yet no scientifically acceptable evidence to support the theory that constipation causes disease through autointoxication.[5]

Management

Lifestyle options

Regular physical activity, increased fluid and a high fibre intake form the basis of non-drug management. Middle-aged inactive subjects with symptoms of chronic constipation who undertake regular physical activity improve both their defecation pattern and rectosigmoid or total colonic transit time.[6]

While increased fluid intake may only be beneficial in somewhat dehydrated persons,[5] a low fluid intake is a recognized factor in the elderly and a significant relationship between liquid deprivation and constipation has been reported.[7] In addition to high fibre foods such as wholegrain cereals, fruit and vegetables, fibre enriched supplements are available. Although fibre as raw bran is not always well tolerated, a fibre-rich porridge has been shown to be effective, well liked and reduced the need for laxatives.[8] Despite it being regularly recommended, adherence to the simple lifestyle measures of an adequate fluid intake, regular exercise and high fibre intake is limited. Pharmacological treatment is frequently required.

Drug options

Laxatives fall into a number of categories. A study of community dwelling elderly persons found that one in 10 subjects used at least one laxative, and stimulants, bulking agents and stool softeners were popular choices.[2] Over-the-counter agents include: bulking agents, e.g. psyllium; natural vegetable powder such as vegetable root extracts; hyperosmotic laxatives, e.g. sorbitol; lubricants, e.g. mineral oil; stimulants, e.g. castor oil, senna; stool softeners, e.g. docusate; saline agents, e.g. milk of magnesium, magnesium citrate, sodium phosphate; and miscellaneous agents such as glycerine.

Bulk and osmotic laxatives are popular choices if dietary fibre is unsuccessful in alleviating symptoms.[9] Hyperosmotic agents are recommended for persons with a low fluid intake.[2] Lactulose, a hyperosmotic laxative, requires prescription and causes flatulence, bloating and abdominal cramping.[10] Provided there are no cardiac or renal comorbid contraindications, saline laxatives are a good option for regular use by the elderly.[9] Nonetheless, dehydration may affect the efficacy of this treatment and is a realistic risk if fluid replacement is not maintained.[7] Both stimulant and saline laxatives increase the risk of electrolyte imbalance and cramping.

Stimulant laxatives, most useful in those instances when constipation is medication related, are used intermittently in patients who do not respond to bulk-forming or osmotic laxatives.[3] It is unlikely that stimulant laxatives, at recommended doses, are harmful to the colon. However, excess use of castor oil may damage the small bowel mucosa and cause steatorrhoea. From the general medical point of view, lubricating agents have become obsolete.[10]

Unfortunately, data are too limited in elderly persons to formally recommend one class of laxative in preference to another or one agent rather than another within each class.[3] Nonetheless, a recent review concluded that there is good evidence to support the use of polyethylene glycol, an osmotic agent, moderate evidence to support use of psyllium and lactulose, and a paucity of quality data regarding the use of many other agents including milk of magnesia, senna, bisacodyl and stool softeners.[11] Moreover, it has been suggested that only polyethylene glycol should be used on a daily basis.[9] Polyethylene glycol has also been shown to relieve faecal impaction in frail patients with neurological disease. It is, however, expensive and should be avoided in patients at high risk for aspiration. In addition to laxatives, the use of suppositories and enemas may be considered in cases with delayed transit and difficult evacuation.[12]

Evidence to suggest rebound constipation results on stopping laxative intake is inconclusive.[5] Laxative habituation may, however, cause diarrhoea and be associated with faecal incontinence. Approximately 3–10% of older people in the community have faecal incontinence.[12] Other causes of faecal incontinence include dementia, an incompetent anal sphincter and faecal impaction. Leakage of feculent brown liquid around impacted stool in a dilated rectum is termed spurious diarrhoea.

GASTRO-OESOPHAGEAL REFLUX (GERD)

Gastro-oesophageal reflux symptoms are common in young and old. In fact, reflux dyspepsia is the most common cause of indigestion in Western society. Polypharmacy in the elderly may aggravate the problem.

A study of elderly Italians found 91.6% took drugs and the mean number of drugs taken was 2.86 per person.[13] One third of subjects reported at least one gastrointestinal symptom; 25% had indigestion syndrome, 16.2% abdominal pain and 14.2% reflux symptoms. Use of nonsteroidal anti-inflammatory drugs, steroids, psycholeptics, diuretics, selective beta-2-adrenoreceptor agonists and antiplatelet drugs was significantly associated with upper gastrointestinal symptoms.

Making a diagnosis

Persons with GERD may be asymptomatic—as many as one in three persons with severe oesophagitis may be symptom free! One study comparing persons under 65 years of age with an older group found heartburn without oesophagitis was present in 28% of the young and in 24% of elderly patients.[14] Another study in which the average age of men was 54 years and that of women 50 years found heartburn without oesophagitis was present in 38% of men and 55% of women.[15] While the former study found prevalence rates, patterns and features of symptomatic GERD were similar in both groups,[13] the latter found women reported significantly higher symptom severity scores for heartburn, regurgitation, belching and nocturnal symptoms than did men.[14] Symptomatic sufferers most often complain of heartburn.[16] However, not everyone who has heartburn has reflux, and not everybody who has reflux has heartburn. Other common complaints are acid regurgitation, excessive belching and dysphagia. Chronic reflux should be excluded whenever elderly persons complain of dysphagia. High-dose treatment trials and ambulatory pH monitoring have become more important than endoscopy in the diagnosis of reflux.

Complications of chronic reflux

Persons with gastro-oesophageal reflux may have symptoms which persist for weeks and years. Chronic reflux can lead to oesophageal erosion, ulceration, fibrosis and oesophageal stricture. It has also been shown to increase the risk of developing adenocarcinoma of the distal oesophagus and cardia.[17] GERD is hypothesized to cause acute mucosal injury, promote cellular proliferation, and induce specialized columnar metaplasia (Barrett's oesophagus) which progresses to invasive adenocarcinoma.[18] Barrett's oesophagus, found in 5–15% of patients with reflux symptoms,[19] is recognized late in the elderly, possibly due to elderly patients with Barrett's oesophagus experiencing significantly less severe symptoms than younger patients. Women appear at lower risk than men.[15] Being overweight and having a hiatus hernia increases risk.[19] Prolonged management of reflux with acid suppression medication may mask symptoms of cancer and delay diagnosis. Periodic endoscopy or imaging studies are therefore recommended for patients with long-standing gastro-oesophageal reflux. Elderly patients with new onset reflux should be actively investigated to exclude cancer of the distal oesophagus or cardia.[20]

Management

Beneficial lifestyle changes include positional changes such as not lying down after eating and not eating or drinking for at least 2 hours before lying down, raising the bed head to encourage drainage and avoiding bending or stooping. Voluntary belching should be avoided as should gastric distension due to overeating or abdominal compression due to tight garments.

Dietary choices can also affect reflux. A cross sectional study reported that, while a high dietary fat intake was associated with an increased risk of reflux symptoms and erosive oesophagitis, a high fibre intake correlated with a reduced risk.[21] A low fat high fibre diet is therefore recommended. In addition to these general recommendations, particular dietary constituents which aggravate reflux should be avoided. These include: chocolates, coffee, spicy foods, tomato-based and citrus foods. A number of medications encourage reflux, including antidepressants and calcium channel blocking agents. It is advisable to quit smoking.

An additional advantage of a low fat high fibre diet is that is likely to be low energy and encourage weight loss. Overweight and obesity are strong independent risk factors for reflux symptoms and oesophageal erosions.[20] One study found obese participants were 2.5 times as likely as those with a normal BMI (<25) to have reflux symptoms or oesophageal erosions.[20] Obesity is furthermore not only associated with a statistically significant increase in the risk for reflux symptoms, it is also associated with an increased risk of erosive oesophagitis and oesophageal adenocarcinoma.[22] The risk for these disorders seems to increase progressively with increasing weight. Management therefore includes weight loss and maintaining a normal body weight.

While these conservative measures are helpful, they do not always relieve symptoms. Self-care remedies include sucking licorice lozenges (380–1140 mg/day). This may slightly reduce inflammation, spasm and discomfort. Prolonged use may, however, lead to pseudohyperaldosteronism; and those with hypertension require deglycyrrhizinated licorice. Another alternative option is slippery elm which may promote tissue healing in doses of 60–320 mg/day taken as 1 teaspoon with water several times a day. Antacids are popular over-the-counter remedies.

When symptoms persist and medical intervention is requested, the mainstays of treatment are acid-suppressing agents, the most helpful of which are proton-pump inhibitors and histamine H(2)-receptor antagonists. Proton-pump inhibitors should be used first.[23] When this fails to relieve symptoms, alternative diagnoses should be considered.[24]

IN PERSPECTIVE

Constipation and GERD are common problems in the elderly and medication may further aggravate bowel motility problems in this age group. Careful monitoring of patients is advisable as symptoms may mask underlying malignancy.

CLINICAL CHALLENGE

An elderly woman presents with faecal incontinence. She is lucid and mobile. She explains she has had to struggle with constipation for many years.

Questions arising

- What is a likely diagnosis?
- How should she be managed?

Clinical considerations

Faecal impaction, laxative abuse and an incompetent anal sphincter need to be considered.

On examination her rectum is found to contain a hard faecal mass.

After relieving her current problem using an enema, refer to Patient Handout 21.2 and guide her through the steps of good bowel hygiene. Discuss the use of laxatives and review her medications with a view to identifying any drugs that may be exacerbating her problem.

Also actively exclude any underlying medical conditions such as hypothyroidism.

PRACTICE GEMS

- ◆ Thyroid disease should be investigated in elderly patients who develop constipation.
- ◆ A good fluid intake, regular exercise, a high fibre diet and responsiveness to the call to stool are important components of conservative management of constipation.
  - ◆ Intermittent use of stimulant laxatives may be necessary for medication—induced or exacerbated constipation.
  - ◆ Polyethylene glycol, psyllium and lactulose are laxatives of choice.
  - ◆ Fluid replacement is an important consideration in elderly persons using laxatives.
  - ◆ Heartburn may be precipitated by chocolate, peppermint, spicy or fatty foods.

- ◆ Reflux sufferers should maintain a low body weight, eat small meals, wear loose clothes and eat several hours before lying down.
- ◆ Bananas and 1 teaspoon of fresh or 0.5 teaspoon of powdered ginger in a cup of boiling water are useful therapy for indigestion; however, ginger increases gastric secretion and may decrease the effectiveness of antacids.
- ◆ Cranberry juice increases vitamin B12 absorption in patients on omeprazole, a proton pump inhibitor used to treat reflux.
- ◆ Sipping 2 or 3 cups of basil tea between meals may ease flatulence.
- ◆ Abdominal massage using essential oils with rosemary, lemon and peppermint helps relieve constipation in the elderly.

References

1. Stessman M. Biofeedback: its role in the treatment of chronic constipation. Gastroenterol Nurs 2003; 26(6):251–260.

2. Ruby CM, Fillenbaum GG, et al. Laxative use in the community-dwelling elderly. Am J Geriatr Pharmacother 2003; 1(1):11–17.

3. Bosshard W, Dreher R, et al. The treatment of chronic constipation in elderly people: an update. Drugs Aging. 2004; 21(14):911–930.

4. Harari D, Gurwitz JH, et al. Bowel habit in relation to age and gender. Findings from the National Health Interview Survey and clinical implications. Arch Intern Med 1996; 156(3):315–320.

5. Muller-Lissner SA, Kamm MA, et al. Myths and misconceptions about chronic constipation. Am J Gastroenterol 2005; 100(1):232–242.

6. De Schryver AM, Keulemans YC, et al. Effects of regular physical activity on defecation pattern in middle-aged patients complaining of chronic constipation. Scand J Gastroenterol 2005; 40(4):422–429.

7. Arnaud MJ. Mild dehydration: a risk factor of constipation? Eur J Clin Nutr 2003; 57(Suppl 2):S88–595.

8. Wisten A, Messner T. Fruit and fibre (Pajala porridge) in the prevention of constipation. Scand J Caring Sci 2005; 19(1):71–76.

9. Pampati V, Fogel R. Treatment options for primary constipation. Curr Treat Options Gastroenterol 2004; 7(3):225–233.

10. Klaschik E, Nauck F, et al. Constipation—modern laxative therapy. Support Care Cancer 2003 Nov; 11(11):679–685.

11. Ramkumar D, Rao SS. Efficacy and safety of traditional medical therapies for chronic constipation: systematic review. Am J Gastroenterol 2005; 100(4):936–971.

12. Potter J, Wagg A. Management of bowel problems in older people: an update. Clin Med 2005; 5(3):289–295.

13. Pilotto A, Franceschi M, et al. Drug use by the elderly in general practice: effects on upper gastrointestinal symptoms. Eur J Clin Pharmacol 2006; 62(1):65–73.

14. Triadafilopoulos G, Sharma R. Features of symptomatic gastroesophageal reflux disease in elderly patients. Am J Gastroenterol 1997; 92(11):2007–2011.

15. Lin M, Gerson LB, et al. Features of gastroesophageal reflux disease in women. Am J Gastroenterol 2004; 99(8):1442–1447.

16. Okamoto K, Iwakiri R, et al. Clinical symptoms in endoscopic reflux esophagitis: evaluation in 8031 adult subjects. Dig Dis Sci 2003; 48(12):2237–2241.

17. Velanovich V, Hollingsworth J, et al. Relationship of gastroesophageal reflux disease with adenocarcinoma of the distal esophagus and cardia. Dig Surg 2002; 19(5):349–353.

18. Casson AG, Williams L, Guernsey DL. Epidemiology and molecular biology of Barrett esophagus. Semin Thorac Cardiovasc Surg 2005; 17(4):284–291.

19. Westhoff B, Brotze S, et al. The frequency of Barrett's esophagus in high-risk patients with chronic GERD. Gastrointest Endosc 2005; 61(2):226–231.

20. El-Serag HB, Graham DY, et al. Obesity is an independent risk factor for GERD symptoms and erosive esophagitis. Am J Gastroenterol 2005; 100(6):1243–1250.

21. El-Serag HB, Satia JA, Rabeneck L. Dietary intake and the risk of gastro-oesophageal reflux disease: a cross sectional study in volunteers. Gut 2005; 54(1):11–17.

22. Hampel H, Abraham NS, El-Serag HB. Meta-analysis: obesity and the risk for gastroesophageal reflux disease and its complications. Ann Intern Med 2005 2; 143(3):199–211.

23. Habu Y, Maeda K, et al. 'Proton-pump inhibitor-first' strategy versus 'step-up' strategy for the acute treatment of reflux esophagitis: a cost-effectiveness analysis in Japan. J Gastroenterol 2005; 40(11):1029–1035.

24. Locke GR. Current medical management of gastroesophageal reflux disease. Thorac Surg Clin 2005; 15(3):369–375.

PATIENT HANDOUT 21.1 – TOWARDS A HEALTHY DIGESTIVE SYSTEM

Elderly persons frequently find they are troubled by constipation and reflux. Living wisely can help to solve both these problems!

A healthy bowel

Eating right can reduce the risk of:

- intestinal infection
- constipation
- non-insulin dependent diabetes
- obesity
- osteoporosis
- colon cancer.

Eating right means having a healthy daily diet rich in:

- whole grains
- vegetables
- fruit
- 4 or more servings of low fat dairy products
- 1 serving of fish or red meat.

Eating better may mean including functional foods in the diet: are these the new wonder foods?

The following groups of functional foods are particularly important for bowel health:

- Prebiotics. Good plant sources of these prebiotics are onions, asparagus, wheat and artichoke leaf. Non-digestible oligosaccharides alter the intestinal flora and stimulate the growth of healthy bacteria.
- Probiotics. These live microbial food supplements provide a rich source of healthy bacteria and improve intestinal microbial balance. You can boost your health by having 250 mL of a low fat yogurt rich in acidophilus and bifidus twice a day. Only fresh products and those specifically stating that they contain *Lactobacilli* and/or *Bifidobacteria* should be used. Freeze-dried powders are another option; these need to be kept dry and refrigerated. Tablets are heat processed and therefore unlikely to contain sufficient viable bacteria to be therapeutic.
- Resistant starch. This form of starch is not readily digested and benefits the large bowel. A daily intake of 20 g is recommended. Foods rich in resistant starch are bananas, potatoes (especially when eaten cold), and processed foods rich in maize or wheat. Certain manufacturers produce bread particularly rich in resistant starch.

PATIENT HANDOUT 21.2 – CONSTIPATION

Constipation is the infrequent passage of a hard stool. Good intestinal hygiene may prevent constipation. It includes:

- regular exercise
- eating a hearty breakfast and allowing time for the gastro-colic reflex to work
- maintaining an adequate fluid intake (1500 ml/day)
- a diet rich in fibre. Eat nuts, wholegrain products, fruit and vegetables
  —good fruit choices are stone fruits, pineapple and citrus fruits
  —good vegetable choices are cabbage, peas, beans, cauliflower and brussels sprouts
- using natural laxatives. Prunes, apricots, figs, rhubarb and kiwi-fruit are good choices.

When constipation persists despite good intestinal hygiene, consider:

- Fibre supplementation. Two tablespoons per day of bran increases stool bulk. Side effects include flatulence, worsened reflux symptoms and anal irritability. Bran is unpalatable.
- A vegetable root extract (e.g. Nu-lux). One teaspoon daily is useful in patients on a high fibre diet whose stool is soft and whose main problem is colonic atony.
- Hydrophilic colloids. Psyllium seeds, sterculia, ispaghula, bassorin and cellulose increase intestinal bulk by increasing the water content of the stool. A daily dose of 6–8 g is required. A warning: intestinal obstruction may occur if insufficient water is taken.
- Synthetic sugars. Lactulose and mannitol act as osmotic laxatives, increasing the water content of the stool. Flatulence and abdominal distention may aggravate reflux. This is an expensive option.

Internet resources

http://www.niapublications.org/engagepages/const.asp
information about constipation

PATIENT HANDOUT 21.3 – REFLUX

Gastro-oesophageal reflux occurs when stomach contents leak into the oesophagus. Suspect reflux if you have:

- heartburn
- regurgitation
- excessive belching.

Reduce the risk of reflux:

- Exercise dietary discretion.
  - —Avoid foods that decrease the tone of the gastro-oesophageal sphincter. Don't eat chocolate, coffee, alcohol or fatty meals, don't smoke.
  - —Eat foods that increase gastro-oesophageal sphincter tone. High protein meals and antacids seem helpful.
- Eat small meals frequently.
- Don't eat or drink for 2 or more hours before going to bed.
- Don't bend or stoop, especially after a large meal.
- Sleep with the head of the bed raised.
- Avoid increased intra-abdominal pressure.
  - —Stay slim/lose excess weight.
  - —Wear loose garments.
  - —Don't wear corsets.

Chapter 22

Chronic pulmonary disease

A 68-year-old man presents for a check up. He says he is well except that last week he missed the bus because he was too out of 'puff' to run to the bus stop. He has a 30-year history of smoking up to five cigarettes a day. His BMI is 23, his blood pressure is normal. He leads a sedentary lifestyle.

- Can this man have dyspnoea in the absence of an underlying cardiopulmonary problem?
- Would exercise be of benefit?
- What can be done to get the man to stop smoking?

INTRODUCTION

Aging involves a progressive decline in the functional reserve of multiple organ systems and an increased prevalence of chronic diseases. Maximal oxygen consumption decreases by 10% in men and 7.5% in women with each decade of adult life.[1] The dominating risk factors for impaired lung disease are increasing age and smoking.[2] Lung capacity is particularly compromised in smokers. Some 50% of elderly smokers develop airflow limitation,[2] and smoking is responsible for about 85% of the risk of developing chronic obstructive pulmonary disease, a condition which the World Health Organization expects to become the fifth major cause of illness by 2020.[3] In this condition lung vital capacity is reduced, peak flow rate is diminished and expiration is prolonged. The maximum peak flow rate is a useful index of best lung function.

A study which followed a group of 60-year-old persons over 15 years found the independent predictors of mortality were cigarette smoking, impaired peak expiratory flow, diabetes, very high blood pressure, physical disability and zero intake of alcohol.[4] Over 15 years, the average reductions in survival time associated with smoking in men and women were 22 and 15 months respectively. For impaired peak expiratory flow they were 14 and 17 months respectively. Peak expiratory flow has been found to provide the highest hazard ratios for predicting time to death in women and the second highest in men.[5]

SMOKING

Use of tobacco is the second leading cause of death in the world.[5] It is responsible for 1 in 10 adult deaths and if current smoking trends continue, it will kill 10 million people annually by 2020. A Chinese study reported that the relative risks of ever-smokers (everyone who at any time has been a smoker) were 1.34 for deaths from all causes, 3.23 for chronic obstructive pulmonary disease, 2.31 for lung cancer and 1.60 for coronary heart disease.[6] The risk amplified significantly as the amount and duration of smoking increased. Even exposure to environmental tobacco smoke is associated with 1.3 times the risk for all respiratory diseases and 1.34 times the risk of lung cancer.[7] This risk is consistently higher for former smokers than for never smokers. Compared with current smokers, former smokers have a lower risk of total mortality and death from heart disease, but a higher risk for death from chronic obstructive pulmonary disease.[6]

While never starting to smoke is preferable, early quitting is highly desirable!

DYSPNOEA

One study of persons 60 years and older found 41% of subjects reported shortness of breath.[8] Another found about 11% of persons 70 years and older had at least one current obstructive pulmonary disease, 12% of whom suffered significant dyspnoea.[9] Dyspnoea, a sensation of laboured and difficult breathing, is by far the most common and debilitating symptom associated with chronic obstructive pulmonary disease.[10] Restrictive ventilatory syndrome, another cause of dyspnea, may result from interstitial lung diseases, muscular weakness, congestive heart failure, diabetes mellitus and obesity.[11] Restrictive syndrome is relatively frequently encountered in the elderly, with a prevalence of about 10–12% after the age of 65 years. While lung disease is the most common cause of dyspnoea in elderly persons,[12] it is also a cardinal symptom of left heart failure.[13] Inspiratory muscle weakness accounts, in part, for this symptom. Patients with diastolic dysfunction adopt a rapid, shallow breathing pattern during exercise and experience dyspnoea at low work loads. Of all respiratory symptoms, dyspnoea alone shows a clear age-related pattern and breathlessness increases with age until 89 years whereupon it starts to decline.[9]

Dyspnoea has a profound impact on the quality of life.

Quality of life

Health-related quality of life is an individual's perception of physical and mental health. Variables that affect the physical health component of health-related quality of life evaluations include breathlessness, physical impairment and reduced activities of daily living; variables that affect mental health are breathlessness, hopelessness and anxiety, and negative affective trait.[14] Breathlessness contributes to both the physical and mental components of health-related quality of life and correlates with fatigue and sleep difficulty in patients with chronic obstructive pulmonary disease.[15]

Asthmatics complain of dyspnoea and wheezing. The quality of life of elderly persons with asthma is substantially lower than others their age—even in those whose asthma has not been diagnosed.[16] One study found 82% of residents in long term facilities report limitation from dyspnoea in daily activities; however, 34% of these individuals failed to show any evidence of cardiac or pulmonary disease.[17] Dyspnoea in older patients does not necessarily imply the presence of cardiac or pulmonary disease.

Aging inevitably reduces resources for adapting to change. Chronic inflammation is involved in the pathogenesis of aging and markers of inflammation such as interleukin-6 are elevated in most geriatric syndromes, ranging from dementia to osteoporosis and sarcopenia. At a biochemical level the concentration of circulating inflammatory markers in older persons predicts the risk of mortality and functional dependence.[18] At a clinical level, the more pronounced the breathlessness, the greater the physical impairment.[14] Dyspnoea predicts variances in functional performance.[15] Frailty results from a critical depletion of physiological reserve, and breathlessness in elderly persons with no apparent cardiac or respiratory disease may be a manifestation of aging.

Dyspnoea is the dominant determinant of health-related quality of life in patients with emphysema. It is, however, not solely responsible. Health-related quality of life is also, to a minor degree, influenced by expiratory muscle strength.[19] Muscle mass in turn appears to be associated with lung function. An increased fat free mass reflecting increased muscle mass appears to be associated with superior lung function and a lesser likelihood of low FEV1–FVC ratio in the elderly.[20] Total body fat and central adiposity are inversely associated with lung function—forced expiratory volume in 1 second (FEV1) was diminished in men with BMI < 22.5 or ≥ 30, but forced vital capacity (FVC) tended to decrease with increasing BMI. Health quality of life, aging and frailty are all interlinked, being affected by multiple factors and numerous interacting processes.

Management

Dyspnoea has a substantial impact on an individual's health quality of life rating. Inactivity itself may induce physical deconditioning. Adoption of a sedentary lifestyle appears to make older subjects less tolerant to exercise and more prone to report dyspnoea even for minimal or moderate efforts. Compared to those in a sedentary control group, persons who did 4 weeks of daily exercise training became less breathless and significantly improved their walking endurance.[17] These outcomes were even documented in persons without overt cardiorespiratory disease.[17] Recent studies indicate that health gains can be achieved with relatively low volumes of exercise.[21] Current data suggest that a cumulative total of 30–50 minutes of aerobic exercise a day performed 3–5 days a week, coupled with one set of resistance exercises targeting the major muscle groups twice a week, can produce significant general health benefits in elderly persons.

Patients with underlying disease may be more difficult to manage. Specific treatment, such as lung resection for bronchogenic cancer or bronchodilation for asthma, is used whenever indicated. In other cases, intervention for pulmonary problems focuses on symptom relief. Patients with chronic obstructive pulmonary disease self-manage their dyspnoea using techniques that range from breathing through pursed lips to modifying their activity both with respect to intensity, e.g. moving more slowly, and quantity, i.e. doing less. As no cure and few effective treatments are available for this progressive disease, these self-help measures are coupled with pulmonary rehabilitation programs in an endeavour to improve the patient's quality of life.[22]

As chronic inflammation is involved in the pathogenesis of this condition, nutritional support to dampen inflammation may be attempted. Supplementation with an omega-3 polyunsaturated fatty acid rich diet (400 kcal/day) over 2 years was found to contribute significantly to a change in cytokine levels.[23] This may provide benefits at several levels as chronic inflammation may represent the common pathway through which different environmental insults hasten the exhaustion of the functional reserve of multiple organ systems.

While treating symptoms and targeting disease processes somewhat alleviates distress, prevention remains the preferred option. The single greatest factor contributing to pulmonary disease is smoking. Never smoking is the prime objective. Failing that, the sooner a smoker quits the better the outcome. This applies regardless of gender even though women find it harder to quit smoking and are more likely to develop aggressive lung cancer at lower levels of smoking.[5] See Patient Handout 22.1.

IN PERSPECTIVE

Smoking is a major risk for pulmonary disease. Decreased lung capacity is encountered in elderly persons even in the absence of lung disease. Dyspnoea has an adverse impact on the health-related quality of life and is best prevented by never smoking and leading an aerobically active lifestyle.

A 50-year-old man presents with a persistent cough. You note he smokes 40 cigarettes a day and has done so for the last 25 years. How could you set about reducing his risk of cancer?

Questions arising

- What needs to be excluded?
- How should the patient be counselled?

Clinical considerations

Bronchogenic carcinoma may present with a cough. In fact, a persistent cough is present in 80% of patients. Single or repeated haemoptysis occurs in 70% of patients. Dyspnoea and weight loss in the absence of anorexia may also be encountered.

Use X-ray, bronchoscopy and bronchial washing to exclude lung cancer.

Persuade the patient to stop smoking:

- See *www.niapublications.org/engagepages/ smoking.asp*—smoking: it's never too late to stop.
- Make the patient aware of the risks of continuing to smoke. See *www.jamisonhealth.com* Handout 14.1.
- Make the patient aware he has a tobacco problem and what benefits can be achieved by quitting. See *www.jamisonhealth.com* Handout 14.2.
- Help the patient to quit. See Patient Handout 22.1.
- This is also a good opportunity to provide the patient with advice on cancer prevention and early detection. See Patient Handouts 23.1 and 23.2.

- ◆ Reduced respiratory reserve is an inevitable consequence of aging.
- ◆ The extent to which dsypnoea impairs the quality of life is influenced by the individual's lifestyle, their smoking habits and the presence of cardiorespiratory disease.

- ◆ The best strategies for maintaining good lung function into old age are regular exercise and avoidance of pollution, particularly that resulting from tobacco smoke.
- ◆ Dyspnoea has a profound influence on physical and mental quality of life evaluations.

References

1. Knight JA. The biochemistry of aging. Adv Clin Chem 2000; 35:1–62.
2. Lundback B, Lindberg A, et al. Not 15 but 50% of smokers develop COPD? Report from the Obstructive Lung Disease in Northern Sweden Studies. Respir Med 2003; 97(2):115–122.
3. Frith PA. Letter. MJA 2005; 182(9):495–496.
4. Murray S. A smouldering epidemic. CMAJ 2006; 174(3). Online.Available:http://www.cmaj.ca/cgi/content/full/174/3/309
5. Simons LA, Simons J, et al. Impact of smoking, diabetes and hypertension on survival time in the elderly: the Dubbo Study. Med J Aust 2005; 182(5):219–222.
6. He Y, Taihing L, et al. A prospective study on smoking, quitting and mortality in a cohort of elderly in Xi'an, China. Zhonghua Liu Xing Bing Xue Za Zhi 2002; 23(3):186–189.
7. Vineis P, Airoldi L, et al. Environmental tobacco smoke and risk of respiratory cancer and chronic obstructive pulmonary disease in former smokers and never smokers in the EPIC prospective study. BMJ 2005; 330(7486):277.
8. Sha MC, Callahan CM, et al. Physical symptoms as a predictor of health care use and mortality among older adults. Am J Med 2005; 118(3):301–306.
9. Hardie JA, Vollmer WM, et al. Respiratory symptoms and obstructive pulmonary disease in a population aged over 70 years. Respir Med 2005; 99(2):186–195.
10. Christenbery TL. Dyspnea self-management strategies: use and effectiveness as reported by patients with chronic obstructive pulmonary disease. Heart Lung 2005; 34(6):406–414.
11. Fimognari FL, Pastorelli R, et al. Restrictive ventilatory dysfunction and dyspnea in elderly subjects. Amer J Med 2005; 118:1300–1301.
12. Pedersen F, Raymond I, et al. Prevalence of diastolic dysfunction as a possible cause of dyspnea in the elderly. Am J Med 2005; 118: 25–31.
13. Arora R. Dyspnea in the elderly. Amer J Med 2005; 118(11):1301–1302.
14. Hu J, Meek P. Health-related quality of life in individuals with chronic obstructive pulmonary disease. Heart Lung 2005; 34(6):415–422.
15. Reishtein JL. Relationship between symptoms and functional performance in COPD. Res Nurs Health 2005; 28(1):39–47.
16. Enright P. The diagnosis of asthma in older patients. Exp Lung Res 2005; 31 (Suppl 1):15–21.
17. Bo M, Fontana M, et al. Positive effects of aerobic physical activity in institutionalized older subjects complaining of dyspnoea. Arch Gerontol Geriatr 2005 Dec 5; [Epub ahead of print].
18. Carreca I, Balducci L, Extermann M. Cancer in the older person. Cancer Treat Rev 2005; 31(5):380–402.
19. Gonzalez E, Herrejon A, et al. Determinants of health-related quality of life in patients with pulmonary emphysema. Respir Med 2005; 99(5):638–644.
20. Wannamethee SG, Shaper AG, Whincup PH. Body fat distribution, body composition, and respiratory function in elderly men. Am J Clin Nutr 2005; 82(5):996–1003.
21. Galloway MT, Jokl P. Aging successfully: the importance of physical activity in maintaining health and function. J Am Acad Orthop Surg 2000; 8(1):37–44.
22. Christenbery TL. Dyspnea self-management strategies: use and effectiveness as reported by patients with chronic obstructive pulmonary disease. Heart Lung 2005; 34(6):406–414.
23. Matsuyama W, Mitsuyama H, et al. Effects of omega-3 polyunsaturated fatty acids on inflammatory markers in COPD. Chest 2005; 128(6):3817–3827.

PATIENT HANDOUT 22.1 – BREATHING BETTER

Shortness of breath is a common problem for elderly people. It may be due to chronic lung or heart disease but it may also accompany pulmonary changes associated with aging.

Exercise

Inactivity is associated with physical deconditioning. This sets up a vicious cycle. The less you exercise, the less able you are to tolerate exercise and the more breathless you are likely to become after minimal or moderate efforts.

Exercise for at least 30–50 minutes on alternate days. Walk, swim or cycle—choose what suits you best.

Regular exercise benefits many aspects of health.

Quitting

The single major avoidable health hazard for the pulmonary system is cigarette smoke. It is best to be a never smoker. Failing that, aim to be an early quitter.

Decide if you are ready to quit:

- Decide whether smoking is a problem. See *www.jamisonhealth.com* Handout 14.3.
- Become aware of the risks you run by smoking. See *www.jamisonhealth.com* Handout 14.4.
- See how soon you could enjoy better health should you decide to quit. See *www.jamisonhealth.com* Handout 14.5.

Tips on how to quit:

- Keep a smoking diary. See *www.jamisonhealth.com* Handout 14.6.
- Explore various strategies for quitting. See *www.jamisonhealth.com* Handout 14.7.
- Evaluate your smoking behaviour and your need for nicotine. See *www.jamisonhealth.com* Handouts 14.8 and 14.9.
- Select a quitting strategy best suited to your needs. See *www.jamisonhealth.com* Handout 14.10.

Review your checklists and set up a quitting program that suits you.

- See *www.jamisonhealth.com* Handout 14.11.

It is never too late to quit!

Internet resources

www.niapublications.org/engagepages/smoking.asp
smoking: its never too late to stop

Chapter **23**

Cancer

CHAPTER CONTENTS

Barry Burns is 60 years old. He is overweight, leads a sedentary lifestyle, smokes 10 cigarettes a day and loves his beer and fries. He recently lost a friend to bowel cancer. He asks if it is too late to reduce his risk of cancer.

- What lifestyle changes could reduce his risk of cancer in general and bowel cancer in particular?
- What strategies are available to diagnose cancer early?

INTRODUCTION

Older persons are at greatest risk of cancer. Data from the cancer registry of 51 countries over five continents show that, except for non-melanoma skin cancer, cancer is almost 7 times more frequent among elderly men and around 4 times more common in elderly women than in younger persons between 30 and 64 years of age.[1] In contrast to the rate in younger persons, elderly men have almost double the cancer incidence rate of elderly women.

Both the incidence and the mortality rate of cancer increase with age. In the USA, 60% of all cancers and approximately 80% of all cancer-related deaths occur in the 12% of individuals aged 65 years and over.[2] The behaviour of cancers may also change with the age of the person. Some cancers, e.g. acute myeloid leukaemia, lymphoma and ovarian cancer, tend to become more aggressive while others, e.g. breast and lung cancer, become more indolent in the elderly.[2]

The prevalence of particular cancers has also changed. Since 1970 the incidence of non-Hodgkin's lymphoma has increased by 80% in individuals aged 60 and older and that of malignant brain tumours has increased 700% in individuals over 70. In the last 10 years, lung cancer-related mortality has increased by almost 50% among those over 80.[2] In contrast with other major causes of death among the elderly, cancer incidence and mortality have not in general declined.[1] However, in Europe the overall prevalence of cancer is highest in countries where both survival and incidence are high.[3]

CARCINOGENESIS

A number of cellular and physiological changes associated with aging have the potential to influence tumour development, metastasis and response to treatment.[2] Carcinogenesis is a multistep process involving impaired differentiation and growth control. Two important phases, those of initiation and promotion, have been identified in the process of tumour development. Initiation involves DNA damage or mutation and is irreversible. For cancer to develop a second phase, the promotion stage of accelerated cell proliferation is required. In phase one, single high level exposure to an initiating agent, e.g. certain viruses, or irradiation, can alter DNA and render a cell susceptible to cancerous change. Thereafter, prolonged exposure to promoting agent(s) is required before cellular proliferation results in cancer. Promoters are only weakly carcinogenic to cells not previously exposed to initiators. Promotion requires prolonged exposure and is reversible in the early stages.

There is a long delay between initiation, the primary causative event and overt disease—a decade or more may pass between the initiation of carcinogenesis and the overt development of cancer. While this long delay makes it difficult to clearly identify causal factors involved in carcinogenesis, it does provide ample opportunity for intervention.

Prevention remains the most effective approach to decreasing mortality. Minimizing lifestyle risks by not smoking and by making prudent exercise and dietary choices can influence the personal risk of developing cancer in all age groups. In fact, given the changes of senescence, environmental factors may be particularly important in carcinogenesis in elderly people. When prevention fails, early detection is important.

Screening is an important diagnostic measure and screening for breast and colorectal cancer is considered beneficial for all individuals with a life expectancy of at least 5 years.[2] Treatment, whether curative or palliative, rather than being determined by chronological age involves consideration of the person's life expectancy, functional reserve and personal and social resources.[2]

CANCER PREVENTION: GENERAL GUIDELINES

As prevention is the preferred approach to intervention, avoidance of risk factors is an important strategy. Globally, of 7 million deaths from cancer in 2001, an estimated 35% were attributable to nine potentially modifiable risk factors.[4] Smoking, alcohol abuse, low fruit and vegetable intake, overweight and obesity all emerged as major global risks. Cigarette consumption followed by obesity are suspected to be the two most common avoidable causes of cancer in Western society.[5]

Of the nine modifiable risks, the two leading hazardous behaviours are smoking and alcohol use. The adverse impact of these risk factors is not limited to cancer. For example, cigarettes and alcohol have also been shown to be independently related to coronary heart disease and injury, the other two main circumstances that contribute significantly to worldwide death and disability.[6] More than 1 in every 5 cancer deaths in the world in the year 2000 is believed to have been caused by smoking.[7]

Nine recommendations of the American Institute for Cancer Research to reduce cancer incidence were applied to a cohort of women aged 55–69 years who had no history of cancer. After 12 years, compared with those who implemented at least six of the recommendations, women who followed one or no recommendation ran 1.35 times the risk of developing, and 1.43 times the risk of dying from, cancer.[8] The nine recommendations were:

1. Maintain an ideal body weight (BMI not to exceed 25) and limit weight gain to less than 11 lbs/5 kg.
2. Take daily moderate and weekly vigorous exercise.
3. Eat 5 or more servings of fruit and vegetables daily.
4. Eat 7 or more complex carbohydrate servings daily; emphasize whole grains and cereals.
5. Limit sugar, salt and processed foods.
6. Limit alcoholic drinks to 1 standard drink daily if a woman and 2 if a man.
7. Limit red meat to 3 ounces or less daily.
8. Limit fatty foods, especially those from animal sources.
9. Eliminate tobacco.

Addressing risk

Smoking

By 2025 one third of all adult deaths are expected to be related to cigarette smoking.[9] Smoking increases the risk of cancer for most sites. It has been implicated in 30% of all cancer deaths and in 87% of deaths attributed to lung cancer. Active and passive smokers inhale carcinogens and precarcinogens. Cancer prevention guidelines are never to start smoking, and having started to stop right away. The threshold risk level for lung cancer in men appears to be 20 pack years, i.e. smoking an average of one packet a day over 20 years. In women the risk threshold is 10 pack years. The relative risk of lung cancer in a two packet a day smoker is 20 times that of the non-smoker. Furthermore, for a fixed number of cigarettes smoked, the risk of lung cancer increases with age.

Quitting changes the outcome. Although the chance of developing lung cancer is 20–40 times higher in lifelong smokers than non-smokers, after quitting the cumulative death risk from lung cancer decreases. For those who are unable to quit, a smokeless tobacco product called Swedish snus may be helpful. Snus is associated with a lower risk than regular cigarettes for all-cause mortality, lung, oral and gastric cancers and for cardiovascular disease.[10] It has been estimated that the impact of primary prevention on the overall incidence of cancer through cessation of tobacco smoking is 18%, through dietary change 4.2% and through alcohol avoidance 2.2%.[11]

Alcohol

Smoking and drinking alcohol are behaviours that frequently coexist, and use of one is associated with higher consumption of the other.[6] While a combination of alcohol and smoking has a multiplicative interaction on the risk of cancers of the oral cavity, larynx, pharynx and oesophagus, alcohol alone is also a recognized cancer risk. In fact, even consuming an 'average' volume of alcohol has been shown to increase, along with other chronic conditions, the risk of a number of cancers including mouth, oropharynx, oesophagus, liver and breast.[12]

Dietary factors may confound the relationship between alcohol and certain cancers.[13]

Dietary choices

Dietary habits have been reported to correlate with around 60% of cancers in women and 40% of cancers in men.[14] Like alcohol, fat is thought to enhance risk whereas there is good evidence that plant foods have preventive potential.[15]

The recommendation of the National Cancer Institute and American Institute for Cancer Research is to eat at least 5–9 servings per day of fruit and vegetables. Raw and fresh vegetables, leafy green vegetables, cruciferae, carrots, broccoli, cabbage, lettuce, and raw and fresh fruit (including tomatoes and citrus fruit) appear particularly protective. Potentially anticarcinogenic substances found in plant foods range from vitamins, e.g. carotenoids, vitamin C, vitamin E, through minerals, e.g. selenium, to dietary fibre and indoles, phenols, allium compounds and plant sterols. Eating whole foods carries the advantage of consuming a number of these agents. Cruciferous vegetables, such as brussels sprouts, broccoli, cauliflower, kale, kohlrabi, turnips, mustard greens and bok choy, for example, contain: flavonoids, some of which reduce the risk of breast cancer by blocking a pathway for oestrogen synthesis; phenols and isthiocyanates, which aid detoxification and may enhance excretion of carcinogen; and dietary fibre, which may reduce the risk of bowel cancer. Members of the allium species, such as garlic and onions, are also protective. Garlic is reported to stimulate immunity and a high intake of both raw and cooked garlic may protect against stomach and colorectal cancers.[16] Nuts appear to offer some protection against colon, prostate and breast cancer. Phytosterols, especially beta-sitosterol, appear to be important ingredients. Roasted peanuts contain 61–114 mg phytosterols per 100 g, depending on the peanut variety, 78–83% of which is in the form of beta-sitosterol.[17] Peanut butter contains 144–157 mg phytosterols per 100 g.

Dietary studies are based upon responses to whole foods, which makes it difficult to identify which constituents are most protective. In theory, single nutrient supplementation could achieve higher intakes and reach therapeutic doses. In practice, the use of supplementation is more complex. Use of high dose single supplements rather than whole foods may precipitate metabolic imbalances, fail to provide unrecognized active constituents and deliver an impotent variant of the supplement. Compared to natural beta-carotene, synthetic beta-carotene lacks cis beta-carotene, the carotene that reduces dysplasia.[18] Furthermore, not all carotenes are equally potent. A case control study found significantly inverse associations of prostate cancer with plasma concentrations of lycopene and zeaxanthin, borderline associations for lutein and beta-cryptoxanthin and no obvious associations for alpha- and beta-carotenes.[19] Lycopene may not be as effective as alpha-carotene against lung cancer. Moreover, large intakes of beta-carotene may increase the risk of lung cancer in heavy long term smokers. Beta-carotene, an antioxidant in non-smokers, assumes the role of a prooxidant in the lungs of smokers. The carotenes are not the only nutrients in which supplementation is problematic. Of the eight isomers of synthesized vitamin E, only one has the RRR configuration of natural vitamin E. The different tocol and tocotrienol derivatives a, b, d, and y also have varied and specific roles with diverse tissue affinities. Y-tocopherol has the unique ability to reduce NO_2, a radical that can initiate carcinogenesis through inducing mutations. The dose of vitamin E determines if it bolsters or suppresses immunity; similarly the dose of L-glycine determines if it protects against cancer or promotes metastasis. Disparity between the clinical outcome achieved by isolated and constitutive isoflavones has also been documented.[20] A diet rich in fruit and vegetables not only provides compounds in desirable biological ratios, it also provides biologically active stereoisomers of the various nutrients.

Food preparation impacts on cancer risk.[21] Cooking may impair the protective effect of plant constituents. Indoles found in cruciferous vegetables are reduced by half when these foods are boiled. While heating may destroy protective constituents, certain cooking methods may produce carcinogens. Barbecuing, especially if meat is charred or coated with splattered fat, broiling and frying animal products produce mutagens. Adding proline or briefly microwaving meat prior to frying or broiling reduces mutagen production. Heterocyclic amines are produced during cooking and a number of heterocyclic amines have been shown to induce cancer of the breast, colon and pancreas. However, formation of heterocyclic amines can be reduced by including soy protein, tea polyphenols and tryptophan in the diet. Food combination is clearly important. A barbecue in which meat and potatoes are cooked over the coals, accompanied by a coleslaw and broccoli salad and washed down with red wine and grapefruit juice has a diverse and complex action on the P-450 enzyme system. Broccoli and cabbage induce certain P-450 enzymes while red wine and protein enhance P-450 catalyzed oxidation. The cytochrome P-450 enzymes are major catalysts involved in the biotransformation of xenobiotic chemicals such as drugs, carcinogens and pesticides, or endobiotics such as steroids, fat soluble vitamins and eicosanoids. Phase II detoxification is vital in cancer prevention. Most endogenous and exogenous chemicals undergo phase I detoxification during which highly reactive and carcinogenic byproducts are produced prior to being passed through phase II for detoxification. The timing of these reactions is crucial to cancer prevention. An overly fast phase I produces a large amount of these byproducts faster than phase II can water-solubilize them. Cigarette smoke, which increases the speed of phase I, is cancer-inducing; broccoli, which speeds up phase II, is protective. Diet and the relative concentration of various constituents impact on this system and other systems.[22–24] Although much remains to be learned about the influence of specific dietary constituents and dietary patterns on cancer risk, it is clear that diet can have a significant impact in cancer prevention and control.[25]

Exercise

While a cause–effect relationship between smoking and cancer is undisputed, and the impact of diet on carcinogenesis is complex and often confusing, the preventive effect of physical exercise on cancer risk remains controversial. Exercise is listed as one of the recommendations for cancer prevention. However, a longitudinal study concluded there were no, or at best weak, inverse associations between physical activity in leisure time and the incidence of cancer.[26] Ovarian cancer was cited as an exception to this generalization. It would appear that the protective effect of exercise, and certain other measures, may be site specific.

CANCER IN THE ELDERLY

The prevalence of cancer increases up to the age of 75–84 years and decreases slightly thereafter.[27] Among elderly women breast, colon, lung and stomach are the common cancer sites.[1] Among elderly men, cancer of the prostate, the lung and colon make up around half of all diagnosed cancers.[1] For all major specific cancer sites except testicular cancer, the incidence rate is significantly higher among elderly than among younger men.

Colorectal cancer

Colorectal cancers usually grow slowly and may take 10–20 years to become malignant. The transition from normal mucosa to adenoma and its subsequent progression to carcinoma are protracted events that offer opportunities for preventive interventions. It has been estimated that primary prevention through dietary modification may reduce the incidence of colorectal cancer by 20% while secondary prevention by procto-sigmoidoscopy may reduce mortality by 55%.[28]

Both lifestyle choices and screening are important.

Lifestyle choices

The 'prudent' dietary pattern, characterized by higher intakes of fruit, vegetables, legumes, fish, poultry and whole grains, appears somewhat protective when compared to the 'Western' dietary pattern with its higher intakes of red and processed meats, sweets and desserts, French fries and refined grains. During 12 years of follow-up, a female study concluded that while the prudent pattern had a non-significant inverse association with colon cancer, the relative risk for this disease was highest in those conforming most closely to the 'Western pattern'.[29] No significant association between dietary patterns and rectal cancer was detected. Indeed, while epidemiological evidence suggests that cancer of the distal colon is linked to fat, that of the rectum appears associated with alcohol consumption. Colorectal cancer may represent three diseases: cancer of the proximal colon, the distal colon and the rectum.[21]

Despite some confusion, dietary choices do influence the risk of colorectal cancer and considerations include the following:

- *Limiting alcohol intake.* Compared with abstainers, current or ex-drinking males double their risk for rectal cancer.[30] In this study light current drinkers who consumed less than 22 g ethanol per day were at slightly lower risk of rectal cancer. Compared with abstainers, regular heavy drinking of 150 or more g of ethanol weekly showed a statistically significant increased risk of colorectal cancer.[31] The risk was dose related with a relative risk of 1.4 on 150–299 g of ethanol per week rising to 2.1 times for those drinking 300 g or more each week. Regular ethanol consumption was not associated with colorectal cancer in women. Another study which confirmed a dose–response relationship between alcohol and rectal cancer reported 41 or more drinks a week increased the relative risk of rectal cancer by 2.2.[32] This study also found the type of alcohol was important. Compared with abstainers, more than 14 drinks of beer and spirits a week increased risk 3.5 fold. However, if wine was included this risk declined to less than double.
- *Having a high dairy food diet.* A diet low in saturated fat has traditionally been advocated. However, a diet rich in dairy foods may be the exception to this rule. Women over 40 years of age who consume at least 4 servings of high fat dairy foods daily reduce their relative risk of colorectal cancer (0.59) when compared with women who consume less than 1 serving daily.[33] Each increment of 2 servings of high fat dairy foods per day corresponded to a 13% reduction in the risk of colorectal cancer. The authors speculated that the protective effect was attributable to potentially anticarcinogenic factors, including conjugated linoleic acid, in high fat dairy foods. Another explanation for the protective effect may be calcium and vitamin D intake.[33] A randomized, single blind, controlled

study found that the proliferative activity of colonic epithelial cells was decreased and markers of normal cellular differentiation were restored by increasing the daily intake of calcium to 1200 mg via low fat dairy food in subjects at risk for colonic neoplasia.[34] If low fat dairy products are indeed beneficial, then a diet low in saturated fat would seem preferable.

- *A high fibre diet.* Diets rich in insoluble fibre prevent constipation and are believed to protect against colon cancer by reducing exposure of the mucosa to carcinogens both through a large stool diluting the concentration of carcinogens and through a faster bowel transit time. A high fibre diet also favours bacteria producing anticarcinogenic substances such as butyric acid. Whole grains and dietary fibre from wheat bran appear protective.[35] Phytochemicals concentrated in the outer portion of grains include phenolic acids, which are natural antioxidants and induce detoxification systems.

- *Including probiotic and prebiotics in the diet.* Eating 250 ml per day of a yogurt rich in lactobacillus and bifidus establishes probiotic-rich bowel flora. Bifidobacteria reside in the caecum, colon and rectum where they produce short chain fatty acids that are antagonistic to gut pathogens and stimulate peristalsis. Putrefactive dysbiosis is strongly implicated in the pathogenesis of colon and breast cancers. Overgrowth of endogenous bacteria and yeasts, exacerbated by gastric hypochlorhydria, a common condition in elderly patients, also increases the risk of gastric cancer. A diet rich in prebiotics (fructo-oligosaccharides) and probiotics (*Lactobacillus acidophilus, Bifidobacterium bifidum*) reduces the risk of gastrointestinal cancers. Good plant sources of oligosaccharides are onions, asparagus, wheat and artichoke leaf.

- *A high resistant starch diet.* Resistant starch is not digested in the small intestine and affects large bowel function. An intake of 20 g per day of resistant starch is recommended. Green bananas, cold boiled potatoes and bread are good sources. Starch increases the stool concentration of short chain fatty acids and butyrate is protective against colorectal cancers.

Chemoprevention

Chemoprevention, to suppress or reverse the carcinogenic process in the colorectum, with non-pharmacological or pharmacological agents, is promising. However, questions remain, including the optimal dosage, timing of initiation and duration of treatment.[36] Regular users of aspirin and other NSAIDs have a lower risk of colorectal cancer than non-regular users.[37] Women who took two or more aspirin daily for longer than 10 years had a 53% lower risk of colorectal cancer than those who did not. Larger doses of aspirin resulted in larger reductions in risk. Another study reported that 100 mg on alternate days failed to offer protection.[38] To reduce the risk of colorectal cancer, 10 years of regular use of large doses of aspirin were required. Another study found that the inverse associations between regular NSAID use and colon cancer, although similar for African Americans and Caucasians, were stronger for women than for men.[39] This study found the inverse associations were slightly weaker for occasional versus regular NSAID use, but they were similar for aspirin and non-aspirin NSAID use. Apart from aspirin, calcium carbonate is the only other agent that has been shown to modestly reduce sporadic adenoma recurrence rates in a randomized trial.

Similar dose, timing and treatment duration issues apply to the nutraceuticals such as calcium, folic acid and selenium given as dietary supplements. Supplemental intakes of vitamins A, C, E, folic acid, calcium, and multivitamins were each associated with a reduced risk of colon cancer.[40]

Screening

The 5-year relative survival rates of digestive tract cancers among patients aged 80 years and older are 12% for stomach cancer, 41% for colon cancer and 37% for rectal cancer.[41] The greater longevity of persons with colorectal cancer is due, at least in part, to earlier diagnosis of the disease. Screening ensures early detection and increases amenability to therapy.

Health authorities recommend screening all persons over 49 years of age for colorectal cancer. Annual faecal occult blood testing or sigmoidoscopy or both is advocated every 3–5 years for everyone between 50 and 70 years of age.[42] However, examination of voided stools for faecal occult blood when feasible, and full colonoscopy every 10 years may represent the more practical approach.[2] Colonoscopy screening provides the greatest benefit but carries the highest risk of complications.

The potential benefit from screening varies widely with age, life expectancy and screening modality. One cancer-related death would be prevented by screening 42 healthy men aged 70–74 years with colonoscopy, 178 healthy women aged 70–74 years with faecal occult blood tests, 431 women aged 75–79 years in poor health with colonoscopy, or 945 men aged 80–84 years in average health with faecal occult blood tests.[43] As the incidence and prevalence of colorectal cancer increases after the age of 80 years, some form of screening appears to be indicated for all persons with a life expectancy of 5 years or longer, particularly as early detection may obviate the need for emergency surgery from obstruction and perforation—complications associated with escalating mortality in those 70 years of age and older.[2]

Breast Cancer

Diagnosis of breast cancer is associated with reduced survival in women aged 50–65, but with an improved survival in those aged 80 years and over.[2] An explanation for this phenomenon is lacking; however, it has been surmised that it may in some way be related to the pathophysiological changes associated with aging. Also perplexing is the multifactorial nature of breast carcinogenesis which has made it difficult to establish clear cause–effect relationships. Nonetheless, attempts have been made to identify and avoid risk factors.

Protective Lifestyle choices

Dietary options
Despite breast cancer being more common in countries where women have a high average intake of total and saturated fat, animal protein and total energy, any overall association between dietary patterns and risk of breast

cancer is unclear.[44] Nonetheless, the prudent pattern appears to have an inverse association with breast cancer risk. Although dietary recommendations for breast cancer prevention have not been definitively formulated, dietary factors postulated to reduce the risk of breast cancer include:[45]

- *A reduced fat intake.* Intakes of both saturated and monounsaturated fat are related to a modestly elevated breast cancer risk.[46] Animal fat, red meat and high fat dairy foods are each associated with an increased risk of breast cancer. However, despite animal studies suggesting fat restriction decreases breast cancer and descriptive epidemiological studies supporting an inverse relationship, case control studies show little effect and cohort studies show few associations.[47] Nonetheless, fat is a carrier of carcinogens and high energy intake predisposes to carcinogenesis: each additional 100 g/day of fat may increase the risk of cancer by up to 25%. An overall fat intake of no more than 20% of total energy and relatively rich in monounsaturated and omega-3 fatty acids would seem prudent.
- *A diet rich in plant foods.* Plant foods rich in vitamins and/or phyto-oestrogens may protect against breast cancer. Premenopausal women who consumed 5 or more servings per day of fruit and vegetables have a modestly lower risk of breast cancer than those who had fewer than 2 servings per day.[48] Inverse associations were strongest for foods rich in alpha-carotene, beta-carotene, lutein/zeaxanthin, total dietary vitamin C and total vitamin A. Eating 30 g daily of fibre appears to promote oestrogen excretion by creating an intestinal environment conducive for gut bacteria to metabolize oestrogen. Soy products e.g. tofu, are particularly rich in phyto-oestrogens. The high content of soybean products in the diet of Asian women has been offered as a possible explanation for their relatively low breast cancer incidence.
- *Limited alcohol intake.* A weak causal relationship, supported by a dose–response relationship, is postulated. A study that found no association between prudent and Western dietary patterns and the risk of breast cancer, found a 'drinker' pattern characterized by intake of wine, liquor, beer, snacks and whole grain was associated with increased risk of breast cancer.[49] This risk was less pronounced in women under 50 years of age. A prospective cohort using lifetime abstainers for comparison found the hazard ratio for breast cancer in women who consumed an average of 40 g or more of alcohol daily was 1.41.[50] A study summarizing the findings of 53 epidemiological studies reported that compared with abstinent women, the relative risk of breast cancer was 1.46 for those consuming on average 45 or more g/day of alcohol.[51] According to the collaborative reanalysis, the relative risk of breast cancer increased by 7% for each additional 10 g/day intake of alcohol. Acetaldehyde, produced by alcohol metabolism, is carcinogenic and mutagenic, binds to DNA and proteins, destroys folate and stimulates hyperproliferation.

Chemoprotection

Folate supplementation may be protective in women with high alcohol consumption. A high folate intake mitigates the excess risk associated with alcohol, despite no direct association between dietary folate intake and risk of breast cancer. The estimated hazard ratio of consuming at least 40 g of alcohol daily was 2.00 for women with intakes of 200 µg/day of folate and 0.77 for those taking 400 µg/day of folate.[50] While an increase in relative risk of 1.19 per 10 g daily alcohol intake was found for women with a daily folate intake below 300 µg, this relationship was lost among women with a folate intake higher than 350 µg.[12] Supplemental folate in doses of 400 µg/day taken for prolonged periods (15 years) seems protective for preventing early tumour progression.

In contrast to folate, there is no evidence that vitamin E supplements confer protection. This despite observational studies suggesting vitamin E from dietary sources may provide women with modest protection from breast cancer. The modest protection derived from dietary vitamin E may be due to effects of the other tocopherols and tocotrienols in the diet.[52] In vitro studies of breast cancer cells indicate that a-, y-, and d-tocotrienol, and to a lesser extent d-tocopherol, have potent antiproliferative and proapoptotic effects that would be expected to reduce the risk of breast cancer. Despite confusion, at least one case control study of postmenopausal women with breast cancer found, compared with non-use, use of supplemental vitamin C and E for at least 3 years was associated with a reduced risk of breast cancer recurrence and breast cancer-related death.[53]

Exercise

In addition to diet, physical activity may affect the risk of breast cancer. One study reported that increased physical activity was associated with a lower risk of breast cancer in postmenopausal women.[54] An hour of moderate or strenuous activity daily provided most benefit. Compared to their inactive peers, postmenopausal women aged 50–79 years who exercised regularly by walking briskly for at least 1.25–2.5 hours per week reduced their risk of breast cancer.[55] An Italian case control study calculated the attributable risk was 12% for low levels of physical activity, and this risk was larger among post- than premenopausal women.[56] This study suggested low levels of physical activity and low beta-carotene intake, <3366 µ/day, accounted for 32% of the breast cancer cases in the overall dataset.

Women diagnosed with breast cancer also benefit from exercise. Compared with women who engaged in less than 3 MET (metabolic equivalent task) hours per week of physical activity, the relative risk of death from breast cancer was 0.80.[57] Risk decreased as physical activity increased, dropping to a low of 0.50 times for 9–14.9 MET hours per week. Three MET hours is equivalent to walking at an average pace of 2–2.9 mph for 1 hour. The researchers recommended that walking 3–5 hours per week at an average pace provided the best cost–benefit outcome for those diagnosed with breast cancer.[56]

Screening

In addition to primary prevention of breast cancer through lifestyle changes, screening provides the option of early diagnosis and successful secondary prevention. Women between the ages of 50 and 69 are likely to benefit most. Although there is insufficient evidence to recommend for or against the use of annual professional breast examination or breast self-examination, routine screening for breast cancer every 1–2 years with mammography is recommended for women from the age of 40 years.[42] Serial mammography, performed 4–7 times, reduced by 20–30% cancer-related mortality in women aged 50–70.[2] It has been calculated that as many as 50% of breast cancer related deaths might have been prevented by continuing screening throughout a person's lifetime.

The benefits of serial screening mammography after age 70 may be inferred from a number of reports. Various studies have shown screening mammography up to age 75 is associated with decreased mortality in women aged 70–75; and breast cancer mortality is reduced for women aged 70–79 undergoing at least two mammographic evaluations after age 70, with the benefits of mammography apparent even in 85-year-old patients with moderate comorbidity.[2]

IN PERSPECTIVE

Cancer is a major cause of morbidity and mortality in elderly persons. Lifestyle choices, chemoprevention and screening deserve consideration regardless of age. The type of intervention is influenced by the nature of the cancer, the person's life expectancy, and capacity to cope with therapy from a physiological and psychosocial perspective.[2]

CLINICAL CHALLENGE

An obese 52-year-old woman detects a lump in her left breast. The lump is rubbery and mobile. She has no associated lymphadenopathy. She does not smoke and drinks 30–40 g of alcohol daily.

Questions arising

- Does this woman have breast cancer?
- Which risk factors would suggest she is at increased risk?
- How should the patient be counselled?

Clinical considerations

Clinical examination of the breast lump suggests a fibroadenoma. Needle biopsy can confirm the result.

Refer to www.jamisonhealth.com Handout 22.4 to review the risk factors for breast cancer.

The patient should be advised to limit her alcohol intake, eat a diet rich in fruit and vegetables and limit her fat intake. Supplementing her diet with 400 µg/day of folate is advisable, particularly if she fails to moderate her alcohol intake. She may also benefit from regular exercise. Advise her to walk briskly for at least 30 minutes on alternate days.

She should also be advised to present for mammography every second year. Regular breast self-examination and professional breast examination annually may be discussed.

As she has some concerns about cancer it may be helpful for her to be provided with a copy of Handout 22.8 from www.jamisonhealth.com.

PRACTICE GEMS

- Stop smoking, or better still never start.
- Limit alcohol intake to no more than 1 or 2 standard drinks daily.
- A plant based diet rich in raw and fresh vegetables, particularly leafy green vegetables, cruciferae, carrots, broccoli, cabbage, lettuce, and raw and fresh fruit (including tomatoes and citrus fruit) appears protective.
- Avoid barbecued, fried and broiled foods.
- Women who gain more than 10 kg as adults double their risk of developing breast cancer.
- Women with low intakes of vitamin A and beta-carotene are at higher risk of cervical dysplasia and carcinoma-in-situ than those with a rich intake of these nutrients.
- A high fibre diet derived from vegetables, grains and fruit, low in fat and rich in calcium, that includes cruciferous vegetables, garlic and onions offers some protection against bowel cancer.
- Eating wholemeal grain bread with fried meat may be protective as heterocyclic amine carcinogens, such as those found in fried meat, may adsorb to insoluble fibre.

- Colorectal cancer must be excluded in patients with a long history of inflammatory bowel disease, especially ulcerative colitis; 1500 mg calcium daily may reduce the risk of colon cancer in these patients.
- Aspirin reduces the risk of colon cancer.
- Limiting the intake of red and processed meats appears to reduce the risk of colon cancer.
- Gastric cancer is a complication of gastric ulcers, especially those linked to Helicobacter infection.
- Nutritional prevention of prostate cancer remains unproven at the level of double blind placebo controlled clinical trials.
- Experimental observations suggest that, rather than inhibiting aetiological factors, low fat diets and soy protein extracts may influence the progression of established prostate tumours.
- Lifestyle choices can reduce the risk of getting cancer; screening offers early diagnosis and treatment and reduces the risk of dying of cancer.

References

1. Hansen J. Common cancers in the elderly. Drugs Aging 1998; 13(6):467–478.
2. Carreca I, Balducci L, Extermann M. Cancer in the older person. Cancer Treat Rev 2005; 31(5):380–402.
3. Micheli A, Mugno E, et al. Cancer prevalence in European registry areas. Ann Oncol 2002; 13(6):840–865.
4. Danaei G, Vander Hoorn S, et al; Comparative Risk Assessment Collaborating Group (Cancers). Causes of cancer in the world: comparative risk assessment of nine behavioural and environmental risk factors. Lancet 2005; 366(9499):1784–1793.
5. Lawrence VJ, Kopelman PG. Medical consequences of obesity. Clin Dermatol 2004; 22(4):296–302.
6. Taylor B, Rehm J. When risk factors combine: The interaction between alcohol and smoking for aerodigestive cancer, coronary heart disease, and traffic and fire injury. Addict Behav 2006 Jan 26; [Epub ahead of print].
7. Ezzati M, Henley SJ, et al. Role of smoking in global and regional cancer epidemiology: current patterns and data needs. Int J Cancer 2005; 116(6):963–971.
8. Cerhan JR, Potter JD, et al. Adherence to the AICR cancer prevention recommendations and subsequent morbidity and mortality in the Iowa Women's Health Study cohort. Cancer Epidemiol Biomarkers Prev 2004;13(7):1114–1120.
9. Ozlu T, Bulbul Y. Smoking and lung cancer. Tuberk Toraks 2005; 53(2):200–209.
10. Roth DH, Roth AB, Liu X. Health risks of smoking compared to Swedish snus. Inhal Toxicol 2005; 17(13):741–748.
11. Armstrong BK. Morbidity and mortality in Australia. In: McNeil JJ, King RWF, et al, eds. A textbook of preventive medicine. Melbourne: Edward Arnold; 1990:1–12.
12. Rehm J, Room R, et al. The relationship of average volume of alcohol consumption and patterns of drinking to burden of disease: an overview. Addiction 2003; 98(9):1209–1228.
13. Tjonneland A, Christensen J, et al. Folate intake, alcohol and risk of breast cancer among postmenopausal women in Denmark. Eur J Clin Nutr 2006; 60(2):280–286.
14. Wynder EL, Gori GB. Contributions of the environment to cancer incidence: an epidemiological exercise. J Natl Cancer Inst 1977; 58:825–832.
15. Potter JD, Steinmetz K. Vegetables, fruit and phytoestrogens as preventive agents. IARC Sci Publ 1996; 139:61–90.
16. Fleischauer AT, Poole C, Arab L. Garlic consumption and cancer prevention: meta-analyses of colorectal and stomach cancers. Am J Clin Nutr 2000; 72(4):1047–1052.
17. Hu FB, Stampfer MJ, et al. Frequent nut consumption and risk of coronary heart disease in women: prospective cohort study. Brit Med J 1998; 317:1341–1345.
18. Werbach M. Nutritional influences on illness. Internat J Altern & Comp Med 1999; 17: 20–21.
19. Lu QY, Hung JC, et al. Inverse associations between plasma lycopene and other carotenoids and prostate cancer. Cancer Epidemiol Biomarkers Prev 2001; 10(7):749–756.
20. Lichtenstein AH. Got soy? Am J Clin Nutr 2001; 73:667–668.
21. Weisburger JH. Dietary fat and risk of chronic disease: Mechanistic insights from experimental studies. J Amer Dietetic Assoc 1997; 97(suppl): S16–S23.
22. Guengerich FP. Influence of nutrients and other dietary materials on cytochrome P-450 enzymes. Am J Clin Nutr 1995; 61:651S–658S.
23. Ferguson LR, Philpott M, Karunasinghe N. Dietary cancer and prevention using antimutagens. Toxicology 2004; 198(1–3):147–159.
24. Weisburger JH. Approaches for chronic disease prevention based on current understanding of underlying mechanisms. Am J Clin Nutr 2000; 71(6 Suppl):1710S–1714S.
25. Greenwald P, Clifford C, et al. New directions in dietary studies in cancer: the National Cancer Institute. Adv Exp Med Biol 1995; 369: 229–239.
26. Schnohr P, Gronbaek M, et al. Physical activity in leisure-time and risk of cancer: 14-year follow-up of 28,000 Danish men and women. Scand J Public Health 2005; 33(4):244–249.
27. Vercelli M, Quaglia A, et al. Cancer prevalence in the elderly. ITAPREVAL Working Group. Tumori 1999; 85(5):391–399.
28. Cardenas VM, Thun MJ, et al. Environmental tobacco smoke and lung cancer mortality in the American Cancer Society's Cancer Prevention Study. II. Cancer Causes Control 1997; 8(1):57–64.
29. Fung T, Hu FB, et al. Major dietary patterns and the risk of colorectal cancer in women. Arch Intern Med 2003; 163(3):309–314.
30. Wakai K, Kojima M, et al. Alcohol consumption and colorectal cancer risk: findings from the JACC Study. J Epidemiol 2005; 15 (Suppl 2):S173–S179.
31. Otani T, Iwasaki M, et al. Alcohol consumption,

smoking, and subsequent risk of colorectal cancer in middle-aged and elderly Japanese men and women: Japan Public Health Center-based prospective study. Cancer Epidemiol Biomarkers Prev 2003; 12(12):1492–1500.

32. Pedersen A, Johansen C, Gronbaek M. Relations between amount and type of alcohol and colon and rectal cancer in a Danish population based cohort study. Gut 2003; 52(6):861–867.

33. Larsson SC, Bergkvist L, et al. High-fat dairy food and conjugated linoleic acid intakes in relation to colorectal cancer incidence in the Swedish Mammography Cohort. Am J Clin Nutr 2005; 82(4):894–900.

34. Holt PR, Atillasoy EO, et al. Modulation of abnormal colonic epithelial cell proliferation and differentiation by low-fat dairy foods: a randomized controlled trial. JAMA 1998; 280(12):1074–1079.

35. Kushi LH, Meyer KA, Jacobs DR. Cereals, legumes, and chronic disease risk reduction: evidence from epidemiological studies. Am J Clin Nutr 1999; 70:451S–458S.

36. Gill S, Sinicrope FA. Colorectal cancer prevention: is an ounce of prevention worth a pound of cure? Semin Oncol 2005; 32(1):24–34.

37. Murray S. Do ASA and NSAIDs reduce the risk of colorectal cancer? CMAJ 2005; 173(10): 1159–1160.

38. Cook NR, Lee IM, et al. Low dose aspirin in the primary prevention of cancer: the Women's Health Study: a randomized controlled trial. JAMA 2005; 294:47–55.

39. Sansbury LB, Millikan RC, et al. Use of nonsteroidal antiinflammatory drugs and risk of colon cancer in a population-based, case-control study of African Americans and Whites. Am J Epidemiol 2005; 162(6):548–558.

40. White E, Shannon JS, Patterson RE. Relationship between vitamin and calcium supplement use and colon cancer. Cancer Epidemiol Biomarkers Prev 1997; 6(10):769–774.

41. Bouvier AM, Launoy G, et al. Trends in the management and survival of digestive tract cancers among patients aged over 80 years. Aliment Pharmacol Ther 2005; 22(3):233–241.

42. Report of the US Preventive Services Task Force. Guide to clinical preventive services. 2nd edn. Baltimore:Williams & Wilkins; 1996.

43. Ko CW, Sonnenberg A. Comparing risks and benefits of colorectal cancer screening in elderly patients. Gastroenterology 2005; 129(4):1163–1170.

44. Adebamowo CA, Hu FB, et al. Dietary patterns and the risk of breast cancer. Ann Epidemiol 2005; 15(10):789–795.

45. Kohlmeier L, Mendez M. Controversies surrounding diet and breast cancer. Proc Nutr Soc 1997; 56:369–382.

46. Cho E, Spiegelman D, et al. Premenopausal fat intake and risk of breast cancer. J Natl Cancer Inst 2003; 95(14):1079–1085.

47. Dwyer JT. Human studies on the effects of fatty acids on cancer: summary, gaps, and future research. Am J Clin Nutr 1997; 66:1581S–1586S.

48. Zhang S, Hunter DJ, et al. Dietary carotenoids and vitamins A, C, and E and risk of breast cancer. J Natl Cancer Inst 1999; 91(6):547-556.

49. Baglietto L, English DR, et al. Does dietary folate intake modify effect of alcohol consumption on breast cancer risk? Prospective cohort study. BMJ 2005; 331(7520):807.

50. Terry P, Suzuki R, et al. A prospective study of major dietary patterns and the risk of breast cancer. Cancer Epidemiol Biomarkers Prev 2001; 10(12):1281–1285.

51. Hamajima N, Hirose K, et al. Alcohol, tobacco and breast cancer—collaborative reanalysis of individual data from 53 epidemiological studies, including 58,515 women with breast cancer and 95,067 women without the disease. Br J Cancer 2002; 87:1234–1245.

52. Schwenke DC. Does lack of tocopherols and tocotrienols put women at increased risk of breast cancer? J Nutr Biochem 2002; 13(1):2–20.

53. Fleischauer AT, Simonsen N, Arab L. Antioxidant supplements and risk of breast cancer recurrence and breast cancer-related mortality among postmenopausal women. Nutr Cancer 2003; 46(1):15–22.

54. Macera CA. Past recreational physical activity and risk of breast cancer. Clin J Sport Med 2005; 15(2):115–116.

55. McTiernan A, Kooperberg C, et al. Recreational physical activity and the risk of breast cancer in postmenopausal women. JAMA 2003; 290(10):1331–1336.

56. Mezzetti M, La Vecchia C, et al. Population attributable risk for breast cancer: diet, nutrition, and physical exercise. J Natl Cancer Inst 1998; 90(5):389–394.

57. Holmes MD, Chen WY, et al. Physical activity and survival after breast cancer diagnosis. JAMA 2005; 293(20):2479–2486.

PATIENT HANDOUT 23.1 – LIFESTYLE CHOICES TO REDUCE THE RISK OF CANCER

Four prudent lifestyle choices are to:

- avoid cigarette smoke
- eat wisely
- limit alcohol cosumption
- exercise regularly.

Avoid cigarette smoke

A major risk factor for cancer is cigarette smoking. Read about:

- the risks of continuing to smoke—see www.jamisonhealth.com Handout 14.4
- the benefits of quitting—see www.jamisonhealth.com Handout 14.5
- strategies to help you quit—see www.jamisonhealth.com Handouts 14.6-14.11.

See also www.niapublications.org/engagepages/smoking.asp—smoking: it's never too late to stop.

Eat wisely

Good dietary advice is to:

- Eat a plant based diet rich in whole grains, fruit and vegetables for fibre, vitamins, and phytochemicals. Be sure to include:
  —cruciferous vegetables, e.g. brussels sprouts, broccoli, cauliflower, kale, kohlrabi, turnips, mustard greens and bok choy
  —umbelliferous vegetables, e.g. carrots, parsley, parsnips and celery
  —allium species, e.g. garlic and onions
  —nuts and legumes, e.g. soybeans
  —ginger and licorice.
- Limit dietary fat, especially animal fat.
- Limit alcohol.
- Maintain an ideal body weight.

Exposure to cigarette smoke increases risk, unwise dietary choices can increase risk but a healthy diet can reduce risk!

Limit alcohol consumption

Drink no more than 1 glass (women) or 2 glasses (men) daily of wine, preferably red. Refer to www.jamisonhealth.com Handout 15.10 for guidelines for safe drinking.

Exercise regularly

Take daily moderate exercise and exercise vigorously weekly.

Information resources

At *www.jamisonhealth.com* Handout 22.8 you will find a self-care cancer risk reduction protocol. Use this to reduce your risk of dying of cancer.

http://www.niapublications.org/engagepages/ cancer.asp
cancer facts for people over 50

http://www.niapublications.org/engagepages/ skin.asp
skin care in later life.

Some Scientific Evidence

Ecological, case control, and cohort studies present convincing evidence that diets rich in fresh fruit and vegetables protect against several common cancers.[1]

Results from 206 epidemiological and 22 animal studies provide evidence that vegetable and fruit consumption protects against a number of cancers.[2]

Garlic, soybeans, ginger, licorice and the umbelliferous vegetables such as carrots, parsley, parsnips and celery are regarded as highly protective.[3]

In addition to being low in fat and high in fibre, plant foods contain a range of protective phytonutrients including allium compounds, vitamin C and E, folic acid, beta-carotene, lutein, lycopene, isoflavones, flavonoids and selenium.[4]

Dietary flaxseed has the potential to reduce tumour growth in patients with breast cancer.[5]

Supplementation with beta-carotene or beta-carotene plus vitamin A appears to increase the incidence and mortality from lung cancer in smokers; it may also increase the incidence and mortality from mesothelioma in high-risk group.[6]

Vitamin E appears to reduce incidence and mortality from prostate cancer and stomach cancer in smokers.[6]

Internet resource

http://www.agingwell.state.ny.us/selfcare/articles/over50.htm
cancer facts for people over 50

References

1. Tavani A, La Vecchia C. Fruit and vegetable consumption and cancer risk in a Mediterranean population. Am J Clin Nutr 1995; 61(6 Suppl):1374S–1377S.
2. Steinmetz KA, Potter JD. Vegetables, fruit, and cancer prevention: a review. J Am Diet Assoc 1996; 96(10):1027–1039.
3. Craig WJ. Phytochemicals: guardians of our health. J Am Dietetic Assoc 1997; 97: S199–S204.
4. Potter JD, Steinmetz K. Vegetables, fruit and phytoestrogens as preventive agents. IARC Sci Publ 1996; (139):61–90.
5. Thompson LU, Chen JM, et al. Dietary flaxseed alters tumor biological markers in postmenopausal breast cancer. Clin Cancer Res 2005; 11(10):3828–3835.
6. Ritenbaugh C, Streit K, Helfand M. Routine vitamin supplementation to prevent cancer: summary of evidence from randomized controlled trials. Agency for Healthcare Research and Quality, Rockville, MD. Online. Available: http://www.ahrq.gov/clinic/3rduspstf/vitamins/vitasum.htm

PATIENT HANDOUT 23.2 – CANCER PREVENTION

Older persons are at increased risk of cancer. Prevention is best, but early diagnosis reduces mortality. Be alert to how you can reduce your risk of cancer and recognize ominous signs early.

You should consult your health professional annually.

Tips for Prevention

Recognize when you are at increased risk and make lifestyle choices that minimize your personal hazard.

Use the following handouts to help you identify if you are at particular risk of some of the cancers common amongst older persons and implement the tips provided to reduce your personal risk:

■ Colorectal cancer—see *www.jamisonhealth.com* Handout 22.2
■ Lung cancer—see *www.jamisonhealth.com* Handout 22.1
■ Stomach cancer—see *www.jamisonhealth.com* Handout 22.3
■ Breast cance—see *www.jamisonhealth.com* Handout 22.4
■ Cervical cancer—see *www.jamisonhealth.com* Handout 22.5
■ Prostate cancer—see *www.jamisonhealth.com* Handout 22.6
■ Skin cancer—see *www.jamisonhealth.com* Handout 22.7.

Screening for early diagnosis

Wise lifestyle choices can reduce the risk of developing cancer, screening detects cancers that are already present and increases your chances of recovery by offering curative intervention.

To increase the chances of early diagnosis of possible malignancy, a prudent screening protocol includes:

■ Annual professional breast examination and mammography (every 1–2 years) for women over the age of 50 years. Mammography detects breast cancers 2–4 years earlier than palpation.
■ Papanicolaou smears every 2 years for women up to the age of 70 years.
■ Annual pelvic examinations for all women over 40 years of age. This is disputed.
■ Rectal examination for prostatic carcinoma in asymptomatic men over the age of 40 years.
■ Annual digital rectal examination to screen for colorectal carcinoma after the age of 40 years.
■ Annual faecal occult blood tests in asymptomatic patients over the age of 50 years.
■ One flexible proctosigmoidoscopy examination at age 55 years; colonoscopy every 10 years thereafter.

Index

Page references in **bold** indicate where a topic is the subject of an entire chapter

Vestibular function, 65–66
Visceral pain, 143–144
Viscosupplementation, 197–198, 200
Vision, 50–51, 65, 70, 113
Vitamin A, 42, 324
Vitamin B
   vitamin B3, 149
   vitamin B6, 121, 149
   vitamin B12, 66, 125
Vitamin C, 6, 7, 11–12, 42, 108–109, 159
   reduced risk of breast cancer with, 319
Vitamin D, 69, 106, 107–108, 111, 113
   oral vitamin D3, 112
Vitamin E, 6–7, 79, 121–122, 124, 159, 207
   breast cancer and, 319
   in disease prevention, 8–9
   insulin action enhanced by, 218
   interactions with drugs and nutrients, 42, 48
   natural and synthetic, 13, 313

platelet aggregation inhibited by, 244
   for reduced cancer risk, 285, 324, 325
   stroke mortality and, 13
   synthesized isomers, 13, 313
Vitamin K, 41, 42, 125, 244
Vitamins
   for cardiovascular disease, 14
   disease prevention and, 8–9, 13–14
   effects of food processing on, 11
   for efficient immune function, 121–123, 124, 126
   vitamin interactions, 42
   see also individual vitamins

W

Waist circumference, 170, 207, 228
   waist-hip ratio, 29, 228, 245
Walnuts, 155
Warfarin, 40, 41, 42, 47

Weight control, 16, 170–183, 194–195, 209
   patient handouts, 187–190
Weight Watchers diet, 172–173
Wheat, 10, 129, 316
Whole grains, 10, 129, 240, 292, 316
Wine, 129, 243, 314
Woman's Health Initiative HRT trial, 77

Y

Yoghurt, 125, 129, 243, 316

Z

Zaleplon, 95
Zinc, 9, 111, 121, 122–123, 124, 159
   prostate cancer risk from, 285
Zone diet, 172

the

FRENCH WOMEN DON'T GET FAT COOKBOOK

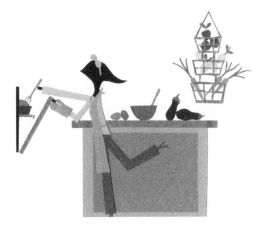

MIREILLE GUILIANO

SIMON &
SCHUSTER

London · New York · Sydney · Toronto

A CBS COMPANY

First published in Great Britain by Simon & Schuster UK Ltd, 2010

This paperback edition first published by Simon & Schuster UK Ltd, 2011
A CBS COMPANY

1 3 5 7 9 10 8 6 4 2

Simon & Schuster UK Ltd
1st Floor
222 Gray's Inn Road
London
WC1X 8HB

www.simonandschuster.co.uk

Simon & Schuster Australia
Sydney

A CIP catalogue record for this book is available
from the British Library

ISBN 978-1-85720-221-5

Designed by Jaime Putorti
Printed and bound in Italy by LEGO SpA

CONTENTS

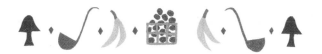

A FEW WORDS BEFORE WE EAT

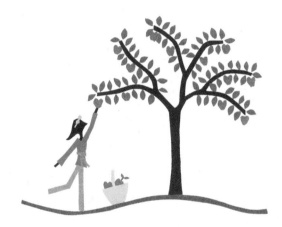

There's a line in my biography that always gets a laugh when I am introduced: "Her favourite pastimes are breakfast, lunch, and dinner." It's all true—people always laugh, and I do take enormous pleasure in and shape my life around meals.

I remember introducing my husband, Edward, to my family in France, an orientation that mostly took place around meals. The smell of a freshly baked breakfast cake would lure him into the kitchen where he'd wake up with some freshly squeezed orange juice (something more American than French, but freshly squeezed to be sure in my parents' house), then a little protein in the form of eggs or cheese or yogurt to go along with the cake and fresh coffee.

Nothing extensive or elaborate, but a healthy start to the day for certain. Before he left the breakfast table my mother would be talking about and preparing lunch, the main meal of the day. It didn't take him long to observe, "You know, your family is always either eating or talking about food." True enough.

Some years later during one of those lunches with my family he asked coyly, "Might it be possible to eat and enjoy this meal before talking about and planning the next one?" It seems we had mastered the art that he had not of enjoying the present while anticipating with all our senses what was to come. That certainly is a French trait. For years now when he and I are in restaurants in France and overhear people enjoying their meal while frequently recounting recent or anticipated meals in other restaurants or sharing recipes and food stories, we give each other a knowing look and shrug.

Yes, breakfast, lunch, and dinner are my favourite pastimes, and that is how I have mostly organized this book of recipes and stories. But the lines of demarcation can be blurry. Some of the same dishes in different portion sizes can be served as the day's main meal, which we normally call dinner, or at the less substantial meal we call lunch if it comes at midday.

I grew up eating my main meal at midday, so is that lunch or dinner? Well, in many areas and throughout much of history, it has been and is called both. Then the last meal of the day is lighter and akin to lunch and is called supper, in part attributable to the French verb *souper,* which relates to soup, common evening fare after a big meal at midday.

And who says you can't have scrambled eggs now and again for dinner . . . at night? So, whether I am offering soups or salads, fish or meat, pasta or vegetables, the recipes that follow are available and inviting for your own *mix-and-match.* In organizing this book I have purposely chosen *not* to always follow conventional logic or be sequential and Cartesian in presenting all the chicken dishes in one spot or all the pasta dishes in another. I've broken these recipes down into three meals, but the rest of the choice is up to you. If you prefer to have your biggest meal midday, feel free to skim the dinner chapter for your lunchtime meal. (Who could argue with pasta for lunch? I've even been known to eat oatmeal at night!)

Of course, I am not suggesting pasta dishes for lunch and again for dinner. I enjoy reading recipes almost every day of my life. For me, reading a single recipe is an intellectual act. For each preparation of, say, chicken, I play it consciously and unconsciously against all the chicken recipes I know, have prepared, or have eaten. I see them—I taste them. I might think this one is like grandma's chicken in a pot, but with x, y, and z added or different. I can taste the differences the way a musician can play a tune in her head from sheet music. (I don't think that's a particularly uncommon trait for anyone who cooks.) And I wish you the mental pleasures of experiencing the recipes presented here in the order that they appear, or in whatever order you wish.

I believe it is important to eat three times a day, to eat in moderation, and to enjoy balanced meals that include protein, fat, and carbohydrates. That's how I live. Breakfast is perhaps the most important meal, and, as simple as it sounds, supplies the fuel for the early stages of the day. In my experience, the people who "don't eat breakfast," or "just have a cup of coffee," are the same ones eating fattening food, primarily carbohydrates, at their desks or in their kitchens at 11 o'clock. Or because they are dehydrated and hungry, they have a fizzy drink as a pick-me-up. And if they get so caught up in a meeting or conference call or whatever and make it to lunch without eating, then, of course, they overdo it. Two or three slices of pizza at lunch isn't the stuff of people who know what they are putting in their body. If any of this rings a bell, don't despair: I promise it is possible to eat for pleasure and modify one's eating patterns. And this book provides what I hope are many tempting meal choices.

So, here's a reminder: eat breakfast. And do not overdose on sugar as a morning stimulant by having oversize portions of fruit juice, sugar-laced cereals, breads, and pastries. Bagels and doughnuts are indulgences, not the core ingredients of a healthy daily meal. With a healthy breakfast, it is possible, if you choose, to have a very modest lunch—but eat something, say some nuts, fruit, yogurt, a soup or salad (half a sandwich? But what to do with the other half?)—rather than pass on lunch altogether, which results in a parallel unhealthy practice of afternoon snacking and/or overdoing it at dinner. "I only eat one big meal a day" is not a motto to live by or be proud of.

Recipes are a personal photo album, a chronicle of who you were and who you are today. My recipes obviously reflect my childhood in France, my adult life in New York and France, and my extensive travels and meals for business and pleasure around America and the world. But mostly they reflect a series of principles on eating for pleasure that I have learned over the years and shared in my two French Women books and on my websites. Almost all are published here in my own interpretations of dishes I've enjoyed with family or friends or "inventions" for the first time. For a little added balance, I include a small selection of a few classic dishes revisited, plus a handful of recipes from my two French Women books that readers have enjoyed.

My philosophy isn't about "dieting" in the conventional sense, but more about eating sensibly and pleasurably. It is partly a cry—okay, more like a whimper—for sanity in an increasingly developed world where, ironically, the abundance of food has become a challenge to good health. Cultural and religious differences as well as the local availability of foodstuffs historically have been the greatest drivers of what we put on our plates, but globalization has meant eating the same genetically modified fruits and vegetables the world over, seasons without end, and spending much less time in the kitchen cooking. As we all recognize, prepared foods, fast food, junk foods abound and people can become overwhelmed by choices (even with yogurts, apples, cheeses, and on and on) and lose touch with what they are putting in their bodies. Cooking is a reality check. Beyond reiterating, expanding, and illustrating the principles that guide my eating and have enabled me to enjoy food and maintain balance and a healthy, consistent weight, I propose to offer—as many of my readers have asked—more meals and recipes that are easy, quick, affordable, and delicious—minimum effort and stress for maximum results.

Yes, I believe in pure and simple recipes. Once in a while I enjoy long hours in the kitchen, but mostly a half hour or even less is enough to put three colours of food on a main plate. (Even my mother's braising and slow cooking required little work once the flame was on—the stove did all the work.)

I like to taste the pure flavours of those balanced ingredients. To me that means buying quality ingredients, which often results in small portions yielding high satisfaction. So, I advise working with foods that taste as good as they look if you want the maximum of pleasure. No matter how great the recipe, tired or tasteless vegetables yield tired or tasteless dishes. And there is no significant correlation between generally tasty and healthy vegetables (or other well-chosen foods) and price. Lots of great things to eat are relatively inexpensive. Work with them.

I like variety in what I eat. Eating fresh foods in season can facilitate this, as well as judicious selection from the freezer section of the supermarket. On the one hand, I like recipes that force good portion control, and on the other, I like it when one preparation can become two meals through a later use of some previously cooked items. So leftovers are for me additional pleasures, and are also in tune with French women's sense of frugality and *débrouillardise* (resourcefulness). I like recipes that work, and all of the recipes in this book have been tested multiple times and on different stoves, since ovens vary according to the changes in the weather and the localized character of the ingredients, such as milk, butter, oil, and the foods themselves. But recipes are guides not laws, so play with them to suit your tastes and kitchen. And most of the recipes I present, for reasons of efficiency, economy, and consistency, serve four. If you are cooking for one, two, or eight, in most cases you should be able to interpolate without a loss in quality. And always have fun.

I especially like recipes that make a meal a sensual experience in that it speaks to all five of our senses—from the look to the texture to the smell and taste, though I confess sound is the least compelling. Of course, recipes need to yield food that tastes good. It is all about pleasures and good health, you'll see.

Chapter One

✳

BREAKFAST
AND *LE BRUNCH*

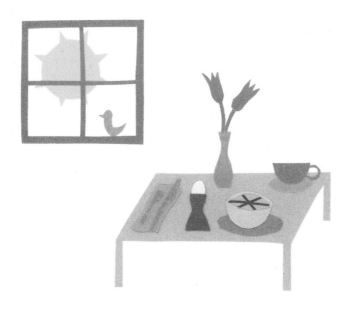

I confess my greatest culinary transformation in life concerns breakfast, and my approach to it continues to evolve. I eat breakfast religiously and, I believe, healthily. That wasn't always the case. Growing up in France, I ate a light breakfast (remember we had our main meal at midday, sometimes not long after I awoke, so I was not always looking to fill up). Generally my breakfast consisted of carbohydrates and coffee. A cup of café au lait and perhaps a piece of bread with butter and preserves (my mother's own). Or a slice of the breakfast cake my mother would make once or twice a week. Once in a while, I ate stale bread in chunks in a *bol*, like a soup bowl, softened and moistened with a soup-size portion of coffee and milk. No protein, no fruit. I was not alone in France. A croissant and coffee, anyone?

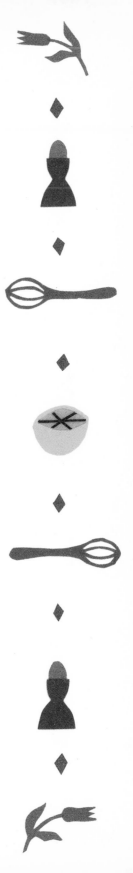

Things did not improve when I came to America as an exchange student. Mostly carbohydrates and coffee again. Once in a while I ingested an egg or two, but with bacon and sometimes potatoes. But those carbs—I discovered doughnuts and bagels, two of which many consider the most delicious albeit fattening and unhealthy foods on earth. Moderation? I only ate one bagel. Who knew that a bagel is loaded with salt and contains as many calories/carbs as a few slices of bread? But, of course, I covered my bagel with cream cheese and jam. Being French, more jam than cream cheese, so I was getting very little protein. And have you noticed the super-sizing of bagels? Not if you were born in the past quarter century. Before that, they actually were what we mostly call mini-bagels today. Plus, being French, I was not then nor am I now into getting my protein or water from a glass of milk. Doughnuts are deep-fried, and I did not restrict myself to just one. The most wonderful discovery of all was muffins, English muffins and blueberry muffins. Who knew? At least they are not fried. I was also introduced to dry cereal in a bowl covered with milk and perhaps with an added banana. And then there was orange juice in a cardboard carton and served in an eight-ounce water glass. But perhaps most memorable of all was that special occasion breakfast: pancakes. Living in New England, I developed a lifelong fondness for maple syrup. No question, I enjoyed and enjoy all of the above, but now in moderation and balance, or better as occasional indulgences.

When I returned to Paris for college, the now plump me drank coffee as my morning stimulant and ate pastry for breakfast (and lunch . . . and dinner). But I lived to tell the tale (in book form). I remember from then through my twenties dismissing German, Scandinavian, even English breakfasts as unappetizing and huge. I wasn't going to eat meat or fish or eggs and cheese and get fat (again). Sausages for breakfast? Please . . .

I am still not a fan of big breakfasts, but am a devotee of and convert to balanced breakfasts (and lunch and dinner): some protein, some carbohydrates, some fat (a holy trinity of sorts), and fluids. I often do eat a slice (or slivers) of cheese. And, I consider breakfast the most important meal of the day. Don't skip it or your wheels tend to come off in a hurry. My true breakfast epiphany occurred just a few years ago when one day a family breakfast speciality, perfected by *Tante* Berthe, and one that I had not thought about or eaten since childhood burst upon my inner eye and palate and changed everything.

Magical Breakfast Cream (with no cream) or MBC

Here's one of my secrets, really *Tante* Berthe's, for some quick and healthy weight loss without dieting. Aunt Berthe had her slow but sure way to lose ten pounds effortlessly each summer. So while most of the French families I knew when I was growing up (and it's still true today) indulged on vacation and came back with a few extra pounds, she came back svelte and *bien dans sa peau*.

I adored my *Tante* Berthe. One of five sisters, she was *Grand-mère* Louise's youngest sister, and although all of the sisters were attractive women with similar features, blue or green eyes, great cheekbones, long hair kept in gorgeous chignons (I used to love to watch Aunt Berthe do her hair), beautiful peachy skin, and a small nose ever so slightly *retroussé*, *Tante* Berthe had that little extra *je ne sais quoi*. Maybe it was her small round glasses or her beautiful smile or her mischievous look that showed in her sparkling eyes. She was also funny, had a great laugh, and sang beautifully while cooking. She always dressed simply with a gray or navy blue long skirt and had the most seductive tops from lovely classic blouses to *charmeuses* in soft cotton, pale colours, and lace, and only a few pieces of classic jewelry. And she loved hats. She was the only sister living by herself, and her status was never discussed although we knew she was not a *veuve* (a widow) since she was addressed as Madame Berthe Juncker. (In France had she been a widow she would have been referred to as Madame Veuve Juncker, like Madame Veuve Clicquot, a famous "widow" from Champagne.) We knew she had some beau, at least we grasped some of that among relatives' hushed conversations. She seemed to have enough money to live without working though she lived rather frugally and would spend the year visiting relatives to help out with children and cooking usually for a week or two at a time and then move on, either go back to her home or travel (some would say disappear) for a week or so. She was also the most gourmande and gourmet and tended to get a bit pleasantly plump particularly at the end of the winter fêtes, but at the end of each summer she was at her best and looked like a movie star. No one could figure out what she had done: Grandma Louise alone knew but surely kept the secret, and we kids had no idea what the secret was and certainly made no connection with her magical breakfast.

She was the favourite aunt of all the grandchildren: Some adults in the family (especially the men) would say because she was the best cook and an incomparable baker; some said because she was single and spoiling us to no end (and she did). I was her very favourite and as such had an added privilege. When she was in town—she lived in Metz—I could visit her once a month on Thursday, the off school day at the time, and believe me I never missed a day between my seventh and twelfth birthdays (before boys started replacing her on my priority list). I would proudly take the one-hour local bus ride by myself (a conversation piece in my town), and she'd be waiting for me at the bus station. Our day together would always start with me going across the street from the station to try the escalator in the Prisunic, a small department store, a novelty I could brag about with my school friends who had never tried or seen one. She would patiently wait as she was scared of that thing. (It is a quaint reminder that there is a first time for everything, and for a seven-year-old in France, where even today escalators are far rarer than in America, an escalator can be an amusement.) After I had gone up and down a few times on the escalator with a great smile on my face, she'd give me signs indicating it was time for lunch at her house. She lived about a ten-minute walk from the store and station, and we could reach her home via an enchanting road along the Moselle River. She had a wonderful little flat, a lovely terrace with a glass-top awning, and wisteria vines. The terrace overlooked residential homes surrounded with gardens. It was country within the city.

Once there, she'd make my favourite lunch, hanger steak with French fries. (You gather by now that she made the best French fries in the world, even better than my mom, and I alone knew her secret; her trick was to make batches in a small, heavy cocotte versus using the typical large deep fryer.) Dessert would always be a seasonal surprise. I loved her for all this. I did not fancy her magical breakfast then or when we were all in the country for the summer. I realize now it was because when she was with us during her week of magical breakfast cream (a week a month, for the two summer months) we would be deprived of the aroma of fresh brioche, *pain aux raisins,* morning cakes, or fruit tarts baking in the wooden stove and perfuming the whole house and the back garden where breakfast would be served. And for a whole week! We couldn't stand it. Complaining and bickering did nothing. She ignored us. We never even noticed that no wine was served during that week. Continued whining didn't change a thing, there was nothing we could do or say to make her change that pattern. Reluctantly, we got used to it and made silly jokes about it. When the regular routine was resumed, she only nibbled at all the goodies but did so discreetly, so that it too went unnoticed. Smart lady.

My recent epiphany and how this episode of my childhood I had sort of forgotten about returned via an early morning telephone call one spring morning while I was working on my business book. Coralie, an old friend's daughter from Eastern France, was telling me how her mother was making my aunt's summer breakfast. Wow. I had not thought of it in decades and thus never made it but instantly visualized the village farmhouse, our summer vacation in a lovely small village near Strasbourg, and the magical mornings eating the summer breakfast in the back of the house watching the fawns come near us (did they like the smell of my aunt's breakfasts?), hearing her grind the nuts and cereal in her mortar and add it to her homemade yogurt base made alternatively from cow, sheep, or goat milk. So, I searched in my recipe boxes and there it was scribbled on a small yellowish piece of disintegrating paper, my *Tante* Berthe's version.

Here's our "family" version that my aunt would make. Beware: it is addictive. It's also extremely easy and quick to make, and one can play and interchange so many ingredients. It is the perfect complete breakfast and will keep you from getting hungry until late lunch. You may have run across Johanna Budwig's variation. A German chemist, pharmacologist, and physicist who lived during much of the twentieth century (and came after my aunt), she promoted a version using cottage cheese as a cancer-fighting breakfast and also part of a nutrition plan. I've made MBC in quite a few versions and can't decide which is my favourite, as it is all a function of where I am, what I feel like, and with whom I share it.

Why do I call it magical breakfast cream? Magical? Something that is a combination of tasty, easy, and so good for your well-being and melts away pounds has to be magical, right? How many pounds? Try a week of MBC for breakfast with a normal but modest lunch and dinner (soup or salad, fish, two vegetables, and fruit), and say good-bye effortlessly to a few pounds, if dozens of converts reporting back from my website are any indication. The trick here is to eat MBC and also to cut two offenders (for me it's bread and wine) and otherwise eat normally. It works splendidly, and your energy and well-being after these few days are remarkable.

Cream, you may ask? There is no cream in it, but the texture looks like cream and cream connotes something utterly sensual such as comfort food and pampering—except in this case you need not worry about the calories. I trust my aunt used the word to make sure we kids would love it and never mentioned the *oil* in the mixture. Smart lady again: no one can taste the oil anyway. That oil, by the way, is preferably flaxseed oil, a superconcentrated source of omega-3 fatty acid that has so many health benefits.

In a variation on a theme dear to me, and a paraphrase of a quote from Lily Bollinger on Champagne, let me say: "I eat it when I am happy and when I am sad. I eat it when I am alone and consider it obligatory when I have company. I trifle with it when I am not hungry and always eat it when I am."

Have fun playing with the range of options and make your own version. Remember, it's like fashion: mix and match to please your own taste buds.

MAGICAL BREAKFAST CREAM

4 to 6 tablespoons yogurt

1 teaspoon flaxseed oil

1 to 2 tablespoons lemon
  juice (preferably
  organic)

1 teaspoon honey

2 tablespoons finely ground
  cereal (with zero sugar
  such as Post Shredded
  Wheat)

2 teaspoons finely ground
  walnuts

1. Put the yogurt in a bowl and add the oil. Mix well. Add the lemon juice and mix well. Add the honey and mix well. (It is important to add each ingredient one at a time and mix well to obtain a homogeneous preparation.)

2. Finely grind the cereal and walnuts (I use a small food processor). Add to the yogurt mixture and mix well. Serve at once.

TIME-SAVER: *You can do a week's worth of grinding cereal/nuts mixture and keep it refrigerated so in the morning it will take just a few instants to mix the yogurt with the oil (have no fear, you will not taste the oil in the final creamy blend), add the lemon juice, honey, and your daily dose of cereal/nut mixture—et voilà.*

NOTE: *I use Post Shredded Wheat Original made from whole grain wheat, adding to this recipe a "health-friendly" mix of 0 grams sugar, 0 grams sodium, and 6 grams of fibre per cup (and I use only 2 tablespoons per serving).*

You can replace the yogurt with ricotta, cottage cheese (beware of high sodium content), *fromage blanc,* or should you be in France, try it with *faisselle.* When using yogurt you can opt for whole or 2% milk. I make my own yogurt and do not like skimmed milk, which tastes like water to me.

You can replace the flaxseed oil with sesame oil or safflower oil.

You can replace the lemon juice with grapefruit juice, orange juice, or blood orange juice. With orange juice, use less honey.

You can replace the honey with maple syrup. As the latter is less sweet than honey, you may want to adjust to your taste.

You can replace the shredded wheat with buckwheat, barley, oatmeal, or any cereal that contains no sugar, a key in this recipe.

You can replace the walnuts with hazelnuts, almonds, or a mixture of both. Pecans, pine nuts, and any other nuts work fine, too.

Finally, you can adjust the doses of the juice (I tend to add more lemon juice when using something thicker than yogurt and because I love it) and the honey (less rather than more). My husband chooses 2 tablespoons of fresh orange juice, which is sweet enough and in his case requires nothing else to compensate for honey, although some times (on Sundays!) he'll add a drizzle of maple syrup (my theory being it is his make-believe for not having pancakes or waffles! Why not?).

You can also add fruit: the obvious is half of a ripe banana mashed with a fork and added after step one or sliced and placed on top of the finished dish. Or top it with any seasonal fruit, especially a mix of berries in summer or dried cranberries, raisins, dried fig or date pieces, or even diced prunes in the cold months. Try it plain, though, as it is simply delicious and in its purest form.

And, as recommended, create your own versions. And a last recommendation: surprise your kids with your favourite concoction as in a blind wine tasting—no details on what it is until after the first taste and a little riddle.

GIOVANNA'S MBC VARIATION

Giovanna, a Roman friend in her early thirties who is nuts about food, particularly French food (don't we always want what we don't have, as so many of us, French and American women, love Italian food?), is someone I have had great meals with at home and in restaurants in Italy, France, and in the United States, mostly New York City. She loves to cook for her family and friends, and during our cooking sessions, we've spent time comparing recipes, making new dishes, and learning from each other when it comes to the presentation of food. We've had lots of laughs in the kitchen and at the table talking about food and wine and making fun of each other's culture and rituals.

She admitted that though she's never had a weight problem and is a tall, pretty young woman, she had applied a few things from my books that she didn't know about or had not yet incorporated in her eating plan, and her body was transformed. She had not really lost weight, well, maybe two to three pounds, but looks like *une belle plante* (a flattering expression French men use when they see a gorgeous woman) and was glad that I said I had noticed . . .

When she stayed with me in Provence, I introduced her to the MBC. I sincerely do not believe I had ever seen anyone enjoy something so simple so much. Eating it, she was *miam miaming* (yum yumming) like a baby. And from then on, we had the MBC every morning. Then she went home and started experimenting. She is not as crazy as I am about lemons (too acidic), so she experimented with orange juice. Here's her latest, and I must say *très réussie* (well done), an Italian interpretation of *Tante* Berthe's basic recipe:

GIOVANNA'S MBC

• •

110g Greek-style yogurt

1 teaspoon flaxseed oil

1 tablespoon finely ground nuts (equal parts walnuts, hazelnuts, and almonds)

1 teaspoon honey

2 tablespoons finely ground old-fashioned oatmeal

Juice and pulp of 2 clementines or tangerines (only available for a couple of winter months) or ½ orange (not quite as delicate)

1. Put the yogurt and flaxseed oil in a cereal bowl and mix well.

2. Add the ground nuts and honey and mix.

3. Add the ground oats on the surface, but don't mix yet. Pour the juice and pulp over and leave for a few seconds, then mix and taste.

And here is her reasoning for her improved version, her treaty on *cuisine moléculaire*! "The small amount of fat in the 2% yogurt is a plus. [We agree on that one.] Oats have fibre and starch, which even in the uncooked version, once in contact with acid substances (citrus food), are practically predigested, and this explains why I prefer to leave the juice on it to be in contact with the oats before mixing it. The acidity level of the clementines is well tolerated by the surface of my teeth and my stomach. Furthermore, for one who loves sugar, it's the type of citrus fruit that is the most delicate; thus when I press the juice, I am careful to pick up any pulp left on the juicer, and so all those little fibres stay in the 'cream,' which is truly fresh, light, thirst quenching, and extra *gourmande*—at least for my taste buds." And apparently my aunt's, too.

And now Giovanna has converted her mother and even her grandmother, who professed not to like yogurt. Here's the account: Giovanna wrote she missed her MBC (due to a rushed day visiting relatives), but made it for a snack in the afternoon while visiting her grandmother. "I made my grandmother taste it, not telling her anything about the ingredients, as she has repeatedly stated to all family members she does not like yogurt and makes disgusted facial expressions when she mentions the word. Here is the surprise: She loved it (my mother was present, knew the ingredients, and was quietly smiling) and looked like a *bébé gourmand*, eating teaspoon after teaspoon to the point when I had to ask whether I should make more or would she leave me some." She finished hers. Imagine if she had liked yogurt!

Eggs

Happy days now that eggs are back in favour—thank you, thank you—not only because they are tasty but because in moderation they are very good for you due to their exceptional nutritional qualities. The egg is actually a small dietetic miracle possessing vitamins A, B, D, E, and K, minerals (notably iron and phosphorus), as well as selenium and iodine. And it's now, *enfin,* confirmed that three eggs a week have no effect on cholesterol (three quarters of which is made by the body itself anyway), since egg is perfectly digestible and well tolerated by our liver. Eggs being a good source of proteins, they are a nice alternative to meat, especially as our body absorbs their nutrients quite easily. As wonderful as the French breakfast of coffee, croissant, and brioche is, (wo)man cannot live by bread alone. How about a little protein added with a yogurt or egg dish?

When I was a student in Weston, Massachusetts, and lived with six very different families during the school year, I was introduced to sunny-side-up eggs (I love the expression, which reminds me of sunflowers) and bacon. One thing these six families shared was fried eggs for breakfast—at some households it was on the breakfast menu three to five times a week. The men in the family would eat three eggs and I dare not remember or mention how many slices of bacon. *Oh la la.* What a shock that was. First, because we never had eggs for breakfast in my family (but ate our dose in prepared salted or sweet dishes). Yet we had omelettes (filled with whatever was in season from mushrooms to asparagus or simply cheese and herbs if there was nothing else in the fridge), but usually for unexpected guests at dinner or some light dinners a couple of times a month, especially on weekends after a multicourse long lunch. Once a week as children we were allowed one *oeuf à la coque,* the soft-boiled egg served in one of *Mamie*'s prize collection of *coquetiers* (eggcups) with *mouillettes,* the little sticks of bread cut into slim rectangles and just toasted, the ones French kids grow up with and the perfect accessory to "wet" the egg yolk with, since it was not proper to let the yolk leak out—it was all in the art of handling the *mouillette*. I came to realize that French and Americans both eat plenty of eggs, just differently.

My reasons for liking eggs go beyond their vitamins and minerals, which make them a great food for any age group. They are inexpensive and keep for a couple of weeks in the fridge, though I'd recommend taking them out 20 minutes before cooking. They are light, easy to digest, and good at any meal and a quick way to make a meal (3 minutes for a soft-boiled egg, a few more for an omelette). Hard-boiled eggs are perfect for an *en cas* (emergency food, in case) or a picnic (I often bring one on the plane for dinner or breakfast on overnight flights, one never knows). They are a saviour for last-minute guests (make sure to always have some cheese in your fridge) showing up hungry. They are also and foremost delicious in desserts from sweet omelettes to French toast, floating island, and the almighty *crème anglaise* not to mention custard, puddings, and soufflés. The textural differences and pleasures one can achieve with eggs are endless.

My houseguests in Provence always tease me when I announce an "English breakfast," which is basically one or two eggs any style, toasted baguette, some local jam, yogurt, a portion of fruit, and a nice cup (or two) of coffee or tea, mixed with a surprise or two like a tomato salad (eh, we are in Provence after all) or a polenta dish for those who want to eat out of the box. Sitting on the terrace and enjoying the first song of the day from our friends the *cigales*, life does not get any better. And the proof is that people linger, relax, converse, and don't want to leave the table; sometimes they stay there until we announce lunch. Maybe my travel to many parts of the world also influenced my way of reassessing breakfast and playing not only with variety but completeness. I'm not up to serving a Chinese breakfast in Manhattan or a Japanese one in Provence, but I like to play on the "when in Rome" dictum, and I love dishes and flavours my guests do and I let them compose their own magical treat. The trick is not to go to the extreme and gorge oneself but carefully pick à la carte. So, generally I pick one of the following recipes for the "staple" breakfast dish.

SOFT SCRAMBLED EGGS

· SERVES 6 TO 8 ·

12 eggs

2 tablespoons butter, cut
  into small pieces

¼ teaspoon salt

2 tablespoons double cream

1. Fill a saucepan with 2 cms of water, place over medium-high heat, and bring to a simmer.

2. Break the eggs into a double boiler insert and place on top of a simmering water bath. Add the butter and salt and cook, whisking constantly, until the eggs thicken, small curds form, and they become very creamy, 5 to 6 minutes.

3. Immediately remove from the heat and stir in the cream, which will stop the cooking process and make the eggs even creamier. Serve immediately.

PROVENÇAL OMELETTE

• SERVES 4 •

3 teaspoons olive oil

3 teaspoons unsalted butter

25 g peeled and chopped shallots

35 g white mushrooms, cleaned and sliced

1 teaspoon lemon juice

35 g broccoli florets, cut into 1 cm pieces

35 g yellow pepper, cut into strips

Salt and freshly ground pepper

10 eggs

55 g grated Gruyère

75 g grated Parmesan

1 tomato, rinsed and diced

75 g baby spinach

20 g fresh basil leaves cut into chiffonade (thin strips)

Baguette for serving

1. Heat 1 teaspoon of the olive oil and 1 teaspoon of the butter in a medium (23 cm) nonstick frying pan over medium heat. Add the shallots and sauté until softened, about 2 minutes. Add the mushrooms, lemon juice, and broccoli and sauté for 2 minutes. Add the yellow pepper and sauté for an additional 2 minutes until crisp-tender. Remove the vegetables from the pan, season to taste, and reserve.

2. In a large bowl, whisk the eggs and season to taste. Heat 1 teaspoon oil and 1 teaspoon butter over medium-high heat in the same frying pan. Add half of the eggs to the pan and shake the pan a bit, lifting the edges of the omelette up to allow the uncooked egg to run underneath. Cook until the top is just set, about 1 minute. Sprinkle the eggs with half of the grated cheeses and place half of the sautéed vegetables, tomato, and spinach on one side of the omelette. Using a large spatula, fold the other side of the omelette over to cover the vegetable filling and allow to cook for 1 minute. Carefully slide onto a platter and repeat with the remaining ingredients for the other omelette.

3. To serve, place both omelettes on a platter and garnish with fresh basil. Serve immediately with slices of a baguette.

TRICOLOUR OMELETTE

• SERVES 4 •

3 tablespoons plus 1
   teaspoon unsalted butter

3 large shallots, peeled and
   finely chopped

10 eggs

Salt and freshly ground
   pepper

2 tablespoons each finely
   chopped fresh parsley,
   basil, and thyme

1 medium tomato, cut into
   5 mm dice

1. Melt 1 teaspoon butter in a small nonstick sauté pan over medium heat. Add the shallots and sauté until softened. Remove the pan from the heat and cool.

2. In a large bowl, whisk the eggs together and season to taste. Divide the eggs among three bowls: in the first bowl, add the herbs, in the second, tomato, and in the third, shallots. Stir each mixture and season with salt and pepper.

3. Melt 1 tablespoon butter in the pan used for the shallots over medium-high heat. Add the egg-herb mixture to the pan, tilting and swirling the pan to evenly distribute the egg mixture. When the top is set, carefully flip the mixture over and cook for another minute. Slide onto a plate and keep warm.

4. Repeat with the remaining two egg mixtures to make three omelettes, stacking the cooked omelettes on top of one another. Garnish with additional herbs if desired, and serve immediately, cut into wedges.

FRIED EGGS, SPANISH STYLE

• SERVES 4 •

20 thin slices chorizo

2 tablespoons olive oil

1 large shallot, peeled and
   sliced

4 eggs

Salt and freshly ground
   pepper

1. Preheat the oven to 200°C/gas mark 6.

2. Place the chorizo on a small baking sheet and cook in the oven for 1 to 2 minutes. Remove from the oven and transfer the slices to a paper towel-lined plate to drain. Reserve.

3. Heat the oil in a medium nonstick frying pan over medium-low heat. Add the shallot and sauté for 3 minutes to infuse the oil. Remove the shallot from the pan and discard. Break 2 eggs into the pan and cook for 1 minute. Baste the eggs with the shallot-infused oil and cook for another minute or until set. Carefully remove the eggs from the pan and place on a paper towel-lined plate to drain and keep warm. Repeat with the remaining 2 eggs.

4. To serve, place 1 egg on a warmed plate, season to taste, and garnish with the warm chorizo slices.

POACHED EGGS WITH SALMON AND SPINACH

1 teaspoon peeled and chopped shallot

1 teaspoon lemon zest

1 tablespoon lemon juice

2 tablespoons olive oil

Salt and freshly ground pepper

150g spinach

½ small shredded fennel bulb

1 tablespoon white wine vinegar

4 eggs

110g thinly sliced smoked salmon

Baguette for serving

1. In a small bowl, whisk together the shallot, lemon zest, lemon juice, and olive oil and season to taste. Place the spinach and fennel in a bowl, add the dressing, and toss well to combine. Set aside.

2. Fill a 25–35 cm frying pan with 6 cm water, add the vinegar, and bring to a simmer over medium-high heat. Break each egg into a small cup and add to the water one at a time. Cook the eggs until the whites are just set, about 1½ minutes. Carefully remove the eggs with a slotted spoon.

3. To serve, place one slice of salmon on each plate. Top with a portion of spinach salad and a poached egg. Season to taste and serve immediately with slices of a baguette.

HAM AND LEEK FRITTATA

• SERVES 4 •

6 eggs

1 teaspoon grainy mustard

Pinch of red pepper flakes

Salt and freshly ground
pepper

2 tablespoons unsalted
butter

1 tablespoon olive oil

1 leek, white part only,
rinsed and thinly sliced

110g baked ham, cut into
small pieces

1. Preheat the grill.

2. In a medium bowl, whisk together the eggs, mustard, and pepper flakes and season with salt and pepper.

3. Heat the butter and olive oil in a large nonstick oven-safe frying pan over medium heat until the butter has melted. Add the leek and cook, stirring, until softened, 3 to 4 minutes. Add the ham and cook, stirring, until warm, about 2 minutes.

4. Add the egg mixture and swirl the pan to distribute the eggs and filling evenly over the surface. Shake the pan gently, tilting slightly while lifting the edges of the frittata with a spatula to let the raw egg run underneath for the first 1 to 2 minutes. Cook until the eggs are almost set, about 5 minutes total, and place the pan under the grill (not too close) for 1 minute. The frittata will puff up and brown slightly. Remove from the oven and carefully slide the frittata out of the pan using a spatula. Cut into wedges and serve hot, at room temperature, or cold.

NOTE: *If desired, sprinkle 50g grated Gruyère on top of the frittata just before placing under the grill.*

COURGETTE AND FRESH GOAT CHEESE FRITTATA

• SERVES 4 •

6 eggs

1½ small unpeeled courgette, rinsed and grated

2 tablespoons fresh thyme (or chopped marjoram)

110g fresh goat cheese (or feta), crumbled

Salt and freshly ground pepper

1 tablespoon olive oil

35g grated pecorino

1 small sprig fresh thyme

1. Preheat the grill.

2. Break the eggs into a bowl and beat slightly with a fork. Add the courgette, thyme, and goat cheese, stir to combine, and season to taste.

3. Heat the olive oil in a large, nonstick, oven-safe frying pan over medium-high heat. Add the egg mixture and swirl the pan to distribute the eggs and filling evenly over the surface. Shake the pan gently, tilting slightly while lifting the edges of the frittata with a spatula to let the egg run underneath for the first 1 to 2 minutes. Lower the heat to medium and cook until the eggs are almost set, 5 to 7 minutes.

4. Cover the frittata with the pecorino and place the pan under the grill (not too close) for 1 minute. The frittata will puff up and brown slightly and the cheese will melt. Remove from the oven, garnish with the thyme, and serve.

Comfort Food

I don't know when I first heard the term comfort food; it probably was only in the last decade, but it hit home immediately. Comfort foods are those security blanket dishes that evoke childhood memories and a sense of well-being. They are extremely cultural as well—from macaroni and cheese to steak and mashed potatoes for some New Yorkers. With the Alsatian cultural influence in my family, desserts rise to the comfort food class from cakes with raisins, ginger, nutmeg, and lots of cinnamon to cookies with anise seeds to sugar tarts with more cinnamon, but also all types of custards—flans and puddings with berries in syrup and fresh fruit tarts being the ultimate, especially those on the sour side with *groseilles* (red currants), *griottes* (a bitter type of cherries), *quetsches* (like some Italian plums), and rhubarb, not everyone's cup of tea but a wonderful reminder of the aroma in the kitchen at baking time.

Can pickles and seaweed be comfort foods for breakfast? Who eats pickles and seaweed for breakfast in the first place? That's right, the Japanese. I will never forget my first Japanese breakfast in a celebrated and ancient *ryokan* in Kyoto many years ago: Edward and I sat on the floor of our matted room, and a very formal attendant on her knees served us grilled fish with *tsukemono* (salty Japanese pickles), steamed rice, nori, *tamagoyaki* (rolled omelette), and, of course, miso soup, plus more things than I can remember now, and tea. No doubt as strange to us for breakfast that first time as some of the dishes in this book or some Alsatian specialities might be to some people. Everyone's comfort foods are individualistic, even solipsistic. Still, that Japanese breakfast and setting made a strong and warm impression on me, and I can easily understand the comfort that a full Japanese breakfast can bring.

Nowadays, it is oatmeal and Cream of Wheat (forms of baby food for grown-ups) that I count among my comfort foods.

OATMEAL WITH LEMON ZEST AND PRUNES

• SERVES 2 TO 4 •

175 g old-fashioned oatmeal

550 ml water

Pinch of salt

2 tablespoons honey

Zest of 1 lemon

1 teaspoon unsalted butter

55 ml 2% milk

90 g pitted prunes, chopped

1. In a medium saucepan, combine the oatmeal, water, and salt and bring to a boil. Cook for 3 to 4 minutes over low heat, stirring occasionally.

2. Add the honey, lemon zest, butter, and milk and mix gently. Cook for another minute and add the prunes, stirring to combine. Serve immediately.

NOTE: *This heats quickly and makes a perfect breakfast-on-the-go during the work week, a nice change from a cold yogurt or toast!*

PEANUT BUTTER BANANA OATMEAL

175 g old-fashioned oatmeal

500 ml water

Pinch of salt

2 tablespoons peanut butter

1 banana, sliced

75 ml whole milk

½ teaspoon butter

1. Combine the oatmeal, water, and salt in a medium saucepan. Bring to a boil.

2. Cook for 5 minutes, stirring occasionally. Add the peanut butter, banana, milk, and butter and mix gently. Cook for another minute and serve.

STRAWBERRY-BANANA OATMEAL SMOOTHIE

• SERVES 1 •

1 banana, peeled and sliced

2 to 4 frozen strawberries

2 tablespoons Greek-style
yogurt

½ teaspoon honey

1 teaspoon old-fashioned
oatmeal

Pinch of cinnamon

1. Place the banana, strawberries, yogurt, honey, and oatmeal in a blender and purée until smooth.

2. Serve in a glass with the cinnamon.

QUINOA WITH ALMONDS, HAZELNUTS, AND APRICOTS

• SERVES 4 •

175g quinoa

2 tablespoons honey

1 tablespoon lemon juice

1 teaspoon butter

75ml milk

Pinch of salt

1 tablespoon finely chopped almonds

1 tablespoon finely chopped hazelnuts

40g dried apricots, diced

1. Cook the quinoa according to the package directions.

2. Stir the honey, lemon juice, butter, milk, and salt into the cooked quinoa and cook for another minute. Serve in individual bowls garnished with chopped nuts and apricots.

PORRIDGE WITH CRANBERRIES AND WALNUTS

75g porridge oats

3 tablespoons brown sugar

Pinch of cinnamon

2 teaspoons lemon juice

1½ tablespoons unsalted butter

35g dried cranberries

30g walnuts, coarsely chopped

1. In a medium saucepan, cook the porridge oats according to the package directions.

2. When the porridge is cooked, stir in the brown sugar, cinnamon, lemon juice, and butter. Mix well and cook for 1 minute.

3. Remove the saucepan from the heat and serve in individual bowls garnished with cranberries and walnuts.

Le Brunch

It does not take a degree in linguistics to recognize the portmanteau nature of brunch, the combination of breakfast and lunch that seemingly connotes a late-morning breakfast or early lunch. Well, today we can forget just the late morning. Walk the streets of Manhattan, for example, on a Sunday morning or early afternoon, and there will be only brunch menus. And certainly restaurants and hotels promote brunch for regular and special occasions such as Mother's Day. Sunday brunch at some hotels is their local signature. Ah, the endless buffets I have seen, with chef stations cooking up omelettes and pancakes and even carving slices of beef.

In New York, in good weather we like to entertain outdoors on our terrace for brunch, which often means telling out-of-town guests to come by at 11 AM, which results in their leaving the table at 1 or 2 PM, so the afternoon is free for sightseeing, shopping, or perhaps a Sunday matinee.

What's better than welcoming friends to your home with a glass of Champagne or sparkling water or a little freshly squeezed fruit juice and heading outside for some conversation, nibbles—say a taste of smoked salmon, cheese, or even miniature croissants—before sitting down for an omelette with vegetables and good breads and coffee or tea.

As I am not a late sleeper—at least not since I left my teens—I generally eat an early breakfast before brunch—but then is it lunch? Sure, just with breakfast foods more often than not. I can taste the ricotta pancakes just thinking about them. When Edward and I truly want to combine breakfast and lunch, we'll head off to, say, Balthazar in New York's SoHo for brunch. We'll skip the onion soup gratinée, thank you very much, but if we are in a breakfasty state of mind we will contemplate the brioche French toast. Otherwise, if the raw bar is open, oysters. Now there's a Sunday morning pick-me-up. Plus, there's moules frites (for me) and steak frites (for Edward) to follow and one of our few French fry indulgences, or frunch for us.

Brunch is a global standard today—a development over just the past perhaps fifteen years—and while the venerable *Académie française* shuns the word *brunch* in the French language, preferring *le grand petit déjeuner,* meaning "big breakfast," *les citoyens* just adore it. The French are crazy about the idea of *le brunch,* even if the menu is not all that different from a bistro lunch with a breakfast basket of pastries (known in French as *viennoiseries,* a combination of croissants, *pains aux raisins,* and *pains au chocolat*).

Le French Snack

For those of us who eat three meals a day, snacks are out or are the exception when dinner is very late or travel plans delay mealtime. *Tartines* are—or at least were—the quintessential snack for hungry French teenagers.

But what strikes me as well suited for brunch fare are *tartines,* those small, open-faced, bread-based French finger foods, so I begin the brunch recipes with them.

The key is to buy some really good bread. *Tartines* are served for breakfast, brunch, lunch, or dinner and at tapas bars and one can make a meal out of them. As great bread lovers, the French invented *tartines* and they used to be included at the start of almost every meal.

The last few years, *tartines* have made a huge comeback (perhaps because we are back to lots of great quality bread and artisan bakers) since they are easy, quick, can be changed indefinitely depending on what you have on hand, what is in season, or simply adapting them to your personal tastes. Lots of small cafés or *salons de thé* in Paris and major French cities offer them as a wonderful meal.

When I grew up, a well-buttered *tartine* with a thin bar of dark chocolate was the *goûter* when we came home from school. It's coming back in schools as well, since I noticed most of the young children in my village in Provence had that very snack versus a more fattening *pain au chocolat* or worse, one of those bars from vending machines, which fortunately have now been banned in French schools. So, it seems it's back to basics: simple, nutritious, yummy, and relatively inexpensive. Here's a variety of *tartines* that can be served as a brunch starter (or dinner hors d'oeuvres), as a small assortment on a plate with a simple green salad for lunch, or as a snack any time of day.

GOAT CHEESE AND HAZELNUT *TARTINES*

• SERVES 4 •

150g fresh goat cheese

4 slices whole grain bread, toasted

35g toasted and coarsely chopped hazelnuts

1 tablespoon honey

1 teaspoon chopped fresh rosemary

Spread the goat cheese on toasts, sprinkle with hazelnuts, and drizzle the honey. Garnish with rosemary and serve.

RICOTTA AND ANCHOVY *TARTINES*

4 anchovies, rinsed and
    drained

1 tablespoon sherry vinegar

2 tablespoons olive oil

110g fresh ricotta, at room
    temperature

Salt and freshly ground
    pepper

4 slices country bread,
    toasted

1. Place the anchovies in a shallow bowl in one layer. Pour the vinegar over the anchovies and marinate for 1 minute. Pour out the vinegar, add 1 tablespoon olive oil to the bowl and set aside.

2. Place the ricotta in a small bowl and season to taste with salt and pepper. Spread the seasoned ricotta on the toasted bread slices. Top each slice with 1 anchovy, drizzle with the remaining 1 tablespoon olive oil, season with additional freshly ground pepper, and serve.

CUCUMBER, PROSCIUTTO, AND PARMESAN *TARTINES*

• SERVES 4 •

3 teaspoons unsalted butter, softened

2 teaspoons grainy mustard

4 slices fresh bread or brioche, lightly toasted

4 slices prosciutto

12 thin slices cucumber

35g Parmesan

Freshly ground pepper

1. In a small bowl combine the butter and mustard and stir until smooth. Spread a thin layer on each slice of toast. Cover each with 1 slice of prosciutto and 3 slices of cucumber.

2. Using a vegetable peeler, shave thin slices of Parmesan and garnish each *tartine* with 1 or 2 shavings. Season generously with fresh pepper and serve.

SARDINE *TARTINES*

• SERVES 4 •

. . . .

100 g can sardines in water, drained

2 tablespoons unsalted butter, at room temperature

1 teaspoon Dijon mustard

1 tablespoon chopped fresh parsley

1 tablespoon chopped fresh chervil

1 teaspoon lemon juice

Salt and freshly ground pepper

4 slices country bread, toasted

1. Remove the bones from the sardines, place in a bowl, and mash with a fork.

2. In a second bowl, combine the butter, mustard, parsley, chervil, and lemon juice and stir until smooth. Add the mashed sardines and mix gently. Season to taste and serve spread on toasted bread.

PEAR AND BLUE CHEESE
TARTINES

• SERVES 4 •

4 slices sourdough bread,
   lightly toasted

50g blue cheese, at room
   temperature

2 pears, rinsed, cored,
   quartered, and thinly
   sliced

¼ cup alfalfa sprouts

2 tablespoons coarsely
   chopped walnuts

Freshly ground pepper

1. Spread each slice of toast with blue cheese and cover with pear slices.

2. Garnish with alfalfa sprouts and walnuts, season with pepper, and serve.

SEA SCALLOP AND
FLEUR DE SEL *TARTINES*

• SERVES 4 •

4 sea scallops, each sliced
    horizontally into 4 thin
    disks

Juice and zest of ½ lemon

4 slices country bread,
    lightly toasted

1 tablespoon olive oil (or
    walnut oil)

½ teaspoon fleur de sel
    (large-grained "flower of
    salt" harvested from the
    sea works magic)

1. Place the scallops in a small bowl with the lemon juice and marinate for 3 to 5 minutes. Meanwhile, brush the toasted bread slices with the olive oil.

2. Drain the scallops and lay 4 scallop slices, overlapping, on each slice of toast, garnish with the lemon zest and fleur de sel, and serve immediately.

PARMESAN POLENTA WITH PROSCIUTTO

• SERVES 4 •

175g polenta
75g grated Parmesan
Freshly ground pepper
1 teaspoon olive oil
4 thin slices prosciutto
4 sun-dried tomatoes
12 black olives

1. Cook the polenta according to the package directions. Add the Parmesan and pepper and mix well. Pour into a buttered 8-inch square baking dish and refrigerate for 1 hour.

2. Heat the oil over medium heat in a large non-stick frying pan. Cut the chilled polenta into four pieces and cook until heated through and slightly crisp, about 1 minute on each side. Reserve on paper towels.

3. Using the same pan, briefly cook the prosciutto over medium-high heat, about 1 minute. Garnish each serving of polenta with 1 slice prosciutto, 1 sun-dried tomato, and 3 olives. Serve immediately.

Special and Luxurious
(as in what a luxury to eat)

These recipes are indulgences, and in our home they are reserved for weekends and for entertaining friends, especially at brunch.

MILK JAM (*CONFITURE DE LAIT*)

• MAKES 100ml •

225ml (2%) milk

75g sugar

1. Place the milk and sugar in a small heavy saucepan and bring to a boil, stirring until the sugar is dissolved. Reduce the heat to low and cook very slowly until the mixture has thickened to the consistency of sour cream and is a light caramel colour.

2. Remove from the heat and serve as a spread for toast, crêpes, or English muffins. Also delicious drizzled over ice cream!

NOTE: *Milk jam may be stored in a sealed jar and refrigerated for up to 2 weeks.*

CLAFOUTIS PROVENÇAL

• SERVES 4 •

We had cherry trees in our garden, and from the time I was eight, I got to climb the ladder (and some branches) and pick cherries. My little girlfriends and I would sometimes overeat the fresh cherries, but there were still enough to bring back to my mom, who used them to make a clafoutis, *baking the fresh fruit in a custardy batter in a round baking dish. The curious name for this dessert comes from the verb* clafir, *"to fill up," because you fill up the batter and mould with fruit, most commonly cherries. Clafoutis usually refers to a dessert preparation, but in Provence it can be a savoury yet still rich dish with cheese, eggs, and bread.*

2 tablespoons olive oil

1 small aubergine, cut into 1 cm dice

1 yellow pepper, seeded and cut into 1 cm dice

Salt and freshly ground pepper

1 slice bread, crusts removed

2 garlic cloves, peeled

225 g ricotta

3 eggs

2 tablespoons fresh basil leaves cut into chiffonade (thin strips)

50 g black olives, pitted and halved

110 g grated Parmesan

Butter, softened, for baking dish

Fresh basil (or mint) for garnish

1. Preheat the oven to 180°C/gas mark 4.

2. Heat the olive oil over medium heat in a frying pan and sauté the aubergine and yellow pepper until softened, about 6 minutes. Season to taste and set aside to cool.

3. In a food processor, combine the bread, garlic, ricotta, and eggs and blend until smooth. Season with salt and pepper and, using a spatula, fold in 1 tablespoon basil, the olives, Parmesan, aubergine, and yellow pepper.

4. Pour the mixture into a lightly buttered 21 cm square baking dish and place in the oven. Bake until lightly golden, 30 to 35 minutes. Remove from the oven and let cool. Serve warm or at room temperature, garnished with basil or mint.

GRAPEFRUIT, AVOCADO, AND CAVIAR MILLE-FEUILLE

• SERVES 4 •

2 pink grapefruit

2 ripe avocados, halved and
  pitted

2 tablespoons lemon juice

Pinch of curry powder

Salt and freshly ground
  pepper

110g domestic caviar

1 teaspoon chopped fresh
  tarragon

1. Prepare the grapefruit segments: Cut slices off the top and bottom of the grapefruit and slice away the peel and pith, top to bottom, following the curve of the fruit. Working over a bowl and using a small, sharp knife, cut between the membranes to release the segments. Chop into small pieces and reserve.

2. Using a spoon, scoop out the avocado flesh and place in a medium bowl. Add the lemon juice and curry powder, season to taste, and, using a fork, mash to obtain a smooth texture.

3. Place an 8cm ring mould in the centre of the first plate and build the mille-feuille. Begin with a layer of grapefruit at the bottom of the mould. Cover with a layer of avocado purée and top with a thin layer of caviar, pressing down slightly before carefully lifting away the ring mould. Garnish with tarragon and repeat on the remaining plates. Serve immediately.

SMOKED SALMON, FENNEL, AND ORANGE MILLE-FEUILLE

• SERVES 4 •

3 oranges (blood oranges
    preferred)

1 fennel bulb, trimmed,
    cored, and finely diced

35 g black olives, pitted and
    coarsely chopped

3 teaspoons olive oil

Freshly ground pepper

220 g smoked salmon,
    thinly sliced

¼ teaspoon fleur de sel

1. Wash and dry the oranges. Grate the zest from 1 orange and then press the juice, reserving the zest and juice. Segment the remaining 2 oranges, one at a time: Cut slices off the top and bottom of the orange and then slice away the peel and pith, top to bottom, following the curve of the fruit. Working over a bowl and using a small, sharp knife, cut between the membranes to release the segments. Chop each segment into small pieces.

2. In a medium bowl, combine the chopped oranges, orange zest, orange juice, fennel, olives, and olive oil, and season to taste.

3. Using an 8 cm ring mould, cut out 8 smoked salmon circles. To serve, place the ring mould in the centre of a salad plate. Place one circle of salmon in the base of the mould and cover with a 1 cm layer of orange-fennel salad, lightly pressing down. Cover with a second layer of smoked salmon and top with 1 cm orange-fennel salad. Lightly press down on the salad and then carefully remove the ring mould. Repeat for the remaining

three plates. Drizzle each with any leftover dressing from the salad and garnish with a sprinkling of fleur de sel. Serve immediately.

NOTE: *Ring moulds can be found at most kitchen supply stores and are a great trick for easily creating restaurant-worthy presentations. You may improvise with a clean tuna fish can by removing the top and bottom and using it as a ring mould.*

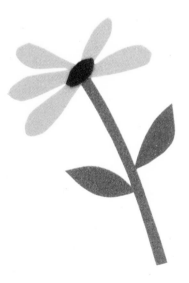

CHEESE-APPLE MILLE-FEUILLE

• SERVES 4 •

75g each of Jarlsberg, Parmesan, and cheddar

2 teaspoons sherry vinegar

2 tablespoons olive oil

Salt and freshly ground pepper

2 apples (any fruity red variety)

1 tablespoon finely chopped fresh parsley

1. Cut each piece of cheese into 5mm-thick slices and each slice into matchsticks. Reserve.

2. Place the sherry vinegar into a small bowl and slowly drizzle in the olive oil while whisking. Season to taste.

3. Rinse and core the apples and cut each horizontally into 6 slices (3 per plate).

4. To serve, place 1 apple slice on each dish and cover with the cheese matchsticks. Cover with another apple slice and continue for each plate. Drizzle the dressing on top of and around each mille-feuille, garnish with parsley, and serve.

FROMAGE BLANC WITH BLUE CHEESE AND CHIVES

• MAKES 600g •

175g blue cheese (Fourme d'Ambert or Roquefort), at room temperature

400g fromage blanc

4 tablespoons chopped fresh chives plus 2cm chive bâtons for garnish, if desired

16 to 20 slices cocktail rye bread, toasted

1. Place the softened blue cheese in a small bowl and mash with a fork.

2. Add the *fromage blanc* and stir until smooth. Add the chives and mix until blended.

3. To serve, spread on rye bread toasts and garnish with chive bâtons, if desired.

LEMON TOASTS

• SERVES 4 •

1 egg white

6 tablespoons sugar

90 g plus 2 tablespoons
ground almonds

Juice and zest of 1 lemon

½ teaspoon orange zest

4 slices brioche

1. Preheat the oven to 190°C/gas mark 5.

2. In a bowl or stand mixer, whisk together the egg white and sugar until creamy. Add the ground almonds, lemon juice and zest, orange zest, and mix until smooth.

3. Place the brioche slices on a greaseproof-lined baking sheet and cover the top of each with an even layer of the lemon-almond mixture. Place in the oven and bake until lightly golden, 8 to 10 minutes. Serve warm.

SAVOURY *FLAMMEKUECHE*

• SERVES 6 TO 8 •

It's said that pizza is the most popular food in the world. Every culture has its variation of flat bread with a local topping. In Alsace, flammekueche *is a famous speciality and pizza variation, a thin dough crust most commonly topped with bacon, onions, and crème fraîche.*

1 egg

1 tablespoon flour

450g fromage blanc (use cottage cheese as a substitute)

Salt and freshly ground pepper

Pinch of freshly grated nutmeg

1 pound puff pastry or pizza dough (store-bought), defrosted if frozen

4 large shallots, peeled and thinly sliced

225g bacon, cut into 1cm pieces

1. Preheat the oven to 200°C/gas mark 6.

2. In a medium bowl, combine the egg, flour, and *fromage blanc*. Stir until smooth and season with salt, pepper, and nutmeg. Set aside.

3. On a floured surface, roll the dough out to fit a 30 × 45 cm baking sheet. Carefully transfer the dough to the baking sheet by rolling the dough around a rolling pin and unrolling it directly onto the pan.

4. Spread an even layer of the *fromage blanc* mixture over the surface of the dough and cover with the shallots and bacon. Fold the edges over, creating a 1 cm border around the tart, and seal by pressing lightly with the tines of a fork. Bake for 30 to 35 minutes or until golden brown. Remove from the oven, let stand for 2 to 3 minutes, cut into squares, and serve.

SWEET *FLAMMEKUECHE*

1 egg

225 g fromage blanc

150 g crème fraîche

1 teaspoon pure vanilla extract

450 g store-bought puff pastry, defrosted according to package directions

4 apples, peeled, cored, quartered, and thinly sliced

4 tablespoons sugar

1 tablespoon Calvados or eau de vie (optional)

1. Preheat the oven to 200°C/gas mark 6.

2. In a medium bowl, combine the egg, *fromage blanc*, crème fraîche, and vanilla. Stir until smooth and set aside.

3. On a floured surface, roll the dough out to fit a 30 × 45 cm baking sheet. Carefully transfer the dough to the baking sheet by rolling the dough around a rolling pin and unrolling it directly onto the pan.

4. Spread an even layer of the *fromage blanc*–crème fraîche mixture over the surface of the dough. Top with overlapping apple slices, arranging them in columns and leaving a 1 cm border all around. Fold the edges over, creating a border around the tart, and seal by pressing lightly with the tines of a fork. Sprinkle 2 tablespoons sugar over the apples and bake in the oven until golden brown, about 30 minutes.

5. While the tart is baking, make a simple syrup, if desired: in a small saucepan, combine the remaining 2 tablespoons sugar with 2 tablespoons water and place over medium heat. Bring to a boil and simmer until the sugar is dissolved, 2 to 3 minutes.

Remove from the heat and carefully pour the Calvados, if using, down the side of the saucepan into the syrup; be careful, as the syrup will start to bubble. Stir and allow to cool. After removing the *flammekueche* from the oven, delicately brush the apples with the syrup using a pastry brush. Cut into large squares and serve warm or at room temperature.

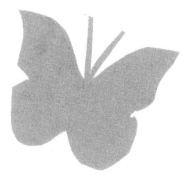

CROQUE MONSIEUR
ERIC RIPERT STYLE

4 slices brioche, crusts
  removed

50g Jarlsberg, cut into 6
  slices

25g domestic caviar

2 slices smoked salmon

2 tablespoons unsalted
  butter

1. Place 2 brioche slices on a work surface and top each with 3 slices of cheese in a single layer. Spread 10g caviar on top of the cheese and cover with a slice of salmon, trimmed to fit the size of the brioche. Top each with a second slice of brioche.

2. Melt 1 tablespoon butter in a nonstick frying pan over medium heat and place the sandwiches in the pan. Cook, pressing down lightly with a spatula, until golden brown, about 3 minutes. Add the remaining tablespoon of butter to the pan and flip the sandwiches, cooking until golden and the cheese has melted, about 2 minutes.

3. Transfer the sandwiches to a cutting board, slice diagonally, and serve immediately.

FRENCH TOAST EDWARD STYLE

4 slices brioche or challah
  (preferably day-old), cut
  2 cm thick

4 teaspoons plus 2
  tablespoons 2% milk

3 eggs

1 egg white

¼ teaspoon cinnamon

Pinch of freshly grated
  nutmeg

1 teaspoon pure vanilla
  extract

4 tablespoons (½ stick)
  unsalted butter

Maple syrup for serving

1. Place the brioche slices in a large, deep, rectangular pan and pour 1 teaspoon of milk on each slice. (This provides moisture at the bread's centre.)

2. In a bowl, whisk together the eggs, egg white, 2 tablespoons milk, cinnamon, nutmeg, and vanilla. Pour over the brioche, turning to coat thoroughly (this step is important so that you end up with a custardy version and not dry French toast), and let stand for about 5 minutes.

3. Heat the butter over medium heat in a large nonstick frying pan and cook the brioche for 2 to 3 minutes per side, first on medium high and then on medium-low until golden brown. Cut each slice diagonally (a trick for giving the illusion of a larger portion) and place on a plate slightly superimposing one on top of the other. Serve with pure maple syrup.

NOTE: *You may also serve French toast garnished with a few grains of fleur de sel and a teaspoon of mascarpone on the side accompanied by fresh berries.*

Chapter Two

SOMETIMES IT IS
CALLED LUNCH

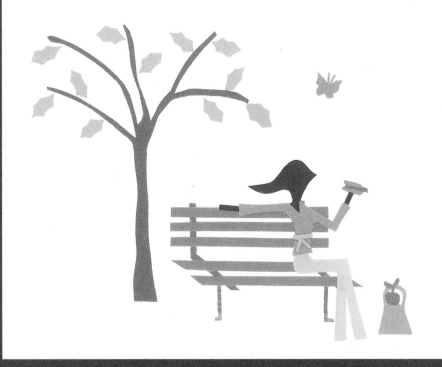

*H*ow are you dealing with ambiguity? Do you ever have cereal for dinner? A snack? Do you ever use recipes for lunch? Cook for lunch? What's a main course versus a side dish? Can sides be lunch or a side dish a main course? In America, many workers buy lunch near their offices or bring a prepared meal to work. Or they eat a somewhat more diversified and usually hot meal at a company or school cafeteria, or a fuller meal when entertaining or being entertained for lunch at a restaurant. For me, the best way to appreciate what we have agreed to call lunch—though that might no longer be the best term—is to consider it the third meal of the day, the meal that supplements and balances breakfast and the larger main meal of the day. So, lunch is really a question of volume and in most cases timing, as it is eaten at midday.

And while there are some classic lunch foods—take sandwiches for an example—almost any dish taken in moderation can be eaten at lunch. Jack up the portion size and suddenly lunch becomes a form of dinner, and the evening meal the smaller meal that balances out the day.

Cereal for dinner? I have a friend in New York who indeed often eats cereal for "dinner," but that's because she eats a big lunch. Healthy and *bien dans sa peau,* Linda is an executive who lives alone, works hard and often late. Every day she has a good, balanced breakfast with protein, fat, and carbohydrates (such as an egg with a piece of buttered toast or yogurt and a slice of toast and always some fresh fruit and coffee) and then regularly has a late business lunch, which she treats as her main meal, including a glass of wine, a few bites of dessert, and no rushing. She works at a large corporation with a staff cafeteria, so when she doesn't go out to lunch, she eats a full, varied meal there. She simply chooses to have her main meal in the early afternoon. After she gets home, at around eight, she is apt to opt for a choice of cereal with perhaps half of a banana or a few blueberries, or sometimes yogurt with a piece of fruit. And she's been known to treat herself to a small piece of dark chocolate (notice the balance in each meal). She enjoys cooking, and it is one of her preferred weekend pastimes. Then she has her main meal in the evening and entertains with passion. Her nutritional and calorific intake per day is balanced. Her two-to-three-day nutritional and calorific intake is regular and healthy. She doesn't worry if she is eating breakfast for dinner or dinner for lunch.

We live in a world that often seems fixated on reducing elements of our lives, singularly and collectively, to ten-second sound bites, to single-word or single-phrase definitions and explanations. It is an ugly sign of superficial times, I fear. What is the reason most French women don't get fat? Easy, I have been told again and again in two words: portion control. (I have also been told many times it is because they smoke so much, but that is nonsense and not supported by any facts.) There is some sound truth, of course, in portion control, but hardly the entire answer.

If you cut your calorific intake in half for each meal, each day for the next three months, you will lose weight regardless of your starting point. You might not enjoy eating as much; you might even develop some health and nutritional deficiencies, and you probably won't find it a sustainable lifestyle, so before year-end you will gain back the weight in yo-yo fashion like so many people who diet instead of adopting a new and informed healthy lifestyle. For me, eating for pleasure is a sustainable approach to learning and maintaining balance (*équilibre*) when it comes to food, and physical routine is another all-important component, at least the equal of portion size.

French women (and men) do eat smaller portions than Americans and many others. A portion of steak might be 4 or 6 ounces, not 8, 10, 12, or more that is common in America. A dish of pasta, as in Italy, is more likely to be a first course than a main course of a meal and to be the portion size of a fist instead of two hands full. And portions especially extend to sugar intake. Dessert portions are not only smaller and more likely to be simply fruit than in America, but the amount of sugar in the recipes for the same type of pies or cakes is significantly less. My recipes reflect a French woman's attitude toward portion proportions.

I want to reemphasize that it is okay to eat more than your body needs as fuel if there is pleasure involved or if a social occasion such as a family holiday or business meal leads to eating a large meal. Balance, however, is what must be remembered and followed. Square your intake over a day or two and be sure to balance your books by the end of the week. Big lunch, then small dinner, and vice versa. Sweet dessert on Monday, perhaps none on Tuesday.

I begin this section on recipes for lunch with soup, the perfect meal by itself: it hydrates well, is more filling than many salads, and is infused with good vitamins, minerals, and other nutrients without piling on the calories. When I know I have a lavish dinner planned, I'll eat a bowl of soup alone for lunch, and feel perfectly satisfied up until dinnertime. However, for a more substantive midday meal, I'll have a cup of soup as an appetizer, and then a main course of fish, chicken, or pasta afterward. Then, of course, I'll strike a balance that evening, enjoying smaller portions or fewer courses for my evening meal. One more observation on soups. When you make them from scratch, you know what's in them, and since they can also be reheated, one preparation can feature more than one appearance in your eating plan over a few days. Beware of the canned or packaged kinds of soups that are often laced with very high doses of sodium, which tend to boost your blood pressure in the afternoon and make you very thirsty—and hungry, just what you don't want at work or play.

A lot of the dishes and recipes that follow can be taken to work the next day or days and reheated or "accessorized" into a different food experience. We live in a world of ubiquitous microwave ovens. One of their advantages is that you can bring vegetables to work uncooked and zap them for a short while and you have a simply cooked vegetable with a very high percentage of its nutrients locked in. Why not a plate of vegetables, typically a side dish, as a meal? As I age, I increasingly order two appetizers instead of an appetizer and a main course. I need less food than some restaurants proffer with their main courses. And why can't a portion of any side dish be the big plate of the day?

And a reminder about portions. The greatest and deepest pleasure in food exists in the first three bites. So, eat with all your senses and then let your brain kick in after three bites. Remember it is your brain not your stomach that controls your hunger once you've sat down for a meal. Do you want or need the next bite? And the next bite?

Soups

ENDIVE AND
AVOCADO GAZPACHO

• SERVES 4 •

. . . .

3 endives, rinsed and sliced

*2 avocados, peeled and
   chopped*

*50g capers, rinsed and
   drained*

6 tablespoons olive oil

Juice of 2 limes

50–100 ml chicken stock

½ teaspoon curry powder

*Salt and freshly ground
   pepper*

Croûtons (optional)

Fresh mint (optional)

1. Place the endives, avocados, capers, olive oil, and lime juice in a food processer and blend until smooth, adding enough chicken stock to obtain the desired consistency. Stir in the curry powder and season to taste.

2. Transfer the mixture to a bowl, cover tightly, and refrigerate for at least 2 hours. Serve chilled, garnished with a few croûtons rubbed with fresh mint, if desired.

BEET AND GINGER GAZPACHO

• SERVES 4 TO 6 •

275 g cooked beets, peeled
and diced

1 tomato, peeled and
chopped

1 garlic clove, peeled and
chopped

1 large onion, peeled and
chopped

1 tablespoon peeled and
grated fresh ginger

1 teaspoon wasabi (or 2
teaspoons horseradish)

1 tablespoon red wine
vinegar

2 tablespoons olive oil

450 ml chicken broth

1 tablespoon crème fraîche

Salt and freshly ground
pepper

1. Place the beets, tomato, garlic, onion, ginger, wasabi, vinegar, olive oil, chicken broth, and crème fraîche in a food processor and purée until smooth.

2. Pass half of the puréed soup through a sieve and combine with the remainder of the soup, season to taste, and chill. Serve cold, garnished with a dollop of crème fraîche, if desired.

BEET AND COURGETTE GAZPACHO

1 tablespoon olive oil

2 onions, peeled and finely chopped

2 medium courgettes, rinsed and sliced

1 celery stalk, rinsed and sliced

4 tablespoons peeled and chopped shallots

1 teaspoon ground cardamom

1 medium beet, cooked, peeled, and sliced

Juice of 1 lemon

Salt and freshly ground pepper

2 hard-boiled eggs, peeled, whites and yolks separated, and finely chopped

4 tablespoons chopped fresh parsley

1. Heat the olive oil in a large pot over medium heat. Add 1 chopped onion, the courgette, celery, and shallots and sauté for 5 minutes.

2. Add the cardamom and 900 ml water and bring to a boil. Simmer for 20 minutes. Remove from the heat and refrigerate until chilled.

3. To serve, add the beet and lemon juice to the chilled soup and season to taste. Pour the soup into individual bowls and garnish with the chopped eggs, the remaining onion, and the parsley.

MAGICAL LEEK BROTH

· SERVES 1 FOR THE WEEKEND ·

This is one of the best-known recipes from my French Women Don't Get Fat, *so I am reprinting it. When that book came out it got lots of press about leeks and I got a lot of emails from readers. I was even cited as the cause of a leek shortage in America. (I am not making this up.) It seems I helped many to discover or rediscover leeks and many professed to love them, while some found leeks dreadful. I admit you have to get used to their odor when they are being cooked, but it is such a sweet vegetable, enjoyed hot or cold, I am surprised when people don't like it. It certainly is good for you and remains one of my favourites. The magical leek broth was/is often misunderstood. It is a fine and light soup for lunch for sure, especially with some of the leek stalk as a side salad with just a drizzle of olive oil.*

I included the broth in that book, however, to kick off a resetting of one's weight and equilibrium, and as a trick French women have traditionally employed, at least in my world. I recommended it for a weekend. First, since it is a mild diuretic, the leek broth helps to flush the blood and kidneys, thus purging the body of various toxins, a so-called mild detox—something I believe in doing every now and again. And since drinking only broth for 48 hours means a sharp decrease in food intake, people tend to lose a pound or two from that exercise and perhaps another pound from water loss. So, voilà, *Monday morning you are two or three pounds lighter. That's a great psychological booster shot toward losing some weight and resetting a desirable body balance. But that was it. It wasn't something designed for a week at a time or every month. (If one vitamin pill is good for you, imagine how good taking ten of them must be!) Just once in a while enjoy a leek broth weekend (or even just for 24 hours) when you feel you need to detox and lose a few pounds quickly toward finding your equilibrium. I am happy that leeks (and not just Magical Leek Broth) have become some people's "new best friend," and it is a pleasure to fill requests for more leek recipes in this book, whether as a salad or with fish, pasta, or simply as a veggie.*

900g leeks

Water to cover in a large pot

1. Clean the leeks and rinse well to get rid of any sand and soil. Cut the ends of the green parts, leaving all the white parts plus a suggestion of green. (Reserve the extra greens for soup stock.)

2. Put the leeks in a large pot and cover with water. Bring to a boil and simmer without a lid for 20 to 30 minutes. Pour off the liquid and reserve. Place the leeks in a bowl.

NOTE: *The juice is to be drunk (reheated or at room temperature to taste) every 2 to 3 hours, a cup at a time. For meals or whenever hungry, have some of the leeks themselves, a few tablespoons at a time. Drizzle with a few drops of extra virgin olive oil and lemon juice. Season sparingly with salt and pepper. Add chopped parsley if you wish. This will be your nourishment for both days, until Sunday dinner, when you can have a small piece of meat or fish (100– 175g; don't lose that scale yet!), with two vegetables steamed with a drizzle of oil and some herbs, and a piece of fruit.*

CARROT SOUP
WITH YOGURT AND KIWI

• SERVES 4 TO 6 •

2 tablespoons olive oil

1 onion, peeled and chopped

900g carrots, peeled and
    chopped, plus 1 carrot,
    peeled and cut into small
    dice, for garnish

2 celery stalks, rinsed and
    chopped

2 tablespoons chopped fresh
    coriander

170g nonfat plain Greek-
    style yogurt

Salt and freshly ground
    pepper

110g boiled ham, cut into
    matchsticks

2 kiwi, peeled and diced

1. Heat the olive oil in a large pot over medium heat and add the onion, carrots, and celery. Sauté the vegetables for 5 minutes; add the fresh coriander and 900 ml of water and bring to a boil. Cover and simmer until the vegetables are tender, about 20 minutes.

2. Carefully transfer the vegetables to a blender or food processer. Purée, adding some of the cooking liquid until the desired consistency is reached. Transfer to a bowl and allow to cool. When cool, stir in the yogurt and season to taste. Cover and place in the refrigerator to chill.

3. Just before serving, cook the ham in a nonstick sauté pan over medium-high heat until hot, 1 to 2 minutes. Place the chilled soup in individual bowls and add the ham and kiwi, garnish with the diced carrot, and serve.

Salads and Vegetables

ENDIVE WITH GREEN TOMATO JAM

• SERVES 4 •

2 tablespoons green tomato jam

2 tablespoons lemon juice

2 tablespoons olive oil

Fleur de sel and freshly ground pepper

4 medium endives, rinsed, trimmed, and cut lengthwise into strips

16 black olives, pitted

10g fresh basil leaves cut into chiffonade (thin strips)

4 baguette slices, toasted and rubbed with mustard

1. In a small bowl, combine the green tomato jam and lemon juice. Whisk in the olive oil and season to taste.

2. Place the endives in a salad bowl and add the dressing, tossing well to combine. Garnish with the olives and basil and serve with toasted baguette slices.

NOTE: *Green tomato jam can be difficult to find. Red pepper jelly is a delicious sweet-tart alternative that goes nicely with the pleasantly bitter flavour of endive.*

MÂCHE, CELERIAC,
AND BEET SALAD

• SERVES 4 •

. . . .

*1 teaspoon mustard
(preferably Dijon)*

2 tablespoons sherry vinegar

5 tablespoons olive oil

*Salt and freshly ground
pepper*

300g mâche

*1 medium (about 450g)
celeriac, peeled and
grated*

*450g red and yellow beets,
cooked, peeled, and
quartered*

1. Combine the mustard and vinegar in a small bowl. Whisk in the olive oil and season to taste.

2. In a large bowl, combine the mâche and celeriac, toss with the dressing, and divide the mixture equally among four plates. Place 3 to 4 beet wedges on each plate and serve.

CARROT AND CELERIAC SALAD

• SERVES 4 •

4 medium carrots, peeled and cut into matchsticks

1 medium celeriac (about 450g), peeled and cut into matchsticks

1 tablespoon whole grain mustard

2 tablespoons red wine vinegar

6 tablespoons olive oil

Salt and freshly ground pepper

35g walnuts, chopped

2 tablespoons chopped fresh parsley

1. Bring a pot of salted water to a boil. Add the carrots and celeriac and blanch for 3 to 4 minutes until crisp-tender. Drain and place the vegetables in a salad bowl.

2. Meanwhile, in a small bowl, whisk together the mustard, vinegar, and olive oil until smooth. Season to taste. Pour the vinaigrette over the warm carrots and celeriac and toss gently to combine. Garnish with the chopped walnuts and parsley and serve.

SHAVED FENNEL
AND CITRUS SALAD

• SERVES 4 •

2 grapefruits

2 oranges

2 fennel bulbs, trimmed and
rinsed

2 tablespoons sherry vinegar

6 tablespoons olive oil

1 tablespoon finely chopped
shallot

½ teaspoon honey

Salt and freshly ground
pepper

225 g frisée, torn into bite-
size pieces

2 tablespoons finely chopped
fresh parsley

1 teaspoon finely chopped
fresh mint

1. Prepare the citrus segments by cutting off the tops and bottoms of the grapefruits and oranges. Cut the peel and white pith from the oranges and grapefruits and, working over a bowl and using a small sharp knife, cut between the membranes to release the segments. Place the citrus segments in a large bowl.

2. Quarter the fennel bulbs lengthwise, then cut crosswise into paper-thin slices using a mandoline.* Add the shaved fennel to the citrus.

3. In a small bowl, whisk together the vinegar, olive oil, shallots, and honey and season to taste. Pour the dressing over the citrus-fennel mixture and gently toss to mix. Arrange the frisée on a serving platter and top with the citrus-fennel salad. Sprinkle with parsley and mint and serve.

*A mandoline is a great addition to your *batterie de cuisine*. The plastic Japanese version is widely available, relatively inexpensive, and makes it incredibly easy to uniformly slice veggies for salads and gratins.

ITALIAN-STYLE FENNEL
AND APPLE SALAD

• SERVES 4 •

. . . .

*2 fennel bulbs, washed,
    trimmed, quartered
    lengthwise, and thinly
    sliced crosswise*

*2 red apples, washed, cored,
    and sliced*

*2 tablespoons lemon juice
    (½ lemon)*

*175 g pecorino, cut into
    matchsticks*

3 tablespoons olive oil

*Salt and freshly ground
    pepper*

35 g pine nuts, toasted

1. Place the fennel, apples, lemon juice, and pecorino in a serving bowl.

2. Add the olive oil and gently toss. Season to taste, garnish with pine nuts, and serve.

NOTE: *Don't peel the apples; the red skin provides a beautiful and colourful contrast in the salad. If you prefer a more acidic flavour, use Granny Smith apples.*

GRATED FRUIT
AND VEGGIE "SLAW"

• SERVES 4 •

· ·

1 lemon

2 tablespoons almond paste
  (not marzipan)

225 g plain yogurt

Salt and freshly ground
  pepper

2 carrots, peeled and grated

2 Granny Smith apples,
  peeled and grated

225 g celeriac, peeled and
  grated

75 g golden raisins

55 g toasted almonds,
  chopped

1. Rinse the lemon, finely grate the zest, and reserve. Press the juice from the lemon into a small bowl and add the almond paste, whisking until smooth. Add the yogurt, season to taste, and reserve.

2. In a large bowl, combine the grated carrots, apples, and celeriac. Add the yogurt dressing and toss. Sprinkle the salad with raisins, almonds, and lemon zest and serve.

SAUTÉ OF PEAS AND PROSCIUTTO WITH FRESH MINT

• SERVES 8 •

1 tablespoon olive oil

55g peeled and thinly sliced
shallots

450g fresh shelled peas or
frozen peas, thawed

450g snow peas, rinsed and
drained

2 tablespoons unsalted
butter

50g prosciutto, chopped

Salt and freshly ground
pepper

1 tablespoon finely chopped
fresh mint

1. Heat the olive oil in a nonstick frying pan over medium heat and add the shallots. Sauté until softened, about 3 minutes. Add the peas and snow peas and cook for about 5 minutes, stirring occasionally, until just tender, being careful not to overcook.

2. Add the butter and prosciutto, mixing delicately, and cover and cook for 1 minute. Season to taste, sprinkle with mint, and serve.

HARICOTS VERTS SALAD WITH PEACHES AND ALMONDS

• SERVES 4 •

450 g haricots verts,
   trimmed

2 peaches (white preferred),
   rinsed, pitted, and thinly
   sliced

25 g almonds, coarsely
   chopped

A few fresh mint leaves,
   finely chopped

Fleur de sel

Freshly ground pepper

Juice of 1 lemon

1 tablespoon olive oil

1. Bring a large pot of salted water to a boil. Add the haricots verts and cook until crisp-tender. Drain and allow to cool.

2. In a medium serving bowl, combine the haricots verts, peaches, almonds, mint, fleur de sel, pepper, lemon juice, and olive oil, tossing gently. Refrigerate for 15 minutes and serve.

ASPARAGUS
WITH YOGURT DRESSING

• SERVES 4 •

450g asparagus, trimmed

10g coarsely chopped fresh
basil

170g 2% Greek-style yogurt

Salt and freshly ground
pepper

2 tablespoons unsalted
butter

1 tablespoon hazelnut oil

1. Bring a large pot of salted water to a boil and blanch the asparagus for 1 minute. Drain and reserve 4 spears. Place the remaining asparagus in a bowl of ice water to stop the cooking process. When chilled, drain and pat dry.

2. Finely chop the reserved 4 asparagus spears and place in a medium bowl. Add the basil and yogurt and stir to combine. Season to taste and reserve.

3. Melt the butter in a large frying pan over medium heat. Add the blanched asparagus and sauté until lightly browned, about 3 minutes. Season to taste, drizzle with hazelnut oil, and place in a serving dish.

4. Spoon the yogurt dressing over the asparagus and serve immediately.

RATATOUILLE

• SERVES 6 •

. . . .

Although there are variations on the number of ingredients in a ratatouille, I keep mine simple and find the flavour of each vegetable more intense as a result. This classic dish from the South of France gained popularity worldwide after the film Ratatouille was released, and many people discovered the word and how to pronounce it. It certainly was not a staple or common recipe in most of the world, after all, but the film as well as interest in a healthy Mediterranean diet spiked curiosity. I was asked to do a demo at many cooking schools and on TV programmes, and people were stunned how easy it is to make and how versatile it is (and add inexpensive considering how you can "stretch" it). A Brazilian TV crew came to my home to tape me making it to share with their weekly magazine's huge audience. What a world! Here's to the frugality of French women! Remember "the least effort for the most pleasure" is a principle to live by—as long as it is healthy.

450 g tomatoes

450 g courgettes

450 g aubergines

4 garlic cloves

2 tablespoons chopped fresh parsley

Salt and freshly ground pepper

Olive oil (optional)

1. Use an equal amount of tomatoes, courgette, and aubergines. Wash and cut into thick slices.

2. Using a large heavy metal enameled pot (such as a Le Creuset cast-iron pot), make layers starting with the aubergines, then the tomatoes, and finally the courgettes and repeat until the pot is almost filled to the edge, adding some garlic cloves and parsley between the layers. Season with salt and pepper. (If you only have a light stainless-steel pot that is not nonstick, brush a drizzle of olive oil at the bottom of the pot so that the first layer of aubergines will not stick.)

3. Cover and cook over very low heat until the vegetables are tender, 1 to 2½ hours.

4. Let it sit for 20 minutes, then serve. Use soup bowls, since at that stage it is more of a soup; the liquid is mostly water from the veggies.

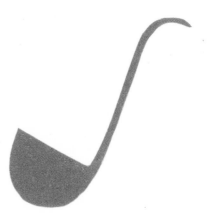

CRIMINI SALAD

• SERVES 4 •

450g crimini mushrooms,
  wiped clean with a damp
  paper towel and sliced

2 tablespoons sherry vinegar

1 tablespoon lemon juice

4 tablespoons walnut oil

Salt and freshly ground
  pepper

2 tablespoons chopped
  walnuts

2 tablespoons chopped fresh
  parsley

2 tablespoons finely chopped
  fresh chives

35g Parmesan shavings

1. Place the mushrooms in a large salad bowl and set aside.

2. In a small bowl, whisk together the sherry vinegar, lemon juice, and walnut oil. Season to taste and add to the mushrooms, tossing to combine.

3. Garnish the salad with the walnuts, parsley, chives, and Parmesan and serve.

Pasta

People don't normally think of pasta as French cuisine, but it is increasingly being served in France: globalization, the economy, and the high cost of food, especially meat, has something to do with that. When I grew up, most families in my town would stick to spaghetti and tomato sauce, and it was usually a dish served at month's end when the food budget was getting short. Occasionally, pasta was used in soups, mostly bouillon or consommé types, and was angel hair, vermicelli, or the fun "alphabet" pastina we used to play with, making those soup dinners endless to our *nounou*'s displeasure. The French also like pasta in gratin dishes, and for that one needs hollow types such as penne or macaroni, which are able to absorb the heavy sauces. In my mother's native Alsace, tagliatelle (also called fettuccine) is often served with fish and cream sauces. Of course, ravioli and lasagna have always been favourites especially when eating out in restaurants. The newest trend in France is for room temperature salads with light noodles such as farfalle or fusilli, something that has been around for a while in America at ubiquitous salad bars.

Because pasta dishes can be eaten at room temperature, added to a salad, or reheated in our take-out, microwave world, they have become a good and nutritious lunchtime meal at work or at home. Some of the "lunch" pastas that follow can certainly figure as "dinner" pasta—again it is a question of portion size and balance. If they are made for dinner, the leftover in some variation (say, add some tuna or vegetables) can become another lunch the next day or so.

PENNE WITH AUBERGINE AND TUNA

• SERVES 4 •

1 medium aubergine, rinsed
   and cut into 1 cm dice

Salt

150g fresh tuna, cut into
   2 cm dice

Freshly ground pepper

1½ tablespoons olive oil plus
   additional for serving

350g penne

75 ml tomato sauce

2 tablespoons capers, rinsed
   in water and drained

10g fresh basil leaves cut
   into chiffonade (thin
   strips)

1. Place the aubergine in a colander and toss with 1 teaspoon salt. Place the colander over a bowl and allow to drain for 30 minutes. Pat the aubergine dry.

2. Season the tuna with salt and pepper. In a large nonstick frying pan, warm up ½ tablespoon olive oil over medium-high heat and quickly sear the tuna, about 10 seconds per side. Remove from the pan and set aside.

3. In a large pot of boiling salted water, cook the penne until al dente, 10 to 12 minutes. Drain.

4. While the pasta is cooking, heat the remaining 1 tablespoon olive oil in the pan over medium-high heat and add the aubergine, sautéing until golden, about 8 minutes. Stir in the tomato sauce, capers, and pasta, tossing to combine. Add the tuna and season to taste. Serve immediately garnished with basil and a drizzle of olive oil.

TAGLIATELLE WITH LEEKS
AND PROSCIUTTO

• SERVES 4 •

700g leeks, white parts only

275g tagliatelle

8 slices prosciutto, cut into
1 cm-wide strips

4 to 6 tablespoons olive oil

55g freshly grated pecorino

115g freshly grated
Parmesan

10g fresh basil leaves cut
into chiffonade (thin
strips)

Salt and freshly ground
pepper

1. Cut the leeks into 1 cm-wide strips, rinse to remove any grit, and steam until softened, about 8 to 10 minutes.

2. Meanwhile, cook the tagliatelle in a large pot of salted boiling water until al dente, 8 to 10 minutes.

3. Drain the pasta and place in a serving bowl. Add the leeks, prosciutto, and olive oil and mix well. Sprinkle with the cheeses and basil, season to taste, and serve immediately.

LINGUINE WITH PRAWNS, TOMATOES, AND BASIL

• SERVES 4 •

350 g linguine

2 tablespoons butter

2 tablespoons olive oil

3 garlic cloves, peeled and chopped

Pinch of red pepper flakes

450 g large raw prawns, peeled and de-veined with tails intact

110 ml dry white wine

400 g tin chopped tomatoes

20 g fresh basil leaves cut into chiffonade (thin strips)

Salt and freshly ground pepper

1. Bring a large pot of salted water to a boil over high heat. Add the linguine and cook until al dente, 10 to 12 minutes.

2. Meanwhile, melt the butter and olive oil in a large sauté pan over medium-high heat. Add the garlic and red pepper flakes and sauté until fragrant, about 1 minute.

3. Add the prawns to the pan and sauté until they start to turn pink and are almost cooked, 2 to 3 minutes. Deglaze the pan with white wine and simmer for 1 minute. Add the tomatoes and juice and simmer for 4 to 6 minutes until slightly thickened.

4. Drain the pasta and add to the pan with the basil. Toss to combine and season to taste. Serve immediately.

FUSILLI WITH SPINACH AND ANCHOVIES

• SERVES 4 •

350 g fusilli

55 ml olive oil

2 tablespoons pine nuts

2 garlic cloves, peeled and chopped

350 g spinach, rinsed and drained

6 anchovies, rinsed and finely chopped

2 teaspoons lemon juice

Salt and freshly ground pepper

1 tablespoon butter

50 g freshly grated Parmesan

1. Bring a large pot of slightly salted water to a boil. Add the fusilli and cook for 8 to 10 minutes.

2. Meanwhile, heat the olive oil in a large frying pan over medium-high heat. Add the pine nuts and cook until golden, about 2 minutes. Remove from the pan and reserve.

3. Reduce the heat to medium-low and add the garlic to the pan. Sauté until fragrant, about 1 minute, add the spinach and anchovies, cover, and cook over medium heat until the spinach is just cooked and slightly wilted. Add the lemon juice and season to taste.

4. When the pasta is cooked, drain and place in a large serving dish. Add the butter and the spinach-anchovy mixture and toss to combine. Sprinkle with the pine nuts and Parmesan and serve immediately.

SPAGHETTI *AL LIMONE*

• SERVES 4 •

350g spaghetti

3 tablespoons olive oil

2 medium onions, peeled
and chopped

110ml dry white wine

Zest and juice of 1 lemon

Salt and freshly ground
pepper

75g watercress, chopped

75g freshly grated
Parmesan

1. Bring a large pot of salted water to a boil over high heat. Add the spaghetti and cook until al dente, about 8 minutes.

2. Meanwhile, heat 1 tablespoon olive oil in a frying pan over medium heat and add the onions. Cook until softened, about 4 minutes. Add the wine, lemon zest, and lemon juice and season to taste. Increase the heat to medium-high and bring to a boil for 1 minute. Reduce the heat to medium and simmer for 5 minutes.

3. Drain the pasta and add to the pan along with the remaining 2 tablespoons olive oil and watercress, tossing to combine. Season to taste and divide among four plates. Serve immediately, garnished with the fresh Parmesan.

SPAGHETTI WITH LIME AND ROCKET

• SERVES 4 •

3 limes

350g spaghetti

2 tablespoons olive oil plus
    additional for pasta

1 garlic clove, peeled and
    chopped

¼ teaspoon red pepper flakes

45g sun-dried tomatoes,
    chopped

1 teaspoon capers, rinsed
    and drained

175g fresh rocket, rinsed,
    patted dry, and roughly
    chopped

Salt and freshly ground
    pepper

35g grated Parmesan

1. Grate the zest of 2 limes and press the juice of 1 of them. Cut the third lime into quarters. Reserve.

2. Bring a large pot of salted water to a boil. Add the spaghetti and cook until just al dente (you want it to be slightly undercooked). Drain, return to the pot, and toss with a drizzle of olive oil. Reserve.

3. In a large frying pan, heat 2 tablespoons olive oil over medium heat and sauté the lime zest for 30 seconds. Add the garlic, red pepper flakes, sun-dried tomatoes, and capers and sauté for 1 to 2 minutes. Add the pasta and cook for 2 to 3 minutes, stirring gently. Add the lime juice and rocket, season to taste, and serve immediately with quarters of lime, a drizzle of olive oil, and grated Parmesan.

FARFALLE WITH YOGURT-BASIL SAUCE

• SERVES 4 •

350g farfalle

1 tablespoon olive oil

55g pearl onions, peeled and thinly sliced

2 garlic cloves, peeled and chopped

Zest and juice of 1 lemon

225g plain Greek-style yogurt

10g fresh basil leaves cut into chiffonade (thin strips)

10g chopped fresh parsley

Salt and freshly ground pepper

1. Bring a pot of salted water to a boil over high heat. Add the farfalle and cook until al dente, about 10 minutes.

2. Meanwhile, heat the olive oil in a large frying pan over medium heat and sauté the onions and garlic until fragrant and soft, 3 to 4 minutes. Deglaze with the lemon juice and cook until the liquid has completely reduced, about 2 minutes. Remove the pan from the heat and stir in the yogurt, lemon zest, basil, and parsley. Season to taste, add the drained farfalle to the pan, and toss to combine. Serve immediately.

From the Sea

Question: If you were at a company cafeteria or if you were taken out to lunch at a restaurant and a fish dish that you like was available, would you order it? Award yourself a health star if you said yes. We all know fish is good for us, and now that we've established that you would eat fish for lunch, let's consider making some for yourself and perhaps anyone eating with you. Okay, granted, a hot fish dish is not the ideal meal to fix or eat at your desk, but plenty of people still order Chinese take-out fish dishes for lunch. I am including fish dishes in my lunch recommendations to encourage people to appreciate that they can be extremely easy to prepare. And a little cooking is enjoyable, even relaxing. Throwing a few sardines or a mackerel or two in a nonstick frying pan for three minutes isn't exactly hard work or haute cuisine, and the result is as healthy and tasty as can be (count squeezing a lemon over them as daily exercise). Why not include them as part of one's regular lunch mix? Hopefully, we all have some days off—holidays, personal days, even birthdays at some companies—and there are weekends, and some people work from home now and again or always. Cooking need not be thought of as a chore but a pleasure. So, ban the excuses and *mange ton poisson.*

On one day of the weekend especially, I like to have a little bit of fish for lunch. If you eat a sandwich for a midday meal on a Saturday, say, then a main meal for dinner, substituting a small portion of fish for the sandwich is a plus. And, again, mix and match. These fish recipes with modest proportions are ideal for lunch and in a bit larger portion work well as a main course at dinner. Because in formal French meals, there is traditionally both a fish and meat course, perhaps I am accustomed to small portions of fish at a meal; so for my purposes now, let's call them lunch-size portions. And try any leftovers cold the next day. Are there lunch fish and dinner fish? There are no rules, perhaps just portion sizes and what appeals to you, but generally I think of larger fish served in steaklike cuts, such as swordfish or tuna, as dinner fish and "softer" and more delicate fish as appropriate for midday. And that is represented a bit in where I chose to place the fish recipes in this book. I also tend to think of fish dishes that take relatively modest preparation or cooking time as lunch friendly. However, how do you know a poem is good or great? You can analyze it again and again in greater depth to support your conclusion, but pretty much you just know a good poem when you read one. I can look at a fish and fish dish and know whether I personally would like it for lunch or dinner. Try it. *De gustibus non est disputandum.*

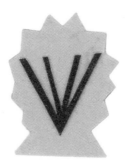

STEAMED MONKFISH
WITH VEGETABLES

• SERVES 4 •

. . . .

40g fresh coriander, washed

50g blanched almonds

*Salt and freshly ground
pepper*

Pinch of cayenne pepper

*4 (150–175g) monkfish
fillets, each about 2cm
thick*

*1 cucumber, washed and
sliced into "ribbons"
using a vegetable peeler
or mandoline*

*2 carrots, peeled and cut
into matchsticks*

*2 courgettes, washed and cut
into matchsticks*

Olive oil for serving

1. Place the coriander and almonds in a food processor and grind into powder. Season to taste, add the cayenne, and place on a large plate.

2. Lightly press the coriander-almond mixture on both sides of the monkfish. Wrap each piece with a single layer of cucumber slices and carefully place, seam side down, in a steamer insert over simmering water. Cover and steam for 7 minutes. Add the carrots and courgettes and continue steaming for 3 to 5 minutes.

3. Place 1 fillet on each plate, season to taste, and drizzle with olive oil. Divide the courgettes and carrots among the four plates and serve immediately.

TILAPIA WITH CUMIN
AND MUSHROOMS

• SERVES 4 •

1 teaspoon ground cumin

4 (75–110g) tilapia fillets

Salt and freshly ground
 pepper

1 tablespoon unsalted butter

2 tablespoons olive oil

150g button mushrooms,
 wiped cleaned and sliced

2 tablespoons chopped fresh
 parsley plus additional
 for garnish

4 lemon wedges (optional)

1. Sprinkle the cumin on both sides of the tilapia fillets and season with salt and pepper. Reserve.

2. Heat the butter and 1 tablespoon olive oil in a large nonstick frying pan over medium-high heat. Add the mushrooms and sauté until softened, about 2 minutes. Season to taste, stir in the parsley, and transfer to a plate and keep warm.

3. Increase the heat to high and add the remaining tablespoon of olive oil to the pan. When the pan is hot, add the fillets and cook for 2 to 3 minutes on each side.

4. To serve, place a portion of mushrooms on each plate and top with a fillet. Garnish with additional parsley and a lemon wedge, if desired.

SEA BASS WITH
CELERIAC-MINT SALSA

• SERVES 4 •

. . . .

4 (110–150g) sea bass fillets

Salt and freshly ground pepper

4 limes, thinly sliced

1 medium unpeeled courgette, sliced and steamed for 2 minutes

225g celeriac, peeled and grated

20g fresh mint leaves cut into chiffonade (thin strips)

2 tablespoons capers, rinsed and drained

Juice of 4 limes

1 tablespoon olive oil

2 leeks, white parts only, sliced into matchsticks, and steamed for 8 minutes

1. Preheat the oven to 180°C/gas mark 4.

2. Place the sea bass fillets on a baking sheet. Season the fillets and cover each with a single layer of lime slices. Top each with a single layer of courgette and season to taste. Bake for 12 to 15 minutes, depending upon the thickness of the fillets.

3. Meanwhile, prepare the celeriac-mint salsa: in a medium bowl, combine the grated celeriac, mint, and capers. Add the lime juice and olive oil, stirring until well mixed. Season to taste and set aside. (This may be made a few hours in advance, covered, and refrigerated.)

4. To serve, place the leeks in the centre of each plate. Top with 1 fillet and spoon the salsa over and around.

BOUILLABAISSE
TWENTY-FIRST CENTURY

• SERVES 4 •

Why twenty-first century? It has no potatoes and much less bread and olive oil than the legions of Marseilles women used in making their speciality for their families in the last century. And since we all don't live near the docks in Marseilles, the fish selection is modified as well.

450 g mixed fish fillets (whiting, cod, halibut, tilapia, or snapper), cut into 2 cm pieces

225 g shellfish (clams, mussels, or prawns in shells)

2 tablespoons Pernod

2 tablespoons olive oil

2 garlic cloves, peeled and chopped

2 small onions, peeled and chopped

1 fennel bulb, washed and sliced

Zest of 1 orange

400 g tinned tomatoes

1.3 litre fish stock

Salt and freshly ground pepper

20 g chopped fresh parsley

4 thick slices country bread, lightly toasted

1. Place the fish and prawns, if using, in a large bowl and add the Pernod and 1 tablespoon olive oil, mixing gently to combine. If using clams or mussels, scrub and remove the beards from the mussels.

2. Heat the remaining tablespoon olive oil in a large, deep saucepan over medium heat. Add the garlic, onions, and fennel and sauté until fragrant and softened, 5 to 6 minutes. Add the orange zest, tomatoes and any juice, and the fish stock. Bring to a boil and cook until the vegetables are soft and the liquid has reduced by half, 20 to 25 minutes.

3. Add the fish and cook for 2 to 3 minutes. Add the shellfish and cook until the shells open or the prawns just turn pink. Correct seasoning. Divide among four bowls, garnish each with parsley, and serve with toasted bread spread with the rouille.

ROUILLE

2 red peppers, roasted and
    peeled
2 garlic cloves, peeled
1 teaspoon lemon juice
Pinch of paprika
Salt and freshly ground
    pepper

ROUILLE

1. Place all the ingredients in a blender and purée until smooth.

2. Season to taste and serve on toast with the bouillabaisse.

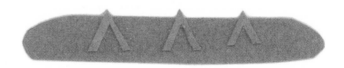

FLOUNDER FILLETS
WITH FENNEL

• SERVES 4 •

. . . .

1 large fennel bulb

1 onion, peeled and diced

2 tablespoons chopped shallots

Pinch of ground cardamom

4 (110–150g) flounder fillets

1 tablespoon tapenade

110ml dry vermouth (or white wine)

1 tablespoon olive oil

Salt and freshly ground pepper

1 tablespoon fresh thyme

4 slices whole wheat bread, toasted

1. Preheat the oven to 200°C/gas mark 6.

2. Remove the fennel stalks and reserve 2 tablespoons fennel fronds. Cut the fennel bulb in half, remove the core, and chop the remaining fennel.

3. In a small saucepan, bring 225ml water to a boil. Add the chopped fennel, onion, shallots, and cardamom. Cover and cook for 15 minutes or until the vegetables are tender.

4. Pat the flounder fillets dry and spread a small amount of tapenade on both sides.

5. Pour the vermouth into a large frying pan and add the fillets. Drizzle with the olive oil and bring to a boil over medium heat. Place the pan in the oven and cook for 10 to 15 minutes.

6. Meanwhile, transfer the fennel, onion, and shallot mixture to a blender and purée. Season to taste and stir in half of the thyme.

7. Remove the pan from the oven and transfer the fish to a plate and keep warm. Place the pan over medium heat and bring the cooking liquid to a boil for 1 to 2 minutes to thicken slightly.

8. To serve, place one slice of toasted bread, spread with the fennel purée, on the plate and top with 1 fillet. Spoon the pan sauce on top of the fish and around the plate, add the remaining thyme, and serve immediately.

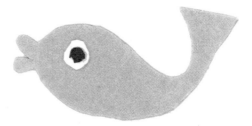

JOHN DORY WITH TOMATOES AND CAPERS

• SERVES 4 •

55 ml olive oil plus
additional for garnish

2 (400 g) tins chopped
tomatoes

2 tablespoons capers in
vinegar, drained

Salt and freshly ground
pepper

4 (175 g) John Dory fillets
(or use cod, monkfish, or
halibut)

4 tablespoons fresh basil
leaves cut into chiffonade
(thin strips)

1. Preheat the oven to 200°C/gas mark 6.

2. Heat 55 ml olive oil in a medium saucepan over medium heat and add the tomatoes and capers. Season to taste and simmer for 5 minutes.

3. Place half of the tomato-caper mixture in a baking dish, add the fillets, and cover with the remaining tomato-caper mixture. Bake until the fish is cooked through, 15 to 20 minutes.

4. To serve, place 1 fillet on each plate and spoon the sauce over. Garnish with basil and a drizzle of olive oil.

And a Little Meat

A little protein at lunch is essential (there's always a few nuts!), and instead of putting slabs of protein between two slices of bread, why not consume it hot or cold in a quick and easy preparation? The argument I made for fish at lunch mostly holds for the meat dishes that follow. Short of eating raw meat, I cannot think of any simpler meat preparation than sautéing thin veal cutlets—as in perhaps three minutes from refrigerator to plate. And cooked chicken, of course, can be refrigerated and enjoyed for a few days, including shredded in a salad. Eating something green along with your meat is always a good idea. And, oh, if you really miss your sandwich bread, have a slice of multigrain bread with your small portion of meat.

VEAL SCALOPPINE
À LA MOUTARDE

• SERVES 4 •

4 (75–110g) veal cutlets,
    pounded thin

2½ tablespoons whole grain
    mustard

1 tablespoon olive oil

1 tablespoon butter

1. Pat the veal cutlets dry with paper towels and spread both sides with mustard.

2. In a large frying pan, heat the olive oil and butter over medium heat. Add the veal and cook until golden, 3 to 5 minutes on each side. Serve immediately.

NOTE: *This works as well with chicken breast or turkey white meat, pounded thin.*

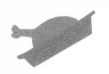

SAUTÉ OF TURKEY
WITH SPRING VEGETABLES

4 turkey cutlets, pounded
thin

2 tablespoons paprika

Salt and freshly ground
pepper

4 tablespoons olive oil

4 small onions, peeled and
thinly sliced

300g frozen peas

300g frozen snow peas

225ml double cream

2 tablespoons finely chopped
fresh coriander

1. Season both sides of the turkey cutlets with the paprika and salt and pepper.

2. Heat 2 tablespoons olive oil in a large frying pan over medium-high heat and add the turkey cutlets. Cook until lightly golden, 3 to 4 minutes per side. Transfer the cutlets to a plate and keep warm.

3. Heat the remaining 2 tablespoons olive oil in the frying pan and add the onions. Sauté until soft, about 4 minutes. Add the peas and snow peas and sauté until warm, about 1 minute. Add the cream and simmer until slightly thickened, about 4 minutes.

4. Add the turkey cutlets back to the pan, correct the seasoning, and add the coriander. Cook for another 2 minutes and serve immediately.

CHICKEN WITH SPINACH
EN PAPILLOTE

• SERVES 4 •

1 tablespoon olive oil

300 g fresh spinach, washed and dried

Salt and freshly ground pepper

2 tablespoons lemon juice

4 (175–225 g) skinless, boneless chicken breasts

4 bay leaves

450 g cherry tomatoes

175 g bulgur, cooked according to package instructions

1. Preheat the oven to 200°C/gas mark 6.

2. Cut four pieces of greaseproof paper into 30 cm × 40 cm rectangles. Place them, stacked on top of one another, horizontally on a clean work surface. Beginning with the top sheet, brush the centre with olive oil and top with 75 g of spinach. Season to taste and sprinkle with ½ tablespoon lemon juice. Place 1 chicken breast, seasoned with salt and pepper, on the bed of spinach and top with 1 bay leaf and 110 g cherry tomatoes. Seal the packet by bringing up the sides to the centre and folding down together tightly. Tuck the top and bottom ends underneath and repeat with the remaining ingredients, creating 4 packets.

3. Place the packets on a baking sheet and bake in a preheated oven for 35 to 40 minutes. Remove from the oven and set one packet on each plate. Carefully open and remove the bay leaf. Spoon some cooked bulgur on top and serve immediately.

CARAMELIZED CHICKEN WITH VEGETABLE "PANCAKE"

• SERVES 4 •

1 carrot, washed and grated

2 medium potatoes, peeled and grated

1 small courgette, washed and grated

1 garlic clove, peeled and chopped

½ teaspoon fresh thyme

3 tablespoons olive oil

Salt and freshly ground pepper

FOR THE VEGETABLE PANCAKE

1. Place the grated carrot, potatoes, and courgette in the centre of a large, clean kitchen towel. Wrap tightly and squeeze as much liquid as possible from the vegetables. Unroll and place the grated vegetables in a large bowl. Add the garlic, thyme, and 1 tablespoon olive oil and mix well.

2. In a large, nonstick sauté pan, heat the remaining 2 tablespoons olive oil over medium-high heat. Add the vegetable mixture to the pan, pressing down so the pancake is about 2 cm thick and cook until golden brown, about 8 minutes. Carefully flip the pancake over (you can invert onto a plate first and slide back into the pan if you are nervous about the pancake falling apart) and continue cooking until the other side is crisp and golden and the vegetables are cooked, another 8 to 10 minutes. Remove from the pan and keep warm. Season to taste.

*1 lemon, rinsed, dried, and
quartered*

*12 small green olives, pitted
and cut in half*

*½ teaspoon hot red pepper
flakes*

2 tablespoons honey

1 tablespoon lemon juice

3 tablespoons olive oil

*4 (175–225g) skinless,
boneless chicken breasts*

*Salt and freshly ground
pepper*

1. In a large bowl, combine the lemon, olives, red pepper flakes, honey, lemon juice, and 1 tablespoon olive oil. Add the chicken breasts, season to taste, and stir to coat.

2. Heat the remaining 2 tablespoons olive oil in a large sauté pan over medium-high heat. Add the chicken-lemon-olive mixture and sauté until the chicken is cooked through and slightly caramelized, about 8 minutes per side. Serve the chicken with lemon and olives and accompanied by a wedge of the vegetable pancake.

CURRIED CHICKEN
WITH CUCUMBER

• SERVES 4 •

1 tablespoon unsalted butter

1 tablespoon olive oil

*4 (175–225g) skinless,
boneless chicken breasts,
cut lengthwise into 1cm
strips*

*Salt and freshly ground
pepper*

110g cup crème fraîche

1 tablespoon curry powder

*2 seedless cucumbers,
washed and cut into 1cm
slices*

Juice of 1 lemon

*Cooked basmati rice for
serving*

1. Heat the butter and olive oil in a large frying pan over medium-high heat. Season the chicken with salt and pepper and add to the pan. Cook until golden, stirring occasionally, about 10 minutes.

2. Meanwhile, in a medium bowl, combine the crème fraîche, curry powder, and cucumber slices and set aside.

3. When the chicken is golden, deglaze the pan with the lemon juice, scraping up all the brown bits from the bottom of the pan. Add the cucumber mixture and stir to combine. Cook for about 3 minutes or until the cucumbers are al dente. Season to taste and serve with basmati rice.

Chapter Three

DINNER

À TABLE

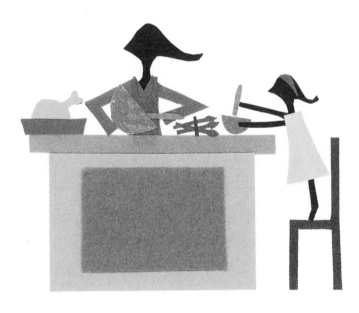

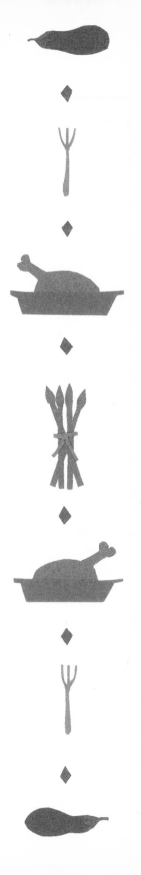

*D*inner hour is a puzzle and a wonder. What time do you normally eat dinner? Does it leave a healthy pause before going to bed? Do you tend to eat a big, bigger, and biggest dinner? How does dinner correlate with your health and with your sleep patterns? For every study and piece of advice I've read or heard, I can point to exceptions that seem to work just fine.

This much I know for myself: the older I get, the earlier and lighter I prefer to eat dinner. Now I can dine at 7:15 or 7:30 PM, compared with the 8:30 PM of most of my years. And the lighter my dinner is, the better I sleep and the better I feel the next morning. That said, in France where I live a good part of the year, try to get a dinner reservation in a restaurant before 8 PM. The French dine at 8:30 or 9 PM. Go to a restaurant that takes an earlier reservation and when the French show up and see people already with dessert, they say to themselves and sometimes out loud, "tourists." And by the way, in France and Germany and the rest of Europe of the same latitude or higher, from mid-spring through summer and mid-autumn, the hours of daylight are far longer than Americans appreciate. Daylight at 9 PM is routine and surely affects the dining hour.

I remember well a different picture during a stay in Bilbao, Spain, when jet-lagged and starving, the earliest reservation we could get for dinner at a top restaurant was 8:30 PM. We arrived at an empty restaurant and ate our entire meal with just one other couple in the dining room. Then as we were getting ready to leave, the Spaniards, legendary for dining late, started to flock in. I always wonder how they can eat and drink so well, so late, and then go to work and function first thing in the morning. Same in Greece. Go figure. In New York in the excess days of the 1980s and 1990s, I recall the poshest restaurants would keep their kitchens open past midnight and take full dinner orders until 11 PM to accommodate the arrival of a wealthy South American crowd around 10:30 PM (and thereby permitting the restaurant to turn tables three times in an evening, starting at about 5:30 or 6 PM when they would open their doors for pre-theatre dinner).

And there is the other extreme. The classic factory worker or physical laborer who comes home depleted and wants and expects dinner on the table shortly thereafter. That surely was the industrial and agrarian age standard and fully understandable, even necessary. And that time fix lingers on. But many of us no longer work long hours toiling in the fields and don't need to refuel our bodies depleted of its reserves so urgently or robustly. In the world's most populous country, China, dinner is relatively early, in my experience 6:30 or 7 PM, even for the fanciest state banquets, which are generally concluded by 9 PM or earlier. In a world homogenized by globalization, it seems dinner customs are slow to change, but they are indeed evolving.

Growing up French, I had the luxury of eating lunch always as the main meal of the day and considered it dinner. Schools and businesses closed from noon to two o'clock (well, fourteen o'clock in Europe) and we sat down at the table 12:30 sharp and did not get up until 1:30 PM. Both my parents worked, and the weekday meals were somewhat formulaic: fish every Friday, steak every Wednesday. Always a main protein dish, two vegetables (usually a type and style of potato was one), a simple green salad, and dessert in the form of fruit unless mother had to make us eat "horse steak," and then a more elaborate dessert was de rigueur as the bargaining power oh so subtly presented to encourage me to eat my steak. (My mother was great at planning—whether shopping the day before or preparing the basics for lunch before work, she was on top of things. It is a wonder how she did it all.)

Starting at age six, my job was to set the table. My father's job year-round was to go to the garden to pick the salad greens and fresh herbs after he had tenderly kissed my mother on her neck while she was attending the stove and putting the final touches to her cooking. The laughter and conversation around the "lunch" table is one of my strongest and best memories of childhood. The food wasn't bad either. The tone and warmth of all the wordplay and punning and silly jokes is hard to forget. (My father would say to me, "How do you make a golden soup?" "Add fourteen carrots.") Following a big lunch, dinner then was "supper," usually a soup (warm and rich in the winter, cold and light in the summer), perhaps some charcuterie such as ham, salami, or pâté, or an omelette, a salad, some cheese, mostly "creamy" such as *fromage blanc* or *petit-suisse*. No baked desserts at supper, only fruit. Dinner was lunchtime on weekends as well, but that was when my mother exercised her cooking skills and passion. It was a *menu dégustation* of sorts with a couple of *amuse* before the *plat de résistance*. The cheese tray was a treat served with wonderful breads. We always had guests and my mother always baked a dessert *and fruit tarts were the predessert!* Also it was the one day (or two) a week when we were permitted French fries!

That dining way of life is increasingly less the practice in France or in our world, though in the warmest climates and in the South of France, for example, shops still close for a long stretch at midday and people go home for a meal and a nap. One advantage of the midday main meal, I've come to realize, is that we get up and go about and the physical activity after lunch allows calories to burn faster and longer at an accelerated pace. It also means not a heavy consumption of alcohol near bedtime, which has the tendency to affect sleep patterns, causing us to awaken in the middle of the night, often dehydrated.

In Paris, my friend Agathe is more the sign of contemporary urban times and has adapted to her married life, and as a young wife who works long hours (and so does her husband, Gilles) her "married" eating pattern is as follows: breakfast is early and a moment where the couple sits down for a few minutes together before going their own way for the day. For both it's a piece of toast with butter and jam (made by Agathe's mother) with a yogurt and a cup of black coffee. Lunch in her case is a salad (sometimes bought in a good little shop near the Madeleine where she works or more often than not prepared by her at home and typically will be greens with seasonal colour—tomatoes or carrots, some protein such as a boiled egg or a few olives, lots of herbs and a lemon juice–olive oil dressing) and a piece of fruit. She has an hour for lunch but will take half of it to eat and the other half to walk and shop in the neighbourhood and often run errands. Dinner is late, about 9 PM, and since they both love to cook, they share the work each week; he does two days, she does two, and midweek they eat in a simple *bon rapport qualité-prix* (good value) bistro in their neighbourhood. Their meals consist mostly of fish with vegetables, a glass or two of wine, and a fruit for dessert, except for the night out when they'll share a dessert. Weekends go in reverse, and they'll get together with friends; the main meal will tend to be lunch on Sunday. In Europe, Sunday lunch is still the regimented meal for family and friends, especially mothers-in-law.

So, what is the point of these observations? It is to "know thyself," and as a function of your lifestyle find the right and healthy balance of time and quantity, then embrace what is a good dinner for you. Dinner comes in all sizes and times, so learn to eat with your head and you will find a winning way. Here's my "contemporary" definition of dinner: the main meal of the day when you sit at a table with knife and fork and eat slowly. *À table, bien sûr.*

One more bit of advice—and forgive me for a true but "self-flattering" portion control story. A friend shared the following: she was eating dinner with her husband in a relatively high-end Manhattan restaurant and two young couples sat next to them. They appeared to be enjoying a special occasion, and the guys ate and drank more than their share. At dessert time they were sent a free extra dessert in addition to the one each had ordered for him or herself. The young women then declared: "Wow, what would Mireille do if she were here?" Well today, I would not finish the desserts, and I would walk away toward home before hailing a taxi. But I confess, in my twenties, I would have eaten the desserts. Nature has a way of forgiving our youthful ways. In our twenty-first-century increasingly urban and pressured society, people tend to overeat at dinner and binge on weekends. So, if a little Mireille in your head can serve as your portion-control and balance conscience, I'm happy.

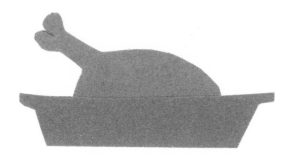

Soups

BUTTERNUT SQUASH SOUP

• SERVES 4 TO 6 •

1 medium (around 1 kg)
   butternut squash, peeled,
   halved, seeds and strings
   discarded

2 tablespoons olive oil

2 tablespoons unsalted
   butter

1 large white onion, roughly
   chopped

2 garlic cloves, peeled and
   chopped

½ teaspoon freshly grated
   nutmeg

3 sprigs fresh thyme

3 fresh sage leaves plus
   additional for garnish

3 carrots, peeled and
   roughly chopped

1 Granny Smith apple,
   peeled, cored, and chopped

around 1 litre chicken broth

Salt and freshly ground
   pepper

1. Cut the butternut squash into 2 cm pieces and set aside.

2. In a large pot, heat the oil and butter over medium-high heat. Add the onion and garlic and sauté until fragrant and softened, about 4 minutes. Add the nutmeg, thyme, and sage and cook for another minute, stirring. Add the squash, carrots, apple, and 800 ml chicken broth. Bring to a boil, lower the heat, and cover. Simmer until the vegetables are tender, about 20 minutes.

3. Remove the thyme sprigs and sage leaves from the soup and carefully transfer the mixture to a blender or a food mill and purée until smooth. If a thinner consistency is desired, add another 200 ml chicken broth. Season to taste and serve hot.

NOTE: *Sage leaves quickly fried in butter are a brilliant complement to the soup's natural sweetness. To prepare, simply melt 3 tablespoons butter in a small sauté pan over medium heat, swirling the pan occasionally. Add whole sage leaves and sauté until brown and toasted, 1 to 2 minutes. Garnish each serving of soup with 1 or 2 leaves and a drizzle of butter.*

POTAGE D'HIVER (WINTER SOUP)

450 g potatoes, peeled and cut into 2 cm pieces

225 g carrots, peeled and sliced

225 g leeks, white parts only, washed and sliced

Salt and freshly ground pepper

2 tablespoons finely chopped fresh parsley

1. Place the potatoes, carrots, and leeks in a large pot and add water to cover. Bring to a boil, reduce the heat to medium-low, and cover. Simmer until the vegetables are tender, about 20 minutes.

2. Remove from the heat and carefully pour the vegetables into a food mill or blender and purée, adding the cooking liquid until the desired consistency is attained. Be sure not to overblend as the starch in the potatoes can make the soup's consistency become "gluey." Season to taste, garnish with parsley, and serve hot.

LENTIL AND CELERIAC SOUP

• SERVES 4 •

1 tablespoon olive oil

1 onion, peeled and chopped

1 garlic clove, peeled and
   chopped

280g green lentils

1 small celeriac, peeled and
   chopped

1.3 litres water or chicken
   stock

Drizzle of red wine vinegar

1 tablespoon crème fraîche

Salt and freshly ground
   pepper

1. Heat the olive oil in a large saucepan over medium heat. Add the onion and garlic and sauté until fragrant and softened, 3 to 4 minutes.

2. Add the lentils, celeriac, and water or chicken stock. Bring to a boil, cover and simmer until the lentils are tender, about 20 minutes. Carefully transfer the mixture to a food processor or food mill and purée until smooth and creamy.

3. Stir in the vinegar to taste and crème fraîche, season to taste, and serve hot.

PUMPKIN AND APPLE SOUP

2 tablespoons olive oil

1 medium onion, peeled and chopped

2 teaspoons peeled and finely grated fresh ginger

around 1 kg pumpkin, peeled, seeded, and chopped

2 Granny Smith apples, peeled, cored, and diced

1 tablespoon honey

Pinch of cinnamon

Pinch of ground cloves

900 ml vegetable broth

Salt and freshly ground pepper

4 sprigs fresh rosemary

1. Warm the olive oil in a large pot over medium heat. Add the onion and ginger and sauté until softened, about 5 minutes.

2. Add the pumpkin, most of the diced apple, the honey, cinnamon, and ground cloves and cook, stirring for 1 minute. Add the vegetable broth and simmer for 10 minutes.

3. Carefully transfer the mixture to a food mill or blender and purée until smooth. Season to taste and serve the soup garnished with the remaining diced apple and sprigs of rosemary.

CREAM OF CELERIAC WITH PEAR AND BLUE CHEESE

• SERVES 4 TO 6 •

700 g celeriac, peeled and
  chopped

2 Comice pears, peeled,
  cored, and chopped

900 ml chicken broth

150 g crème fraîche

Salt and freshly ground
  pepper

4 tablespoons finely chopped
  fresh chives

50 g blue cheese, crumbled,
  at room temperature

1. Place the celeriac, pears, and chicken broth in a large pot over medium-high heat and bring to a boil. Cover, reduce the heat, and simmer until the celeriac is tender, about 15 minutes.

2. Meanwhile, using a stand or hand mixer, whip the crème fraîche until soft peaks form. Season to taste and fold in the chives. Cover and refrigerate.

3. Carefully transfer the celeriac, pears, and chicken broth to a blender and purée until smooth. To serve, pour the hot soup into bowls and garnish with the crumbled blue cheese and whipped crème fraîche.

Pasta, Perché No?

ORECCHIETTE WITH BROCCOLI RABE AND SAUSAGE

• SERVES 4 •

275g orecchiette

450g broccoli rabe, stems trimmed and roughly chopped

2 tablespoons olive oil

1 garlic clove, peeled and chopped

1 small onion, peeled and finely chopped

225g hot Italian sausage, split lengthwise down the middle and removed from casings

225ml tomato sauce

Salt and freshly ground pepper

50g grated pecorino

50g grated Parmesan

2 tablespoons chopped fresh parsley

1. Cook the orecchiette in a large pot of boiling salted water until they begin to soften, about 8 minutes. Add the broccoli rabe and cook until the pasta is just tender but still firm to the bite (al dente), about 3 minutes. Drain and reserve.

2. While the pasta is cooking, heat the olive oil in a large sauté pan over medium heat. Add the garlic and onion and cook until fragrant and softened, about 3 minutes. Add the sausage, breaking it up with a wooden spoon, and cook until browned, 5 to 8 minutes.

3. Add the cooked pasta and broccoli rabe to the sauté pan and toss until fully incorporated. Stir in the tomato sauce and cook for 1 to 2 minutes until heated through. Taste and correct the seasonings. Sprinkle with the grated cheeses and parsley and serve immediately.

SPAGHETTI CARBONARA

• SERVES 4 •

· ·

You will find two spaghetti carbonara recipes that follow, and I like them both because they have brought hours of heated discussions on what to put or not to put in the carbonara. And discussed with Italian, French, American, or Spanish friends, no one agrees. Cream is a big debate. So is the cheese: pecorino or Parmesan or both. The brand of spaghetti and fresh versus packaged. What size do you cut the pancetta? When and how do you add the egg yolks? The amount of water in the pot (the Italians put too much, and I put the minimum and it works). And on and on. Here is one of my favourites, though as a French woman I like Edward's because of the cream, which many Italians consider blasphemy, though quite a few have loved it when we served it to them, but then they were eating it in New York and not in Italy. So when in Rome, you know what you have to do.

350g spaghetti

2 medium eggs plus yolk of a
   third medium egg, beaten

115g freshly grated
   Parmesan

35g freshly grated pecorino

Salt and freshly ground pepper

1 teaspoon olive oil

110–225g bacon, cut
   crosswise into 1cm pieces
   or 5mm cubes (or 150g
   pancetta, chopped)

2 garlic cloves, chopped

1 tablespoon finely chopped
   fresh parsley

1. Bring a large pot of salted water to a boil over high heat. Add the spaghetti and cook until al dente, about 8 minutes. While the pasta is cooking, whisk the eggs and egg yolk with the Parmesan and pecorino in a medium bowl. Season to taste and set aside.

2. Warm the olive oil in a large sauté pan over medium-high heat. Add the bacon and cook until lightly browned and the fat has rendered. If there seems to be an excessive amount of fat, remove a bit, reserving 4 to 5 tablespoons in the pan. Reduce the heat to low, add the garlic, and quickly sauté until fragrant, being careful not to brown it, about 45 seconds.

3. Drain the spaghetti and reserve a little of the cooking water. Slowly whisk in half of the reserved cooking water to warm the egg and cheese mixture.

4. Add the hot spaghetti to the pan with bacon and toss well over medium heat. Remove the pan from the heat, add the egg mixture, and toss quickly until the pasta is evenly coated and the sauce has thickened, about 1 minute. If the sauce is too thick, thin with some of the reserved pasta cooking water. Divide the pasta among four plates, season to taste, and garnish with parsley.

SPAGHETTI CARBONARA
ALLA EDOARDO

• SERVES 4 •

I never stayed in the kitchen when Edward prepared his version, until I had to for this book, as I needed the specific amounts of ingredients. What amazes me and amuses me the most when he makes this dish is the state of the kitchen—almost as if a hurricane had gone through. But then we sit down and savour it with a great glass of Brunello di Montalcino, truly a cherished pleasure I will never tire of.

350g spaghetti

2 medium eggs plus yolk of a third medium egg

150ml double cream

100g freshly grated Parmesan

1 teaspoon olive oil

Sliver of butter (about ½ teaspoon)

150g pancetta, diced in 2cm-long and 5mm-wide pieces

Freshly ground pepper

1. Bring half a litre of water to a boil in a heavy pot over high heat. Add a pinch of salt and the spaghetti. Cook for 8 minutes or until al dente. While the pasta is cooking, whisk the eggs, egg yolk, double cream, and Parmesan in a bowl until combined.

2. Heat a large, heavy frying pan over medium heat and add the olive oil and butter, and sprinkle with the pancetta pieces. Cook until the pancetta is lightly coloured, 3 to 4 minutes, and some of the fat has been rendered; the pancetta should remain soft. (Drain off some of the fat if there seems to be an excessive amount.)

Pinch of piment d'Espelette
  (available at gourmet
  stores) or red pepper
  flakes for a stronger
  flavour
2 tablespoons finely chopped
  fresh parsley

3. Drain the pasta and reserve a little of the cooking water. Add the spaghetti to the pan with the pancetta. Mix gently over medium heat, shaking the pan for a minute or so. Add the egg mixture and toss until well incorporated, coating the pasta but not scrambling the eggs. Thin the sauce with the reserved water if necessary. Season to taste with a good dose of pepper and a pinch of *piment d'Espelette*, a mild pepper from Spain, and garnish with parsley. Serve *pronto*.

MACARONI WITH RICOTTA AND WALNUTS

• SERVES 4 •

275g macaroni

135g walnuts, coarsely chopped

20g fresh basil leaves cut into chiffonade (thin strips)

280g fresh ricotta

75g freshly grated Parmesan

Salt and freshly ground pepper

1 to 2 tablespoons walnut oil

1. Bring a large pot of salted water to a boil. Add the macaroni and cook until al dente, 8 to 10 minutes.

2. Meanwhile, combine the walnuts, basil, ricotta, and Parmesan in a bowl and season to taste.

3. To serve, drain the cooked pasta and place in a serving bowl with the walnut oil, tossing well. Add the ricotta mixture to the pasta and toss to combine. Serve hot or at room temperature.

TAGLIATELLE WITH TURKEY "BOLOGNESE"

• SERVES 4 •

2 tablespoons olive oil

2 celery stalks, rinsed and
diced

2 carrots, peeled and finely
diced

½ large onion, peeled and
finely chopped

2 garlic cloves, peeled and
chopped

1 teaspoon chopped fresh
rosemary

Pinch of paprika

1 boneless, skinless turkey
breast half (about
225g), diced

110 ml red wine

400g tin chopped tomatoes

350g tagliatelle

115g freshly grated
pecorino

1. Heat the olive oil over medium heat in a large, heavy saucepan and add the celery, carrots, onion, garlic, rosemary, and paprika. Sauté, stirring occasionally, until softened and fragrant, about 4 minutes. Add the diced turkey and sauté until golden, 2 to 3 minutes.

2. Add the red wine and tomatoes, stirring to scrape any browned bits at the bottom of the pot. Cover, reduce the heat to medium-low, and cook for 30 minutes, stirring occasionally and adding a bit of water if the sauce becomes too dry.

3. While the sauce is simmering, bring a large pot of salted water to a boil. Add the tagliatelle and cook until al dente, about 10 minutes.

4. Drain the pasta and serve with the sauce, garnished with the pecorino.

Adding the Colours of Vegetables

POTATO AND FENNEL PURÉE

• SERVES 4 •

2 large fennel bulbs

4 medium potatoes, peeled and chopped

4 tablespoons olive oil plus extra for serving

75 ml chicken broth

Salt and freshly ground pepper

1 tablespoon chopped fresh dill

1. Remove the stalks from each fennel bulb and reserve 1 tablespoon fronds. Remove the outer "envelopes" of each fennel bulb, slice in half to create cups, rinse, and reserve. Discard the stalks and core and chop the remaining fennel.

2. Place the fennel cups, chopped fennel, and potatoes in a steamer insert set over simmering water and cook for 20 minutes or until tender.

3. Remove the fennel cups and reserve. In a blender, combine the olive oil, chicken broth, and steamed chopped fennel, and purée until smooth. Pass the steamed potatoes through the fine plate of a ricer or food mill into a large bowl and add the fennel purée. Stir until smooth and season with salt and pepper.

4. Place one fennel cup on each plate, season with salt and pepper, and fill with the purée. Garnish with fresh dill, fennel fronds, and a drizzle of olive oil and serve.

QUINOA WITH PEAS AND BROAD BEANS

175g quinoa

225g peas, fresh or frozen

225g broad beans, peeled

110g snow peas, chopped

2½ tablespoons unsalted butter

1 tablespoon olive oil

½ teaspoon ground cumin

½ teaspoon ground coriander

Salt and freshly ground pepper

1. Cook the quinoa according to the package directions.

2. Meanwhile, place the vegetables and beans in a steamer and steam over medium to high heat until crisp-tender and bright green, 8 to 10 minutes. Be careful not to overcook.

3. Place the cooked quinoa in a serving bowl, add the butter, and mix well. Add the vegetables, olive oil, cumin, and coriander and season to taste. Serve hot or at room temperature.

CAULIFLOWER PURÉE

• SERVES 4 •

550 ml chicken or vegetable broth

1 head cauliflower, stems and stalks trimmed, florets chopped

1 tablespoon unsalted butter

2 tablespoons sour cream (or fromage blanc)

1 tablespoon grated Parmesan

Pinch of paprika

Salt and freshly ground pepper

1. In a large saucepan, bring the chicken or vegetable broth to a boil over high heat. Add the cauliflower, cover, and simmer until very tender, about 12 minutes.

2. Reserve 170 ml of the cooking liquid and carefully place half of the cauliflower in a blender. Add about 50 ml of the cooking liquid and purée until smooth. Add the remaining cauliflower and blend, adding just enough liquid to produce a silky purée. Finish the purée by adding the butter, sour cream, Parmesan, and paprika and blending just until incorporated. Season to taste and serve hot.

POTATO RAGOÛT WITH PEPPERS, LEMON, AND OLIVES

• SERVES 4 •

5 tablespoons olive oil

2 large potatoes, peeled and cut lengthwise into quarters

1 red bell pepper, seeded and cut into strips

4 garlic cloves, peeled and chopped

1 lemon, rinsed and sliced

225 ml green olives, pitted

Salt and freshly ground pepper

20 g fresh coriander, finely chopped

1. Preheat the oven to 190°/gas mark 5.

2. Heat 3 tablespoons olive oil in a large oven-safe pan over medium heat. Add the potatoes, red pepper, and garlic and sauté until fragrant, about 2 minutes. Add the lemon slices and olives, season to taste, and place the pan in the oven. Bake until the potatoes are golden and tender, 40 to 45 minutes.

3. Remove from the oven and transfer the vegetables to a serving bowl. Add the remaining 2 tablespoons olive oil and the fresh coriander, gently toss to combine, and serve.

ROASTED CARROTS AND PUMPKIN WITH HERBS

• SERVES 4 •

700g small carrots, peeled
   and green tops trimmed
   to 1 to 3 inches

900g pumpkin, peeled,
   seeded, and thinly sliced

Butter, softened, for baking
   dish

75ml olive oil

1 garlic clove, peeled and
   chopped

½ teaspoon ground cumin

½ teaspoon ground coriander

Salt and freshly ground
   pepper

2 tablespoons finely chopped
   fresh parsley

2 tablespoons finely chopped
   fresh mint

1. Preheat the oven to 190°/gas mark 5.

2. Place the carrots and pumpkin in a buttered baking dish. Add the olive oil, garlic, cumin, and coriander and toss to combine. Season to taste and place in the oven. Bake for about 40 minutes, stirring occasionally, until the vegetables are tender and very lightly caramelized.

3. Remove from the oven, sprinkle with parsley and mint, and serve.

SWEET POTATO FRENCH FRIES

• SERVES 4 •

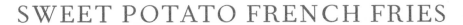

Olive oil

4 medium sweet potatoes,
   unpeeled

Salt and freshly ground
   pepper

Sea salt for serving

1. Preheat the oven to 230°C/gas mark 8 and brush a baking sheet with olive oil.

2. Halve the sweet potatoes lengthwise and cut each half into 3 to 5 spears. Place the spears on the prepared baking sheet, season to taste, and bake, turning the spears once, for 15 to 20 minutes until crisp. Remove from the oven, sprinkle with sea salt, and serve hot.

MUSHROOMS AND SWISS CHARD

1 tablespoon olive oil

1 tablespoon unsalted butter

1 large shallot, peeled and
  chopped

450g Swiss chard, centre
  ribs discarded and leaves
  coarsely chopped

350g mixed mushrooms
  (use a variety such as
  portobello, shiitake, and
  button), wiped clean and
  chopped

Salt and freshly ground
  pepper

1. Heat the olive oil and butter in a large frying pan over medium-high heat. Add the shallot and sauté until fragrant and softened, 1 minute.

2. Add the Swiss chard and cook, stirring, until tender, 5 to 7 minutes. Add the mushrooms and sauté for 3 minutes. Season to taste and serve immediately.

NOTE: *In addition to being a delicious side dish, this makes a fabulous sandwich. Place a layer of mushrooms and Swiss chard on a slice of baguette or other good, crusty bread. Top with a few slices of fresh mozzarella and place under the grill until melted. Sprinkle with salt and serve immediately.*

LEEKS MOZZARELLA

• SERVES 4 •

900g leeks, white parts only

40g fresh basil leaves

225g mozzarella

1 to 2 tablespoons olive oil

1 teaspoon wine or sherry
vinegar

Salt, preferably freshly
ground fleur de sel
(large-grained "flower of
salt" harvested from the
sea works magic), and
freshly ground pepper

4 slices country bread

1. Preheat the grill.

2. Clean the leeks thoroughly and boil in salted water for 6 to 10 minutes, until cooked but still firm, then drain.

3. Put the leeks in a baking dish and cover with a layer of basil leaves. Cut the mozzarella into 5 mm slices and place atop the basil layer. Put the dish under the preheated grill and watch carefully. In 3 to 5 minutes the cheese should start to melt and brown; at this point, remove the dish.

4. Mix the oil and vinegar and drizzle over the mozzarella. Season with salt and pepper to taste. Serve immediately with a slice of country bread.

QUINOA AND BEET SALAD

• SERVES 4 TO 6 •

2 tablespoons red wine
vinegar

2 tablespoons lemon juice

6 tablespoons olive oil

Salt and freshly ground
pepper

175 g quinoa, cooked
according to the package
directions

450 g red beets, boiled,
peeled, and quartered

225 g mushrooms, cleaned
and chopped

1 avocado, pitted, peeled,
and diced

2 yellow peppers, seeded,
sliced into thin strips,
and steamed

20 g red onion, peeled and
finely diced

2 tablespoons coarsely
chopped almonds

10 g chopped fresh parsley

1. In a small bowl combine the vinegar and lemon juice. Slowly drizzle in the olive oil while whisking and season to taste.

2. Place the quinoa in a large bowl and add the beets, mushrooms, avocado, yellow peppers, onion, and almonds. Pour the dressing over the salad and gently toss. Sprinkle with parsley and serve.

BLACK OLIVE POTATO SALAD
WITH BROAD BEANS

• SERVES 4 •

350g red potatoes, unpeeled

2 tablespoons black olive tapenade (store-bought)

3 tablespoons olive oil

Salt and freshly ground pepper

450g broad beans, shelled, peeled, cooked for 1 minute in boiling, salted water, and drained

90g sun-dried tomatoes, coarsely chopped

1. Place the potatoes in a pot of salted cold water. Bring to a boil and cook for 10 minutes or until a fork can easily pierce the potatoes. Drain and quarter.

2. Meanwhile, in a small bowl combine the tapenade and olive oil and season to taste.

3. Place the potatoes, broad beans, and sun-dried tomatoes in a large bowl. Pour the tapenade mixture over the salad, toss well, and serve at room temperature.

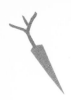

Omega-3 to the Rescue:
Toujours Poissons

SARDINES WITH CARROTS AND LEEKS

• SERVES 4 •

3 tablespoons olive oil

175 g carrots, peeled and
 thinly sliced

Salt and freshly ground
 pepper

275 g leeks, white parts
 only, thinly sliced

2 tablespoons chopped
 shallots

1 tablespoon unsalted butter

12 medium fresh sardines
 (about 700 g)

1 tablespoon chopped fresh
 oregano

Juice of 1 lemon

1. Preheat the oven to 180°C/gas mark 4.

2. Warm 2 tablespoons of the olive oil in a large frying pan. Add the carrots and cook over medium heat for 5 minutes. Add 75 ml water, season to taste, and stir in the leeks and shallots. Cover and cook for 5 to 7 minutes, stirring occasionally, until the vegetables are tender. Add the butter and cook a minute or two more.

3. Put the sardines in one layer in a shallow 25 cm × 40 cm baking dish. Drizzle the remaining 1 tablespoon olive oil over them, season to taste, and sprinkle with oregano. Bake 5 to 7 minutes on each side. Drizzle with the lemon juice and serve with the carrots and leeks.

MACKEREL WITH CARROTS AND LEEKS

• SERVES 4 •

3 tablespoons olive oil

4 tablespoons chopped fresh
rosemary

2 tablespoons chopped
shallots

Juice of 1 lemon

700g mackerel fillets

Salt and freshly ground
pepper

Carrot-leek mixture from
Sardines with Carrots
and Leeks (page 136)

1. Make a marinade by combining 2 tablespoons of the olive oil with the rosemary, shallots, and lemon juice. Pour over the mackerel and marinate for 10 to 20 minutes.

2. Warm the remaining tablespoon olive oil in a large frying pan and cook the mackerel over medium heat, about 3 minutes on each side.

3. Season to taste (be careful not to oversalt, since mackerel is already salty) and serve with the carrot-leek mixture.

FRIED OYSTERS

• SERVES 4 •

• •

Life is filled with surprises. I love oysters, and never imagined what I learned from my books, websites, and appearances: that so many people had never tasted oysters and/or did not want to taste oysters. (I'll spare you the adjectives describing those poor molluscs.) And also that so many people are allergic to shellfish and seafood, and for that I have compassion—you are missing one of the most sensual foods on earth or as Léon Paul Fargue said, "Eating oysters will always be like kissing the sea on the lips."

Here is an easy introduction to the oyster via a recipe (the only oyster recipe in this book). I truly hope a few more readers will be adventurous and taste oysters. I like oysters best raw, but what I've learned (similar lessons with Champagne, broccoli, and fish) is don't try the raw stuff first. Manipulate: coat it, "cajole" it, hide it. Since most of us like fried foods, and fried oysters are made quickly, here is one of my favourite "non raw" ways of eating oysters.

Vegetable oil, for frying

80 g flour

130 g cornmeal

1 egg, beaten

1 dozen oysters, opened, removed from shells, and patted dry

Salt

Lemon wedges or Quick "Aïoli," page 140 (optional)

1. Heat the oil in a deep, heavy saucepan over medium-high heat until the oil is 190°C; the oil should be at least 8 cm deep.

2. Meanwhile, place the flour and cornmeal on separate plates and place the egg in a small bowl. Dredge 1 oyster in the flour and shake off the excess. Dip in the egg, remove with a fork, and roll in cornmeal until well coated. Shake off any excess and set on a plate. Repeat with the remaining oysters.

3. When the oil is ready, carefully deep-fry the oysters, three at a time, until golden, about 2 minutes. Be sure to monitor the temperature of the oil: if the oysters brown too fast, reduce the heat, and if they cook too slowly, increase the heat. Carefully remove the oysters with a slotted spoon and set on a paper towel–lined plate. Sprinkle with salt and serve immediately with lemon wedges or aïoli, if desired.

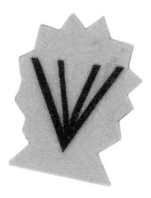

QUICK "AÏOLI"

• MAKES 1 CUP •

· ·

*200g good-quality
mayonnaise*

*1 large garlic clove, peeled
and finely chopped*

1 teaspoon lemon juice

*1 tablespoon finely chopped
fresh basil*

Combine all the ingredients and serve.

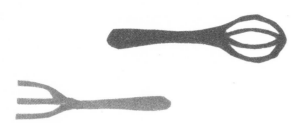

MACKEREL WITH CURRY AND LEEKS

• SERVES 4 •

1 tablespoon olive oil

2 tablespoons unsalted
  butter

450g leeks, washed
  carefully to remove grit,
  halved vertically, and cut
  into thin strips

2 shallots, peeled and finely
  chopped

450g potatoes, peeled,
  washed, cut into 5mm
  dice, and reserved in a
  bowl of cold water

1 bouquet garni (a bundle or
  small sachet of mixed
  herbs)

1 teaspoon curry powder

4 (110g) mackerel fillets

Salt and freshly ground
  pepper

1. Preheat the oven to 200°C/gas mark 6.

2. Heat the olive oil and 1 tablespoon butter in a saucepan over medium-low heat and sauté the leeks and shallots until fragrant and softened, 10 minutes.

3. Add the potatoes and just enough water to cover them, along with the bouquet garni and curry powder. Bring to a boil, cover, and cook over medium to low heat for 10 to 12 minutes or until the potatoes can be pierced with a fork.

4. Carefully pour the potatoes and cooking liquid into a baking dish. Top with the mackerel fillets, season to taste, and dot the fillets with the remaining tablespoon of butter. Bake for 15 minutes and serve immediately from the baking dish.

FLOUNDER FILLETS WITH PAPRIKA SAUCE

• SERVES 4 •

4 medium carrots, peeled

110g haricots verts, trimmed

4 (110g) flounder fillets (may also use snapper or sea bream)

2 tablespoons olive oil

Salt and freshly ground pepper

1 tablespoon butter

300ml double cream

2 teaspoons paprika

½ teaspoon sugar

2 tablespoons chopped chives

1. Slice the carrots into matchsticks as long as the width of the fillets, about 8cm. Cut the haricots verts to the same length.

2. Place the haricots verts in a steamer insert set above simmering water and steam for 2 minutes, covered. Add the carrots, cover, and steam for an additional 6 minutes or until crisp-tender. Remove from the heat and reserve.

3. Lay the fillets vertically on a work surface and pat dry. Brush the top of the fillets with 1 table-spoon olive oil and season to taste. Place one bundle of carrots and haricots verts at the bottom of a fillet and roll up, securing with a toothpick. Repeat with the other fillets.

4. Heat the butter and the remaining tablespoon olive oil over medium heat in a large frying pan and add the fillets. Cover and cook for 4 to 6 minutes on each side.

5. Transfer the fillets to a plate and keep warm. Add the cream, paprika, and sugar to the pan and whisk to combine. Increase the heat to medium-high and simmer until thickened, about 5 minutes. Remove from the heat, stir in the chives, and correct the seasoning.

6. Place each fillet on a plate, spoon the sauce over and around, and serve immediately.

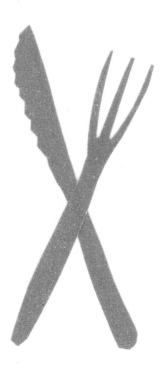

TUNA WITH GREEN SAUCE

• SERVES 4 •

One of the ways to increase your fish intake—at least one of the ways I increase mine—is to make two meals out of one-time cooking. Tuna and salmon in particular are two cooked fish I enjoy eating cold the next day or two as part of a salad. So, I tend to make steaklike fish for my evening meal, not only because they are bulkier and fall into the American pattern of lighter meals that culminate in a more substantial main meal at dinner but because I cook a small extra portion to supply the protein for my lunch salads. And while a cold fish is not my idea of dinner, it is quick and appealing for lunch.

20 g fresh parsley, chopped

1 green pepper, rinsed, seeded, and chopped into 5 mm dice

50 g green olives, pitted and chopped

2 tablespoons capers, rinsed and drained

1 teaspoon fresh thyme

2 tablespoons olive oil

Juice of 1 lemon

150 ml white wine or dry vermouth

1 (450 g) tuna steak, cut into 4 pieces

Salt and freshly ground pepper

1. Preheat the oven to 190°C/gas mark 5.

2. In a bowl, combine the parsley, green pepper, olives, capers, thyme, 1 tablespoon olive oil, lemon juice, and wine. Pour into a baking dish, place in the oven, and bake for 10 minutes.

3. Lower the heat to 180°C/gas mark 4. Remove the baking dish from the oven, add the tuna, spoon the sauce over, drizzle with the remaining tablespoon olive oil, and season to taste. Return the baking dish to the oven and cook for 10 to 15 minutes or until the tuna is done to taste. Remove from the oven and serve immediately.

Meat

PORK CHOPS WITH APPLES

• SERVES 4 •

4 medium pork chops

4 whole cloves

110g dry white wine or
   vermouth

4 celery leaves

2 bay leaves

4 celery stalks, washed and
   finely diced

1 tablespoon butter

2 apples, cored and coarsely
   sliced

1 tablespoon brown sugar

110g Swiss or Jarlsberg
   cheese, coarsely grated

1. Preheat the oven to 190°C/gas mark 5. Butter a baking pan and place the pork chops in it.

2. Press a clove into each chop. Add the white wine, celery leaves, and bay leaves and put the pan in the preheated oven. Bake the chops for 30 minutes.

3. While the pork chops are baking, in a frying pan, sauté the diced celery in the butter for 5 minutes, then add the sliced apples and sprinkle with the brown sugar. Continue cooking over very low heat for 10 minutes, or until the apples are tender but not mushy.

4. Finish the pork chops by removing the bay and celery leaves and sprinkle the cheese over the top of each chop; baste and then grill for a few minutes to brown the top.

5. Serve the celery-apple mixture on the plate as an accompaniment to the pork chops. Use a few spoons of the pan juices to further flavour the celery-apple mixture.

ROSEMARY LAMB MEATBALLS

• SERVES 4 TO 6

(MAKES ABOUT THIRTY 3 cm MEATBALLS) •

4 slices whole wheat bread, crusts removed

450g minced lamb shoulder

1 medium onion, peeled, grated, and excess moisture removed

1 garlic clove, peeled and chopped

2 tablespoons finely diced sun-dried tomatoes

2 tablespoons finely chopped fresh rosemary

1 tablespoon olive oil plus additional for baking sheet

1 teaspoon quatre épices*

Salt and freshly ground pepper

Buttered noodles or cooked brown rice for serving

1. Preheat the oven to 220°C/gas mark 7. Soak the bread in a small amount of water for 5 minutes. Firmly squeeze the bread to remove any excess water, discard the water, and place in a large bowl with the ground lamb. Add the onion, garlic, sun-dried tomatoes, rosemary, 1 tablespoon olive oil, and quatre épices. Season to taste and mix well.

2. To form the meatballs, wet your hands with cold water (to prevent sticking) and form 3 cm balls.

3. Arrange the meatballs on a large, heavy oiled baking sheet and bake until firm and cooked through, 12 to 15 minutes, turning once halfway.

4. Serve hot over buttered noodles or brown rice.

NOTE: *These meatballs would also be great made smaller, skewered, and served with mint-yogurt dip as an hors d'oeuvre, or make a delicious sandwich tucked inside a pita with chopped tomato and mint-yogurt dip. To make mint-yogurt dip, combine 450g plain Greek-style yogurt with 10g finely chopped fresh mint and 75g peeled and grated cucumber, and season to taste.*

*Often used in France, quatre épices is a spice blend that usually consists of ground pepper, cloves, nutmeg, and ginger or cinnamon.

CHICKEN EN CROÛTE
FIONA STYLE

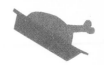

• SERVES 4 •

Zest of 2 lemons

Zest of 2 oranges

3 garlic cloves, peeled and
chopped

6 tablespoons chopped fresh
parsley

4 teaspoons chopped fresh
rosemary

150g grated Parmesan

2 teaspoons olive oil

Salt and freshly ground
pepper

2 eggs

4 (150–175g) skinless,
boneless chicken breast
halves, pounded to 1cm
thickness

1. Preheat the oven to 200°C/gas mark 6. Cover a baking sheet with aluminum foil and set aside.

2. In a shallow bowl or pie plate, combine the zests, garlic, parsley, rosemary, Parmesan, and olive oil and season to taste. In a second shallow bowl, whisk the eggs with a pinch of salt.

3. Dip each chicken breast in the egg, allowing any excess to drip off, and then dip in the citrus-herb-Parmesan mixture, pressing to lightly coat each side. Place the chicken breasts on the prepared baking sheet and transfer to the oven. Bake for 20 minutes or until the chicken is done.

4. Remove from the oven and serve immediately with lemon slices and a green salad.

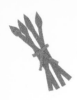

ITALIAN-STYLE CHICKEN

• SERVES 4 •

1 tablespoon olive oil

4 (150–175g) skinless,
   boneless chicken breasts,
   cut lengthwise into 1 cm
   strips

Salt and freshly ground
   pepper

45g sun-dried tomatoes,
   soaked in hot water for
   10 minutes, drained, and
   chopped

8 black olives, pitted and
   quartered

1 tablespoon capers, rinsed
   and drained

Pinch of cayenne pepper

Sautéed spinach for serving

1. Heat the olive oil in a nonstick frying pan over medium-high heat. Season the chicken pieces with salt and pepper and cook, stirring often, until golden, about 10 minutes. Remove the chicken from the pan and reserve.

2. Deglaze the pan with 2 tablespoons water and reduce until syrupy, about 1½ minutes. Add the tomatoes, olives, capers, and chicken and cook until heated through, about 1 minute. Correct the seasoning and add the cayenne. Serve immediately over spinach sautéed with garlic and lemon.

CHICKEN *À LA TUNISIENNE*

• SERVES 4 •

. . . .

1 tablespoon butter

1 tablespoon olive oil

4 shallots, peeled and chopped

700g boneless, skinless chicken breasts, cut into 2cm dice

1 (400g) tin apricots in their juice

½ teaspoon cinnamon

2 tablespoons crème fraîche

Salt and freshly ground pepper

Couscous for serving

1. Heat the butter and olive oil in a large, heavy saucepan over medium heat. Add the shallots and cook until softened, 2 to 3 minutes.

2. Add the chicken and cook, stirring, until the meat is golden. Stir in the apricots and their juice and the cinnamon. Cover, reduce the heat, and cook for 20 minutes. Remove the cover, increase the heat to medium-high and allow the cooking liquid to reduce slightly, about 10 minutes. Before serving, stir in the crème fraîche and season to taste. Serve with couscous.

CAREFREE CHICKEN

• SERVES 4 •

1 tablespoon olive oil

1 tablespoon unsalted butter

1 (1.3–1.8 kg) free-range
chicken, cut into 6 pieces
(2 breasts, 2 legs, 2
thighs), wings not
included

1 large onion, peeled and
chopped

75 ml water

1 teaspoon curry powder

1 teaspoon ground
cardamom

½ teaspoon freshly grated
nutmeg

1 chicken bouillon cube

Pinch of paprika

225 g tinned tomatoes

Salt and freshly ground
pepper

Rice for serving

1. Heat the olive oil and butter in a large frying pan over medium-high heat. Add the chicken pieces and brown on all sides. Remove from the pan and reserve.

2. Using the same pan, add the onion and cook until soft, 4 to 5 minutes. Deglaze the pan with the water, scraping up any browned bits.

3. Add the curry powder, cardamom, nutmeg, bouillon cube, paprika, and tomatoes. Stir well and return the chicken pieces back to the pan and season to taste. Cover and simmer over medium-low heat for 1 hour. Serve with basmati rice.

Chapter Four

EAT YOUR FISH AND VEGETABLES

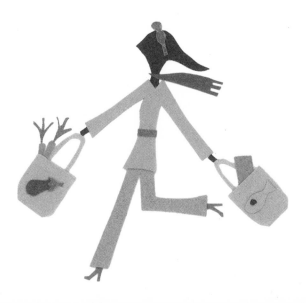

*I*t's no secret that men and women have different tastes in food. In 2008 the results of the most extensive study of gender differences in eating habits found that men were more likely to eat meat and poultry, especially duck, beef, and ham. Women were more likely to eat vegetables, especially carrots and tomatoes, and fruits, especially strawberries, blueberries, raspberries, and apples. Women also preferred dry foods, such as almonds and walnuts, and were more likely to consume yogurt.

But just because men (or you) *tend* to favour steak over asparagus doesn't mean they can't learn to appreciate a delicious ratatouille or sardines with carrots and leeks, two of the most popular recipes in *French Women Don't Get Fat* and *French Women for All Seasons* respectively and reprinted in this book.

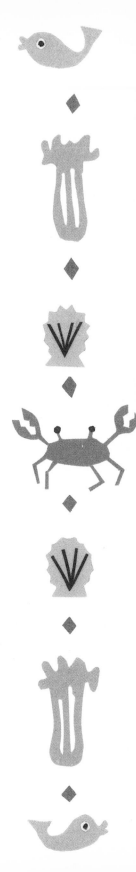

But first things first: you should eat more fish and vegetables. Short of overdosing on mercury-toxic big fish (especially if you are pregnant), they are good for you. So, by design, I've included this chapter of additional fish and vegetable recipes to inspire readers to be adventurous and to tempt them to a path that marries health with happiness and pleasure. (*Ménage à trois?*) New dishes and preparations and presentations can mean new appeal and new habits, even new health. You probably know the reasons and recommendations for eating your fish and vegetables. The benefits of eating fish two to three times a week is to cover your protein (lunch or dinner) needs with food that is low in fat and high in good fat and antioxidants, which help reduce the risks of heart disease and alleviate many conditions from inflammation to depression. In addition, fish is versatile in its varieties (shellfish, white fish, oily fish, etc.) and preparations (steam, bake, sauté, poach, *en papillote*, grill). As for vegetables, they are about the best food on the planet (nuts are competitors) and eating two to four portions a day is healthy to get your fibre, which fill the stomach but also because vegetables are low in fat like fish. The vitamins and minerals in vegetables are an energy booster, their low sodium content means less water retention and, of course, they, like fish, are loaded with antioxidants and protect against heart disease, cancer, and much more. Along with water, the fibres in veggies (also in fruit and grains) act as a digestive tract stimulant. So, it was often said at our table when I was growing up "*Mange tes légumes,*" eat your veggies. Your metabolism will love it. As for preparations from raw to cooked, the ways are infinite and the mixing a true pleasure plus an easy way not to waste what's in the fridge.

Unless you are the rarity who dines all the time in restaurants (where you can order individually what you want) or you normally eat alone, you, like most people, dine with a companion or family members in a communal meal. Thus, you generally eat what is prepared for everyone *ensemble*. If your dining companions are "meat and potato" types, you may need to do a little missionary conversion. It is for your own good as well as theirs. Whether you are breaking poor eating habits, attempting to slim down, or just exploring a new culinary lifestyle, having co-explorers along to support you is a proven benefit. Having conscientious objectors along for the ride is proven not to be a good thing.

I converted my husband into a fish eater. It just took a little exposure and education. The conversion started during one of our very first "dates." I've written elsewhere how we met on a bus in Istanbul. That led to a reconnection in Athens, where we decided to go to the port of Piraeus for a fish dinner. The restaurant turned out to be literally out on a dock and ordering meant you walked into the area next to the kitchen and pointed to the fish you wanted to eat among dozens either still swimming in tanks or chilling on ice. Fresh as fresh can be. I'd spent quite a bit of time in Greece and spoke the language and knew the practice. There are Greek restaurants in New York that offer fish in the same wonderful manner. And top Chinese restaurants the world over do the same. For Edward, it was a revelation.

Though he had grown up a few miles from the ocean and ate fish every Friday in a Catholic household, he could not identify a single fish outside the goldfish bowl. Okay, I exaggerate, only slightly: he could identify mackerel and I expect swordfish (in a picture book). He had no idea what he was looking at in that seaside Greek restaurant. That evening he told me a story I have never forgotten.

Until he left for college, he mostly ate fish that looked and tasted like cardboard. So, it was no surprise he was shy on fish. It seems his mother only bought frozen fish (which meant to her fresh and no cleaning). He recalls blocks of frozen flounder fillet and now and then cod. Once they were thawed, she would mostly wash the fillets in egg batter, smother them in bread crumbs (from a can), and then panfry them in oil into an advanced state of rigor mortis. Occasionally a neighbour would deliver some freshly caught and cleaned fish, but then they, too, were inflicted with the same disguise and cooked to death. When he went off to college in New England, he occasionally tasted fish that were soft and tender, but mostly he acquired a taste for lobster.

So that evening in Piraeus, a whole fish, brushed with olive oil and lightly grilled to tender perfection, was an unusual treat and taste for him. Subsequently I (and my mother) used a little seductive French sauce as a "flavour enhancer" on delicately poached or grilled fish. Cooked tender and moist and not overdone. For him, it was like discovering a new food category. Correction: it was in fact discovering a new food category. And fish accompanied by potatoes or rice, what was not to like? Nowadays, I mostly avoid disguises, and twice a week at least we enjoy simply steamed or grilled fresh fish, and only sometimes with potatoes or rice, but always with something green (okay, once in a while orange or red).

If you need to convert a companion or children to diversify their meat and potatoes fixation, here are a few simple "tricks."

■ Effect a transition and remember balance. What if the kids want chicken fingers and French fries and you want them to eat fish? Don't shock them by serving salmon over a bed of spinach. Remember *peu à peu*, little by little. Serve a small portion of salmon with their favourite side dish, even if it's French fries. It may not be the perfect combo in your mind, but you'll have a much better chance of persuading picky eaters to eat something new if it's sitting next to something they enjoy. And you don't have to eat more than a few French fries yourself (hard, I know, but this is only the first half of the transition).

■ Add one vegetable at a time. Start by making a vegetable phobic try (just try) one green at dinner, or one new vegetable. Learn what flavour combinations your dining companion(s) like and serve the veggies that way. My friend and associate Erin learned that her meat-and-potatoes fiancé loved lemon-butter-garlic sauce. So she started introducing things he'd usually turn his nose up at (broccoli rabe, asparagus, courgette) in lemon and butter with chopped garlic. It was a big hit. Soon he was not only happily scarfing down loads of greens, he was requesting them for dinner! Little by little she started reducing the amount of butter as his palate developed a taste for greens. She now only uses olive oil (no butter) and he never even knew the difference.

■ Create "secret" vegetable delivery systems (SVDS?). Soup is the time-tested secret of the French and the most efficient way to get vegetables into a finicky eater's diet. When made from scratch, soup is generally low in calories, high in water, and bursting with nutrients, not to mention a great first course. Omelettes filled with veggies are another option. Serve with a small salad and/or potatoes. This is another great alternative for hungry men who usually go for bacon and eggs on Saturday mornings.

You can modify eating habits little by little. The key is to find a way to present new and healthy foods in a fun and delicious manner. Mothers of children who refuse to eat vegetables and fruits would be thrilled to know that another recent study found that when salad bars were placed in school lunchrooms, students took advantage, doubling their daily fresh produce intake. This "proves that kids will indeed eat more fruits and vegetables if offered in an appetizing and accessible manner" remarked the head of the study. I agree. You may not see improvement or acceptance at first; remember this is a process that will take a bit of time. And though you may get resistance, it doesn't mean the message is not sinking in. Maria, a community member on my website, shared with me, "I've always been one to prepare and enjoy good meals. For many years my daughter said everything was 'too fancy, too weird, too spicy, too something.' Who is the epicurean now? My daughter has a palate and natural talent for cooking that equals most foodies I know. It really seems that what she saw, as opposed to what she agreed to eat, as a child prevailed. Also, both my husband and his brother went through similar stages and are both refined eaters now." So remember, take the complaints in stride, stick to your guns, and, above all, remember to have patience. Good things often take time.

My additional fish dishes are all cooked *en papillote* because to me it's the most versatile way of serving fish: You have the choice to prepare it ahead (great time saver whether for a family meal or entertaining), it cooks fast and is fool-proof (no worry to have under or overdone fish), you add your veggies in the package, it saves use and cleaning of another pot (you actually have no dish to clean by using the greaseproof paper), and the presentation is unusual. And to top it all it is the safest and best way to keep the nutrients. To me it's a win-win anytime, oh, and did I forget to say that kids love to help preparing the papillotes? Make it a fun activity. Once you have practiced on a few fish you can pick your favourite and match it with your favourite veggies. They are all interchangeable. *Merci*, Juliette, for introducing me to *en papillote* years ago and sharing so many recipes with me over the years. (And now they are particularly popular in France.) I think of you every time I prepare them.

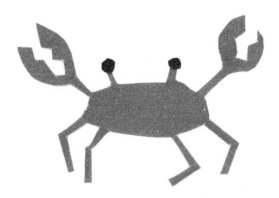

COD WITH FENNEL AND ORANGE *EN PAPILLOTE*

• SERVES 4 •

4 tablespoons olive oil plus additional for greaseproof paper

4 (110–150g) cod fillets

Salt and freshly ground pepper

1 fennel bulb, stalks removed, cored, and thinly sliced

1 orange, cut into 4 thick slices

1 teaspoon slightly crushed fennel seeds

2 teaspoons grated orange zest

Pinch of fleur de sel

1. Preheat the oven to 200°C / gas mark 6.

2. Cut four pieces of greaseproof paper into 30 cm × 40 cm rectangles and brush the centres with olive oil. Place 1 cod fillet in the centre of the greaseproof paper and season to taste. Top with sliced fennel and 1 slice of orange and season again. Seal the packet by bringing the sides up to the centre and folding them down tightly. Seal the ends by folding each in tightly. Repeat with the remaining ingredients, creating four packets.

3. Place the packets on a baking sheet and bake for 15 to 20 minutes (the packets will be puffed and lightly browned). Remove from the oven and place one packet on each plate.

4. Meanwhile, place 4 tablespoons olive oil in a small saucepan with the fennel seeds and orange zest and warm over low heat until fragrant, about 7 minutes. Remove from the heat and pour into four small ramekins.

5. Serve each papillote accompanied by a small ramekin of olive oil and some fleur de sel.

SALMON WITH ENDIVES AND ORANGES *EN PAPILLOTE*

• SERVES 4 •

3 oranges

1 teaspoon olive oil plus
    additional for
    greaseproof paper

2 medium to large endives,
    washed and cut into thin
    strips

4 (150–175 g) salmon
    steaks

2 teaspoons peeled and
    finely grated ginger

2 teaspoons honey

Salt and freshly ground
    pepper

1. Preheat the oven to 200°C/gas mark 6.

2. Remove the zest of 1 orange in long strips and julienne; reserve the orange. Place the julienned strips of orange zest in a small pot of cold water and bring to a boil. Drain the zest and set aside.

3. To prepare the orange segments, cut slices off the top and bottom of the remaining 2 oranges and then slice away the peel and pith, top to bottom, following the curve of the fruit. Working over a bowl and using a small, sharp knife, cut between the membranes to release the segments and juice of all 3 oranges.

4. Cut four pieces of greaseproof paper into 30 cm × 40 cm rectangles and brush the centres with olive oil. Place one quarter of the endive in the centre of the first rectangle and top with 1 salmon steak. Add the orange segments, orange zest, ginger, and a drizzle of olive oil and honey. Season to taste and seal the packet by bringing up the sides to the centre and folding them down tightly. Seal the ends by tightly folding each in. Repeat with the remaining ingredients, creating four packets.

5. Bake for 15 minutes and remove from the oven; the packets will be puffed and lightly browned. Allow to rest for 5 minutes before placing each packet on a plate and serving. Allow guests to open their packets.

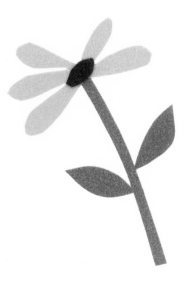

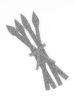

SALMON WITH LEEKS AND ASPARAGUS *EN PAPILLOTE*

3 oranges

2 teaspoons sesame oil

2 medium carrots, peeled
  and grated

1 leek, white part only, cut
  into thin strips

8 asparagus tips, cut in half
  (reserve asparagus stalks
  for a salad)

4 (150–175 g) salmon
  steaks

Salt and freshly ground
  pepper

1 tablespoon chopped fresh
  coriander

1 teaspoon chopped fresh
  dill

1. Preheat the oven to 200°C / gas mark 6.

2. Remove the zest of 1 orange in long strips and julienne; reserve the orange. Place the julienned strips of orange zest in a small pot of cold water and bring to a boil. Drain the zest and set aside.

3. Prepare the orange segments: cut slices off the top and bottom of the remaining 2 oranges and then slice away the peel and pith, top to bottom, following the curve of the fruit. Working over a bowl and using a small, sharp knife, cut between the membranes to release the segments and juice of all 3 oranges.

4. Cut four pieces of greaseproof paper into 30 cm × 40 cm rectangles and brush the centres with sesame oil. Place one quarter of the carrots, leeks, and asparagus tips in the centre of the first piece of greaseproof paper and top with 1 salmon steak. Add the orange segments, blanched orange zest, ¼ teaspoon sesame oil, and 1 teaspoon orange

juice. Season to taste and seal the packet by bringing up the sides to the centre and folding them down tightly. Seal the ends by folding each in tightly. Repeat with the remaining ingredients, creating four packets.

5. Place the packets on a baking sheet and cook in the oven for 18 to 20 minutes. Remove from the oven (the packets will be puffed and lightly browned) and allow to rest for 5 minutes before placing each packet on a plate and serving. Allow guests to open their packets and garnish with coriander and dill.

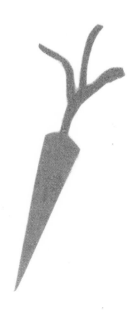

SEA BASS WITH SWEET SPICES
EN PAPILLOTE

1 tablespoon olive oil plus additional for greaseproof paper

2 yellow peppers, rinsed, seeded, and sliced lengthwise

2 medium courgettes, rinsed and cut into matchsticks

2 star anise

Pinch each of ground ginger, cinnamon, and paprika

Salt and freshly ground pepper

3 tablespoons balsamic vinegar

4 (110 g) sea bass fillets

2 tablespoons chopped fresh coriander

1. Preheat the oven to 200°C/gas mark 6.

2. Heat 1 tablespoon olive oil in a large frying pan over medium heat. Add the yellow peppers, courgette, star anise, and spices and sauté until the vegetables are crisp-tender, about 5 minutes. Season to taste and transfer the vegetables to a plate, removing the star anise. Deglaze the pan with the balsamic vinegar and 2 tablespoons water over medium heat, allowing the liquid to simmer for 1 to 2 minutes and reduce slightly.

3. Cut four pieces of greaseproof paper into 30 cm × 40 cm rectangles, brush the centres with olive oil, and place one quarter of the vegetables in the centre of the greaseproof paper. Top with 1 fillet, season, drizzle with a bit of the deglazing liquid, and sprinkle with ½ tablespoon chopped coriander. Seal the packet by bringing the sides up to the centre and folding them down tightly. Seal the ends by folding each in tightly. Repeat with the remaining ingredients, creating four packets.

4. Place the papillotes on a baking sheet and bake for 15 minutes. Serve immediately.

Veggies on the Side
or in the Middle

As for veggies, these recipes evolved from experimenting with young friends and guests who have travelled and like to play with curry, capers, confit, and more.

VEGETABLE CURRY

• SERVES 4 TO 6 •

2 tablespoons olive oil

1 tablespoon unsalted butter

1 medium red onion, peeled and finely chopped

1 courgette, washed and chopped into 1 cm cubes

1 aubergine, washed and chopped into 1 cm cubes

4 medium potatoes, peeled and chopped into 1 cm cubes

1 tablespoon curry powder

1 cinnamon stick

Salt and freshly ground pepper

450 ml water or chicken broth

1. In a large sauté pan, heat the olive oil and butter over medium-high heat. Add the onion and cook until softened, about 4 minutes. Add the courgette, aubergine, and potatoes and mix well. Add the curry and cinnamon stick and season to taste.

2. Add the water or chicken broth, cover, and cook over low heat for 20 minutes. Remove the cover, increase the heat to medium, and cook for an additional 10 minutes, allowing the cooking liquid to thicken slightly. Season to taste and serve warm or cold.

ROASTED VEGETABLES
WITH CUMIN

• SERVES 4 •

4 turnips, peeled and cut
    into quarters

4 carrots, peeled and sliced
    on the bias

4 onions, peeled and sliced
    into 1 cm wedges

2 fennel bulbs, stalks and
    core discarded, cut into
    1 cm wedges

3 tablespoons olive oil

1 teaspoon cumin seeds

Salt and freshly ground
    pepper

1. Preheat the oven to 220°C/gas mark 7.

2. Place the turnips, carrots, onions, and fennel in a large bowl. Add the olive oil and cumin seeds and toss to coat.

3. Arrange the vegetables in a single layer on a baking sheet and season generously. Place in the oven and roast for 30 to 40 minutes, turning the vegetables occasionally, until they are tender and caramelized.

4. Remove from the oven and serve warm or at room temperature.

PUMPKIN AND APPLE GRATIN

• SERVES 4 TO 6 •

2 tablespoons unsalted
butter plus additional for
baking dish

900g pumpkin, peeled,
seeded, and cut into 5cm
pieces

3 baking apples, peeled,
cored and cut into wedges

1 tablespoon lemon juice

Salt and freshly ground
pepper

170g crème fraîche

Pinch of cinnamon

1 medium onion, peeled and
finely chopped

150g pancetta, thinly sliced
into strips

1 tablespoon chopped
walnuts

170g feta cheese, crumbled

1 teaspoon fresh thyme

1. Preheat the oven to 180°C/gas mark 4.

2. Butter a 25 cm × 35 cm baking dish and add the sliced pumpkin and apples. Sprinkle with lemon juice, dot with 1 tablespoon butter, and season to taste. Place in the oven and bake for 20 minutes.

3. Meanwhile, in a medium bowl combine the crème fraîche and cinnamon and set aside. Melt the remaining tablespoon of butter in a nonstick pan over medium heat and add the onion and pancetta. Sauté until the onion is softened and the pancetta has browned a bit, about 3 minutes. Remove from the heat and stir in the walnuts, feta, and thyme. Add the onion-pancetta mixture to the crème fraîche and stir to combine. Pour over the pumpkin and apples and return to the oven.

4. Continue cooking until the vegetables are tender and the top is golden, 20 to 30 minutes. Remove from the oven and serve immediately.

NOTE: *If pumpkin is not available, butternut squash makes a fine substitution.*

POÊLÉE PROVENÇALE

• SERVES 4 •

2 tablespoons olive oil

2 courgettes, washed and
sliced into 5mm-thick
rounds

2 garlic cloves, peeled and
chopped

1 teaspoon chopped fresh
thyme

3 peppers (yellow, red, and
orange), washed,
seeded, and cut into thin
strips

Salt and freshly ground
pepper

Warm the olive oil in a large sauté pan over medium-high heat. Add the courgette and cook, stirring, for 6 minutes. Add the garlic, thyme, and peppers and continue cooking until fragrant and the peppers are crisp-tender, about 3 minutes. Season to taste and serve warm or cold.

CARAMELIZED ENDIVES

1 tablespoon unsalted butter

1 tablespoon olive oil

4 endives, rinsed and quartered lengthwise

35 g walnuts, coarsely chopped

1 heaped teaspoon sugar

Salt and freshly ground pepper

1. Heat the butter and olive oil in a large sauté pan over medium-high heat. Add the endives and cook, stirring, until golden, about 5 minutes.

2. Add the walnuts and sugar and continue cooking, gently stirring, until caramelized, about 3 more minutes. Remove from the heat, season to taste, and serve.

ROASTED CAULIFLOWER WITH RAISINS AND CAPERS

• SERVES 4 •

50g golden raisins

2 tablespoons red wine vinegar

1 large head cauliflower, trimmed and cut into small florets

5 tablespoons olive oil

Salt and freshly ground pepper

1 tablespoon capers, drained and chopped

3 tablespoons pine nuts

1 tablespoon finely chopped fresh parsley

1. Preheat the oven to 200°C/gas mark 6.

2. Combine the raisins and vinegar in a small bowl and allow the raisins to "plump" for about 30 minutes.

3. Place the cauliflower florets on a baking sheet and drizzle with 2 tablespoons olive oil. Season to taste and roast in the oven for 25 minutes, turning occasionally.

4. In a medium bowl, combine the raisins and any remaining vinegar, capers, pine nuts, parsley, and the remaining 3 tablespoons olive oil. Season to taste.

5. Remove the baking sheet from the oven and pour the raisin-caper mixture over the cauliflower, tossing gently. Return the baking sheet to the oven and continue roasting for an additional 15 minutes or until the cauliflower is tender and caramelized. Remove from the oven, place in a bowl, and season to taste. Serve warm or at room temperature.

AUBERGINE WITH CURRY AND HONEY

• SERVES 4 •

2 large shallots, peeled and chopped

1 lemon confit, drained and diced

4 teaspoons honey

Juice of 1 lemon

4 tablespoons olive oil

1 teaspoon curry powder

4 medium aubergines, rinsed and quartered lengthwise

Salt and freshly ground pepper

1. Preheat the oven to 190°C/gas mark 5.

2. In a medium bowl, combine the shallots, lemon confit, honey, lemon juice, olive oil, and curry powder.

3. Place the aubergine on a baking sheet in a single layer. Season to taste and pour the lemon-curry-honey mixture over the aubergine, tossing gently to coat evenly.

4. Bake for 10 minutes, lower the temperature to 150°C/gas mark 2, and baste with the lemon-curry-honey mixture. Continue cooking for 1 hour or until the aubergine is slightly caramelized and soft, turning occasionally.

ENDIVES *CONFITES* WITH BLUE CHEESE CROSTINI

• SERVES 4 •

6 tablespoons butter

4 medium to large endives, rinsed and cut lengthwise into thin strips

2 tablespoons honey

110 ml whole milk

Fresh thyme to taste

Fleur de sel and freshly ground pepper

4 slices whole wheat bread, toasted

175 g blue cheese, at room temperature

1. In a large frying pan, melt the butter over medium-low heat. Add the endives, honey, milk, and thyme. Bring to a simmer, reduce the heat, cover, and cook until the endives are tender, about 30 minutes.

2. To serve, season the endives with fleur de sel and pepper and serve immediately in a soup dish with a slice of toasted bread spread with blue cheese.

ONION *POÊLÉE* WITH APPLES

• SERVES 4 •

50g bacon, diced

4 tablespoons unsalted
butter

450g onions, peeled,
halved, and thinly sliced

3 apples, peeled, cored, and
sliced

Salt and freshly ground
pepper

1. Cook the bacon in a nonstick frying pan over medium heat until golden and crisp. Transfer to a paper towel–lined plate to drain.

2. Add the butter to the pan and melt over medium heat. Add the onions and cook until softened, stirring occasionally, about 10 minutes. Add the apples and bacon and season to taste. Continue cooking for another 10 minutes, stirring occasionally and adding a bit of water if the apples and onions stick. Remove from the heat and serve immediately.

CARROT PARSNIP PURÉE

• SERVES 4 •

450g carrots, peeled and chopped

2 parsnips, peeled and chopped

1 medium sweet potato, peeled and chopped

3 tablespoons chilled unsalted butter

Pinch of sugar (optional)

Salt and freshly ground pepper

1 teaspoon freshly grated nutmeg

2 tablespoons crème fraîche

1. In a medium saucepan, combine the carrots, parsnips, sweet potato, 1 tablespoon butter, and a pinch of sugar, if using, and season to taste. Add 110 ml water, cover, and cook over medium-high heat for 15 minutes. Uncover and cook for an additional 10 minutes or until the vegetables are very tender and the cooking liquid has reduced and become syrupy.

2. Remove the saucepan from the heat and carefully transfer the vegetables to a blender. Add the remaining 2 tablespoons butter, nutmeg, and crème fraîche and purée until smooth. Season to taste and serve immediately.

LENTIL, FENNEL, AND ORANGE SALAD

900 ml water or vegetable broth

225 g lentils

2 oranges

2 tablespoons red wine or sherry vinegar

½ medium shallot, chopped (about 1 tablespoon)

1 teaspoon peeled and finely grated fresh ginger

4 tablespoons olive oil

1 fennel bulb, washed, trimmed, quartered lengthwise, and thinly sliced crosswise

Salt and freshly ground pepper

1. Bring the water or vegetable broth and lentils to a boil in a large saucepan. Reduce the heat and simmer, uncovered, until the lentils are just tender, about 20 minutes. Drain and reserve.

2. To prepare the orange segments, cut slices off the top and bottom of the oranges and then slice away the peel and pith from the oranges, following the curve of the fruit. Working over a bowl and using a small sharp knife, cut between the membranes to release the segments and juice.

3. In a separate small bowl, whisk together the vinegar, shallot, ginger, and olive oil. In a large bowl, combine the lentils, fennel, and orange segments and juice. Add the vinaigrette and mix well. Taste, correct the seasoning, and serve.

LEEK AND COURGETTE SALAD

• SERVES 4 •

8 medium leeks, white parts
only, quartered and
rinsed in cold water to
remove any grit

4 small courgettes, cut
crosswise into 5 cm pieces
and quartered

1 teaspoon Dijon mustard

1 teaspoon acacia honey

2 tablespoons lemon juice

2 tablespoons olive oil

Salt and freshly ground
pepper

2 tablespoons chopped fresh
dill

1. Bring a pot of salted water to a boil over medium-high heat. Add the leeks and cook for 7 minutes. Add the courgettes and cook until crisp-tender, about 2 minutes. Drain and let cool.

2. In a medium bowl, whisk together the mustard, honey, lemon juice, and olive oil. Season to taste. Add the leeks and courgettes and toss gently to combine.

3. Serve garnished with dill.

SWEET-AND-SOUR CARROT SALAD

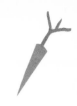

• SERVES 4 •

Juice of 1 orange

Juice of ½ lemon

Pinch of cinnamon

1 teaspoon honey

3 tablespoons olive oil

Salt and freshly ground
pepper

450g carrots, washed and
grated

1 apple, peeled and grated

25g walnuts

1. Mix the orange and lemon juices, add the cinnamon and honey, and slowly drizzle in the olive oil, whisking to combine. Season to taste.

2. Place the grated carrots, apple, and walnuts in a large salad bowl. Add the dressing, toss gently to combine, and serve.

Chapter Five

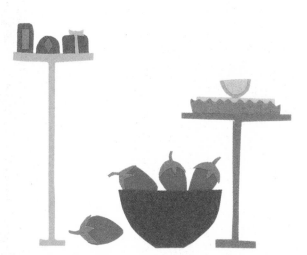

CLOSURES—SWEET, CHOCOLATE, AND OTHERWISE

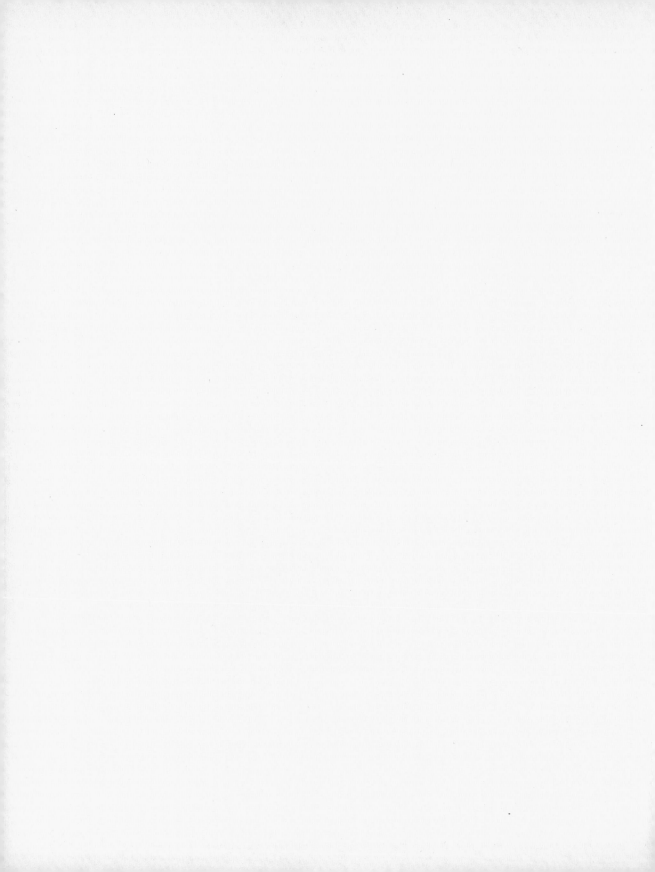

I love sweets. Did I need to say that? Growing up with a mother, grandmother, aunt, and many relatives who loved baking, the sweet smell and taste of something in the oven invaded my childhood. Desserts and things sweet are mildly addictive—the more you get, it seems, the more you need to feel fully satisfied. Okay, for some of us sweets are fully addictive. It took my year in Weston, Massachusetts, and gaining too many kilos, to later understand the power of sugar and its control of our brain. But to borrow from *Alice,* "The question is," said Humpty Dumpty, "which is to be master—that's all."

For me a little something sweet at the end of a meal, even one bite of chocolate, clicks shut the lunch pail oh so perfectly, achieving a balanced closure. I should emphasize, a *little* something at the end of the meal (remember portion proportions), and also that perfectly ripe fruit in season is nature's best way to round out a healthy and satisfying meal. Sweet, fresh fruit—berries or globes of fruit—is not an acquired taste. When they are ripe and sweet, people adore them. They are an acquired habit, however. One that advertisers of gooey desserts have defended against. A fresh peach or slice of melon or a cupcake?

If you are looking to ban a few food offenders, I implore you to reconsider, for one illustrative seductress, the cupcake. I know: I am asking for a lot. It is covered with a lot of childhood memories. But the reality of most cupcakes' unnecessary and excessive sweetness was brought home to me twice in the past year. (I am citing the cupcake, but you can come up with apt alternatives that will bring the eat-with-your-head-as-well-as-your-senses point home.)

There's a bakery in our Greenwich Village neighbourhood in New York City that was made famous via the *Sex and the City* TV series. The series may be no more—though everywhere around the world in reruns—but the bakery is very much alive in the present with hordes of people lining up to buy its cupcakes. It is a quaint little bakery on a charming tree-lined street, and it is nothing to see twenty or thirty people on line stretching around the corner to gain access to the privilege of purchasing one of these coveted treats. What is their magic? My husband grew up on cupcakes, so once I bought him one of this store's famous "cakes" for his birthday. Surprise: he couldn't finish it and did not enjoy it. He said it was so sweet it was what we call *écœurant* (the extreme opposite of appetizing).

The second surprise came when I was passing by the shop early in the morning (before the lines) with a young foreign friend who wanted to take a picture of it. We talked with one of the staff to ask about the icing and colouring and he said, "You don't want to know or you wouldn't touch the stuff." We explained that we had no intention of buying, even less eating them, but were just taking pictures for a New York photo album. Then he added, "The icing is bad enough, but the inside is just as bad." (Now how's that for a loyal and helpful employee? Or should I say former employee . . .)

The store is such a curiosity that I've also watched on many occasions, particularly on weekend afternoons, people emerging victorious after their twenty minutes on line with a cupcake or more and then devouring it in under two minutes (more like one minute) flat out right there on the street outside the shop. Forget the pleasure factor; that's not savouring or experiencing pleasure. That's a quick fix. And what does that do to your body? I suspect you'll be craving sweets for days. It surely sends the wrong message to your brain, and yet so many of us wonder about our cravings. Enough studies have proved that sugary treats trigger mood swings tied to our soaring blood sugar levels and prime us for energy crashes followed by more cravings for sweets. What a vicious circle. Sweets are tough to walk away from, so it's up to you to come up with the tricks that work for you: don't walk by the pastry shops (that's one of mine), don't bring home more than a reasonable portion of dessert or you'll eat the whole thing, avoid strange encounters of the sugary kind at work—walk away.

Enough. This chapter is a celebration of desserts and the pleasures they bring (really) and not a discourse on their evil ways. One of the things I have been implicitly highlighting, and now explicitly, is that desserts and other sweets should not exist often in isolation. Okay, an ice cream cone now and again is a pleasure not a crime. At the end of a meal laden with protein and varied food groups, a dessert is a perfect and healthy closure. Enjoy it. Just remember portion size and balance over a few days.

Prufrock may have "known them all already, known them all:—/have known the evenings, mornings, afternoons,/. . . have measured out my life with coffee spoons . . ." Well, I have tasted them all, eaten them all. I have measured out my life with chocolate mousse, apricot tart, cannelé, tiramisù, crème brûlée, éclair, blueberry tart, opéra, mille-feuille. No regrets. My weight is still normal. (I should have mentioned coffee ice cream.)

Here then for your pleasure, I offer desserts that are mostly made with fresh fruits plus the occasional tart or cake and, *bien sûr*, a little chocolate that will satisfy you with a mini portion. Enjoy.

APPLE COMPOTE
WITH PISTACHIOS

• SERVES 4 •

. . . .

*4 Golden Delicious apples,
peeled, cored, and cut
into small dice*

1 tablespoon lemon juice

*2 tablespoons unsalted
butter*

3 tablespoons sugar

1 cinnamon stick

*2 tablespoons pistachio nuts,
chopped*

1. Combine the apples and lemon juice.

2. Melt the butter in a medium sauté pan over medium-low heat. Add the apples, sugar, and cinnamon stick and cook for 20 minutes, stirring occasionally. Add the pistachios and cook for an additional 10 minutes. Remove the apple compote from the pan and serve at room temperature, garnished with the cinnamon stick.

PEAR AND DATE AU GRATIN

• SERVES 4 •

3 ripe Comice pears, peeled, cored, and thinly sliced

8 dates, julienned

4 egg yolks

⅛ teaspoon wasabi (this Japanese horseradish adds a touch of spicy heat and flavour)

110g crème fraîche

1. Preheat the grill or set the oven to 200°C/gas mark 6 and grease four individual ramekins with butter.

2. Divide the sliced pears and dates equally among four ramekins.

3. In a stand mixer and using a whisk attachment, mix together the egg yolks and wasabi. Add the crème fraîche and mix until combined.

4. Pour the crème fraîche mixture over the fruit and place under the grill for 4 minutes (or place in the oven for 8 minutes). Remove from the oven and serve warm.

FRUIT SALAD WITH QUINOA

• SERVES 4 TO 6 •

· ·

175g quinoa

*110ml freshly squeezed
grapefruit juice*

3 tablespoons honey

½ teaspoon lime zest

*450g mixed fruit (such as
strawberries, grapes,
melon, blueberries, and
raspberries)*

Fresh mint sprigs

1. Cook the quinoa according to the package instructions. Drain and cool.

2. In a small bowl, whisk together the grapefruit juice, honey, and lime zest. Set aside.

3. Prepare the fruit: slice the strawberries and grapes in half; peel and dice the melon. Place all the fruit in a serving bowl and add the cooled quinoa. Add the grapefruit juice mixture and toss gently to combine. Garnish with mint and serve.

Smoothies and Verrines

Verrines are those small, clear glass containers—some only a bit taller and a bit bigger than shot glasses and other glass sizes—the French have fallen in love with to serve savoury or sweet food. Go to one of those grand three Michelin–star restaurants and wannabes and the pricey menus include additional free goodies, often including one, two, or three miniature verrines as preappetizers and also sometimes as predesserts. It has been an increasing trend for at least a decade. Nowadays, home cooks are getting the hang of serving an appetite opener or modest tasting in a glass as they have been featured in magazines, pastry shops, television cooking programmes, and small cookbooks dedicated exclusively to the art of the verrine.

To me, their first and best appeal is visual. The layers (often three), colours, textures, and top garnish make them look like a small piece of art, and three in a row on an oblong dish can easily look like a miniature painting that you can actually eat. I've been serving them for years, especially in the summer in Provence and the "wow" sign is a given when they appear on the breakfast table, a buffet, a party, or a sit-down meal. Bringing the same food in a bowl or dish just does not create that surprise.

The concept is also a practical one (no doubt a reason French women love it) as verrines can be prepared in advance, eaten anywhere from a terrace (yours or a café), a bench in a park, a picnic, or any party where people can move around eating or drinking. And the portions are small: It really is all in the three bites, *n'est-ce pas?*

Smoothies—a big, very big, cousin of sorts (a few times removed) of verrines—gained popularity in America first before becoming globalized (no doubt every culture will have some claim on their origin; blended fruits and vegetables are hardly new, but the widespread availability of electric blenders is). The best are those freshly made and consumed before the vitamins and other elements start to degrade. Beware of those in supermarkets, where additional sugars of the strange kind are added. And beware of preservatives and artificial ingredients in the processed variety.

RED BERRY SMOOTHIE

75g fresh strawberries,
rinsed and hulled

100g frozen raspberries

150g plain Greek-style
yogurt

110ml apple juice

Place all the ingredients in a blender and purée until smooth. Serve at once.

RASPBERRY-BANANA SMOOTHIE

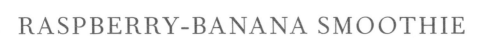

• SERVES 2 •

150g plain Greek-style
    yogurt

110ml 2% milk

100g frozen raspberries

1 ripe banana, peeled and
    sliced

Place all the ingredients in a blender and purée
until smooth. Serve at once.

RHUBARB SMOOTHIE

• SERVES 2 •

225g rhubarb, cut into
    small pieces

1 teaspoon honey

Zest and juice of 1 orange

1 banana, peeled and sliced

2 to 4 fresh or frozen
    strawberries

1. In a small saucepan, combine the rhubarb, honey, and orange zest. Add 55 ml water, cover, and cook over low heat until the rhubarb is very tender, about 20 minutes.

2. Remove the saucepan from the heat and cool (this may be done in advance).

3. Place the rhubarb in a blender with the orange juice, banana, and strawberries and purée. Serve immediately.

RASPBERRY-BLACKBERRY RICE PUDDING VERRINES

150 g raspberries, rinsed and patted dry with paper towels

150 g blackberries, rinsed and patted dry with paper towels

150 g sugar

250 g pudding rice

300 ml milk, whole or 2%

1 teaspoon pure vanilla extract

4 egg yolks

50 g butter

150 g strawberries, rinsed, patted dry with paper towels, and cut into halves

Fresh mint sprigs

1. Put the raspberries and blackberries in a salad bowl and cover with 25 g of sugar. Reserve in the refrigerator.

2. Bring 225 ml water to a boil. Add the rice and cook for 2 minutes in boiling water. Drain and reserve.

3. Bring the milk to a boil in a heavy saucepan. Add the rice, the remaining 110 g sugar, and the vanilla. Cook over low heat for 30 minutes and stir gently a couple of times. It is important to watch this process so that the rice does not get gluey. Off the heat, add the egg yolks one at a time, add the butter, and over low heat combine and cook for 1 minute. Let the mixture cool.

4. Add 2 tablespoons water to the raspberry-blackberry mixture and put through a sieve to obtain a coulis. Cover the bottom of the verrines with the coulis. Top with the rice pudding. Garnish with the strawberries and fresh mint.

PINEAPPLE, YOGURT, AND CHOCOLATE VERRINES

1 fresh pineapple

Zest and juice of 1 orange

Pinch of saffron

100 g dark chocolate, chopped (70% to 80% cacao preferred)

3 tablespoons 2% milk

225 g plain Greek-style yogurt

1 tablespoon crème fraîche

1. Peel and core the pineapple, then cut into small dice. In a medium bowl, combine the pineapple, orange zest and juice, and saffron. Reserve.

2. Place the chocolate in a bowl. Pour the milk into a small saucepan and bring to a simmer. Remove from the heat, pour the milk over the chocolate, and let stand for 2 minutes before stirring the chocolate until smooth. Allow the chocolate to cool until just warm to the touch.

3. When the chocolate has cooled, add the yogurt, crème fraîche, and 1 to 2 tablespoons of juice from the chopped pineapple and stir until combined. Refrigerate for at least 15 minutes and up to 6 hours.

4. To serve, alternate layers of pineapple with a small amount of juice and the chocolate-yogurt mixture in individual serving bowls or small glasses. Serve at once.

CHOCOLATE-COFFEE VERRINES

• SERVES 6 TO 8 •

FOR THE COFFEE MOUSSE

4 egg whites

Pinch of salt

3 tablespoons strong
   espresso

150g sugar

FOR THE CHOCOLATE MOUSSE

350g dark chocolate (70%
   to 80% cacao preferred)

110g butter, at room
   temperature

2 egg yolks

5 egg whites

35g sugar

FOR THE GARNISH

Little squares of high-
   quality milk chocolate

Fresh mint sprigs

TO MAKE THE COFFEE MOUSSE

1. Beat the egg whites with a pinch of salt until very firm. Add the coffee and sugar while continuing to beat. Refrigerate for 2 hours.

TO MAKE THE CHOCOLATE MOUSSE

2. Melt the chocolate over a pot of simmering water. Remove from the heat and add the butter and egg yolks, mixing gently. Beat the egg whites with the sugar into soft peaks. Incorporate a third of the chocolate-butter mixture, mix, and add the rest, mixing delicately. Refrigerate for 2 hours.

3. To serve, put a layer of coffee mousse at the bottom of each verrine, top with a layer of chocolate mousse, and decorate with a square of milk chocolate and a sprig of mint.

CRÊPES

My New England friend, Sarah, who loves things French and studied cooking in Paris, lived on crêpes when she was a student there. She continued the practice as a busy stagiaire *in restaurants in France. Now that she's back in New England, this is her basic crêpe recipe.*

110g flour
280ml 2% or whole milk
2 eggs
2 tablespoons butter, melted
¼ teaspoon salt
Butter for pan

1. Combine the flour, milk, eggs, melted butter, and salt in a blender and mix just until combined, about 10 seconds (make sure the flour is fully incorporated).

2. Refrigerate the crêpe batter for at least 1 hour and up to 2 days before cooking.

3. Heat a small nonstick pan over medium-high heat and brush the surface with butter. Pour a small amount of batter onto the centre of the pan and swirl the pan to evenly distribute in a thin layer. Cook for about 30 seconds; the top of the crêpe will appear dry and the edges will start to crisp. Loosen the edges and flip with a spatula. Cook for another 10 seconds and carefully slide the crêpe onto a plate. Repeat with the remaining batter, brushing the pan surface lightly with butter each time. Crêpes may be stacked on top of one another and kept warm. Serve immediately.

VARIATIONS

SAVOURY: *Mix 2 tablespoons finely chopped chives (or another favourite herb) into the batter.*

SWEET: *Add 2 tablespoons of your favourite liqueur to the batter or 1 tablespoon citrus zest.*

For serving, try these toppings:

- *butter and sugar*

- *shaved bittersweet chocolate*

- *butter, lemon juice, sugar*

- *sliced fresh fruit and yogurt*

- *grated cheese, boiled ham*

- *Parmesan and grated apple*

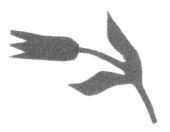

MANGO LASSI, THE FRENCH WAY

Tusshar, my French friend's companion, likes to drink mango lassi (a South Indian drink), but he used canned mango with syrup and added sugar. Not our cup of tea, we said. We like ours thicker and less sweet, and we serve it at the end of a meal. Kids love it. So here is our Frenchie version.

1 mango, peeled and diced

225 ml fromage blanc *(or buttermilk)*

225 ml water

2 teaspoons honey

Pinch of salt

Combine the mango with the *fromage blanc*, water, honey, and salt in a blender and purée at medium speed until smooth. Serve immediately.

YOGURT AND NUT "COCKTAIL"

• SERVES 2 •

330g plain Greek-style
yogurt

2 tablespoons chopped
almonds

2 tablespoons pine nuts

2 ice cubes

1 teaspoon cinnamon

3 teaspoons honey

1. Place half of the yogurt along with the almonds, pine nuts, and ice cubes in a blender and purée until smooth.

2. Add the remaining yogurt, cinnamon, and honey and blend again until smooth and frothy. Serve at once.

YOGURT AND FRUIT SALAD

• SERVES 4 •

1 pear, peeled, cored, and
  diced

2 kiwi, peeled and sliced

2 peaches, rinsed and cut
  into small dice

2 tablespoons sugar

25g pistachio nuts, coarsely
  chopped

1 banana, peeled and thinly
  sliced

450g plain goat milk yogurt
  (or cow's milk yogurt)

2 teaspoons strawberry or
  raspberry jam

1. Place the pear, kiwi, and peaches in a bowl and sprinkle with 1 tablespoon sugar. Mix gently, cover with plastic wrap, and refrigerate for 30 minutes.

2. Mix the remaining tablespoon of sugar with the pistachios and set aside.

3. To serve, add the banana slices to the fruit salad and gently toss. Divide the fruit salad among four clear glass bowls. Top with a layer of yogurt and sprinkle with pistachios. Garnish with a dollop of jam and serve.

YOGURT AND OATMEAL CAKE

225 ml boiling water

100 g old-fashioned oatmeal

Butter, softened for baking dish

150 g brown sugar

110 g granulated sugar

8 tablespoons (1 stick) unsalted butter, melted

2 eggs

150 g plain yogurt

1 teaspoon pure vanilla extract

165 g unbleached white flour

1 teaspoon baking powder

1 teaspoon baking soda

½ teaspoon salt

1 teaspoon cinnamon

½ teaspoon ground allspice

¼ teaspoon freshly grated nutmeg

1 teaspoon orange zest

Coffee ice cream (optional)

1. Pour the boiling water over the rolled oats and let stand for 15 minutes.

2. Preheat the oven to 180°C / gas mark 4. Butter a 20 cm × 30 cm baking dish and set aside.

3. In a large bowl, mix together the sugars and melted butter. Add the eggs and whisk until well blended. Stir in the yogurt and vanilla and set aside.

4. In a separate bowl, combine the flour, baking powder, baking soda, salt, and spices. Add half of the flour mixture and the oats to the wet ingredients and stir until blended. Add the remaining flour mixture and orange zest and mix gently until combined. Pour the batter into the baking dish and bake for 25 minutes or until a knife inserted all the way comes out clean. Remove from the oven and cool before cutting and serving. Serve with a scoop of coffee ice cream, if desired.

PANNA COTTA

• SERVES 8 •

· ·

My Tuscan friend, Emiliana, first introduced me to this moulded chilled dessert ages ago in a small, unpretentious restaurant in Forte dei Marmi, near Lucca. It was love at first sight and taste, and I'd never reveal how many times I've made panna cotta for added culinary entertainment. Guests often think it takes a great dessert maker to produce this—not at all. It's about the easiest, fastest dessert that has chutzpah, and it's impossible to blow it. I tell them so, but no one believes me. Try it.

1 tablespoon unflavoured gelatin

2 tablespoons cold water

225 ml 2% or whole milk

450 ml double cream

110 g sugar

1½ teaspoons pure vanilla extract

1. In a small saucepan, sprinkle the gelatin over the water and let soften for about 1 minute. Heat the mixture over low heat until the gelatin is dissolved. Remove from the heat.

2. In a large saucepan, bring the milk, cream, and sugar just to a boil over moderately high heat, stirring once in a while. Remove the pan from the heat and whisk in the gelatin mixture and vanilla. Divide the mixture among eight ramekins and cool to room temperature.

3. Cover with plastic film and chill for 4 hours or overnight.

4. To unmould, just before serving, dip the ramekins one at a time in a bowl of hot water for a few seconds. Run a thin knife around the edge of each ramekin and invert on the centre of a dessert plate.

NOTE: *Serve with fresh mixed berries (strawberries and blackberries or raspberries and blueberries) in the summer, an apple-pear compote or cranberry chutney in the winter, or make a fruit coulis with a mango. The choice of accompaniment is infinite. Place a mint or basil leaf in the middle of the panna cotta (this adds a nice colourful touch).*

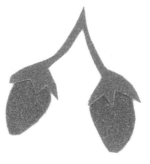

LEMON CURD

After tomatoes and strawberries, lemon is probably my favourite fruit (today at least, but cherries or apricots don't count as their season is, alas, so short). I use lemon with abandon for my magical breakfast but also with fish, veggies, salads, and in citron pressé *as a thirst quencher. Then, there are desserts, and a French lemon tart (oh so tart and tangy) is one of my favourite things. You can keep the meringue. Here is a curd I often make and use to make* tartines *for visiting kids or to make a last-minute tart and garnish a pâte brisée mould or make small individual tarts. Of course, you can also use the curd in a verrine with a dollop of cream and store-bought tuile cookies.*

150 ml lemon juice (about 3 lemons, preferably organic)

2 teaspoons lemon zest

6 egg yolks

150 g sugar

¾ teaspoon butter

1. In a stainless-steel bowl over simmering water, combine the lemon juice, lemon zest, egg yolks, and sugar and whisk continuously until the mixture is smooth and has thickened to the consistency of sour cream, 8 to 10 minutes.

2. Remove the bowl from over the water, add the butter and continue whisking until smooth and the curd has cooled a bit. Cover with plastic wrap and refrigerate for 24 hours.

NOTE: *Curd will keep for 1 week, chilled and covered. Since it's addictive, you may want to double the recipe next time you make it. Save and use the egg whites for omelettes or frittatas.*

(EGGLESS) CHOCOLATE MOUSSE WITH CARDAMOM

• SERVES 4 •

6 cardamom pods, slightly crushed

450 ml double cream

150 g dark chocolate (70 to 80% cacao preferred), chopped

1 tablespoon pistachio nuts, shelled and toasted

1. Place the cardamom and 110 ml double cream in a small, heavy saucepan and bring to a boil. Meanwhile, place the chopped chocolate in a large bowl. Remove the saucepan from the heat and pour the cream through a fine-mesh sieve over the chopped chocolate. Allow the chocolate to melt for 2 minutes, then stir until smooth; cool until the chocolate-cream mixture is just warm to the touch.

2. Whip the remaining chilled double cream until stiff peaks form (be careful not to overwhip). Gently fold half of the whipped cream into the chocolate mixture to lighten and then incorporate the remaining whipped cream; the mousse will be a bit soft. Spoon the mousse into serving dishes, cover, and refrigerate for at least 2 hours. Before serving, garnish with pistachio nuts.

MADELEINES AU CHOCOLAT

Madeleines, those cookie-size, shell-shape cakes, may make you reread Proust's Remembrance of Things Past *(although dunking madeleines in tea is not my way of enjoying them, stale or not). My childhood memories are filled with eating freshly made madeleines by* Mamie. *None of my girlfriends' mothers ever made them since the local pâtisserie carried them. Apparently,* Mamie's *versions were better or shall we say different, freshly made and eaten only when warm. Usually, she made standard madeleines, although once in a while she would surprise us with our favourite,* les madeleines au chocolat. *The ritual was always the same: They were served for the* goûter, *afternoon snack after school, and I could bring a friend. In the spring, we would go outside and eat them at the garden table, and in wintertime, in our large kitchen, at the table, sometimes with hot chocolate. Just as Proust's madeleine started his journey of recollection, these "cookie-cakes" always remind me of a story from my own childhood (which my family referred to as* de la souris et des madeleines).*

When I went to primary school (age six) I made a new friend, Danielle, whom I invited home on a cold, snowy December day. Mamie *was working in the front of the house and announced that the madeleines were just out of the oven and cooling off in the kitchen. By then, I knew what to do (I never waited until they were at room temperature as I liked them best a touch warm). That day, however, as we entered the kitchen we spotted a mouse on the floor near the work area where the madeleines were resting. We were both equally scared of mice and jumped on the kitchen table speechless and paralyzed. Time passed, not a word was spoken, and neither of us would go down from the kitchen table while the mouse was wandering about ignoring us (fortunately not going near the madeleines but sniffing the aroma for sure). I don't remember how long we stood on that table (I can still see myself on the table), it felt like hours, but suddenly Mother came in wondering why there was such silence, and seeing us in that position started laughing her head off. She scared away the mouse. We blushed, and that day the madeleines did not taste the same, but it was not because they were completely cold. For years, every time my mother wanted to illustrate the gourmande I was, she would tell whoever was there the story de la souris et des madeleines. I still love chocolate madeleines best, and I still don't care for mice in the house. And who doesn't love chocolate?*

100g dark chocolate (70% to 80% cacao preferred)

6 tablespoons unsalted butter, cut into small pieces

55g plus 3 tablespoons all-purpose flour

1 teaspoon baking powder

2 large eggs

110g sugar

1. Combine the chocolate and butter in a bowl set over a pot of simmering water and melt, stirring until smooth. Remove the bowl from the heat and let cool.

2. In a small bowl, sift together the flour and baking powder and reserve.

3. In a stand mixer, whisk the eggs until frothy. Gradually add the sugar and continue whisking until the mixture is pale yellow and has thickened, 2 to 3 minutes. Add the cooled chocolate-butter mixture, folding it in gently until well combined. Carefully fold in the flour mixture and mix just until combined. Cover the batter and refrigerate for 3 hours.

4. Preheat the oven to 200°C/gas mark 6. Spoon the chilled batter in (preferably) nonstick madeleine moulds, filling them three quarters full. Bake for 11 to 13 minutes until they are puffed and spring back to the touch. Do not overbake. Remove from the oven and unmould directly onto a cooling rack. Serve slightly warm or at room temperature. Madeleines can be kept for 2 to 3 days in an airtight container.

SPICED CHOCOLATE MOUSSE

• SERVES 4 •

200g dark chocolate (70 to 80% cacao preferred), chopped

4 eggs, separated, at room temperature

75g plus 2 tablespoons sugar

110g crème fraîche

Zest of 1 orange

Zest of 1 lemon

Pinch of cinnamon

Pinch of freshly grated nutmeg

1 teaspoon pure vanilla extract

1. In a double boiler insert set over barely simmering water, melt the chocolate, stirring until smooth. Remove from the heat and let the chocolate cool slightly. It should feel warm but not hot to the touch.

2. Meanwhile, place the egg whites and a pinch of sugar in the bowl of a stand mixer and whisk for 2 to 3 minutes on medium-high speed while gradually incorporating half of the sugar. When the egg whites almost form stiff peaks, add the remaining sugar and beat until glossy. Remove the whipped egg whites and place in a large bowl. Clean the mixing bowl and add the crème fraîche, citrus zests, cinnamon, nutmeg, vanilla, and egg yolks and mix for 20 seconds on medium-high speed. Add the warm chocolate and beat until smooth.

3. Carefully fold the chocolate mixture into the egg whites and gently mix. Serve, garnished with additional crème fraîche and orange zest, if desired, or refrigerate, covered, until ready to serve. This may be made one day in advance (let stand at room temperature for 20 minutes before serving if chilled).

Chapter Six

PUTTING IT
ALL TOGETHER

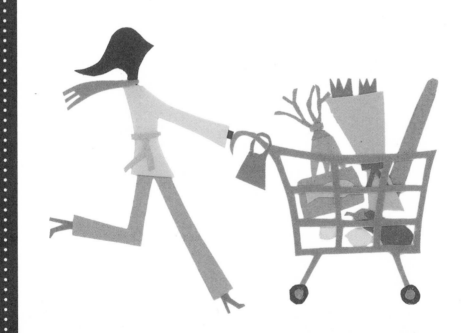

I love the phrase "putting it all together." It implies a little mental and manual dexterity, and in a world where so many things take so long to come together (ever move to a new house or apartment? Or renovate a kitchen or bath? Or write a marketing plan?) that they bring discomfort not comfort, open-endedness not closure.

Planning and making a dish and planning a menu can be highly satisfying activities. Almost instant gratification. (Note I did not include cleaning up afterward.) I used to go to the office day after day and plug away on this campaign or that challenge only to return the next day and the next to continue the task. Cooking, however, is where you can get your hands dirty and in short order eat your efforts. That's satisfaction. What's not great and healthy about that?

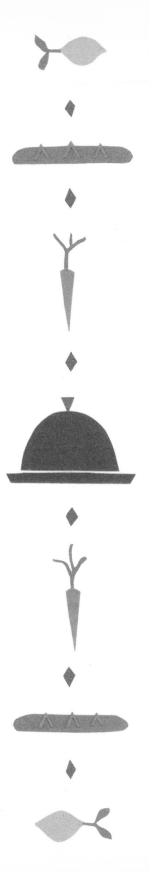

As a CEO I used knowledge and experience more than intellect. Perhaps intellect got me where I landed, but my value to my company was that I knew what to do immediately in a host of challenging situations. I knew how to read the tea leaves and react favourably. There is no substitute for experience or a knowledge base learned by fire. But I did not use the same brain cells that I did the first time I read Pascal. Sure, I gained satisfaction when I was part of a solution or part of a winning action, but mostly these played out over time, often months, regularly a year or more. In the kitchen, I had and have to plan, organize, and then juggle three things at once, be ready to adjust on the fly, and use brain cells—I would say intellect and focus—as challenging in the moment as I found in a corner office. And the reward—almost immediate. What a healthy sense of achievement when the dish comes out of the oven or is plated appealingly for dinner. Cooking is a form of mental health—at least for me.

And that's why I like "putting it all together." Besides, it is the title of a musical revue of Stephen Sondheim music that plays in my head when I say the phrase.

What follows are some basic menus and some not so basic entertainment menus. Think of them as a starting point, a stimulation point, perhaps a launching point. I like to read recipes, menus, and watch cooking shows. I almost never reproduce what I mentally ingest. But they are warm-ups for me and stimulate me to imagine what I would and indeed do in the kitchen. Perhaps what follows will do the same for you. But they might also help you break old habits and reinvent what you eat—to try something new and to learn a new song. Sometimes we all need a little easy follow-along guidance to move on down the road.

Here are a few more divergent thoughts on menus, consumption, and balance. First is to remember the phrase "exceptions prove the rule." I believe in a three meals a day rule, with the following exception. Sometimes, two will have to do. That happens, say, when you are traveling in different time zones. Or you sleep exceedingly late on vacation, in another time zone or not, then brunch is the order of the day. Remember to balance your intake over time so you don't run down or overeat later. When you are down to two meals, add some protein such as eggs, ham, or even some smoked salmon to your initial meal. Then to pace your body and energy level, you'll need some sort of "snack" before dinner (three meals), even just a few nuts (and I really mean a few as in three to five); for me, a good choice is always a mix of plain yogurt with fruit.

Beware of too much raw veggies at any time, particularly in the summer months. The fashion for eating raw did not last very long in the United States and for good and obvious reasons. If raw vegetables fill you up due to their water and fibre content, you'll eat less of a main course but risk getting hungry a few hours later and a call for fat or sweet stuff (read cupcake or cereal bar, or fill in the blank) will be waiting for you. They also may get boring in taste and texture and chewing action, inhibiting diversity of experience and pleasure.

As for sweet stuff, the best placement is to eat dessert at the end of a meal. No news there. But why? This way they assimilate better and more slowly than if eaten by themselves in the middle of the day outside mealtimes. And with dessert you give your body its "sweet" craving dose on a semi-full stomach with *you* controlling (and capable of controlling) the portion.

In putting it all together, remember to avoid fried foods as much as possible and when included in a meal to really remember portion sizes (that small apple is a normal portion rule). You also need to be sensitive to your intake of fatty and overly salty food. Salt makes you want to eat more, which easily explains why crisp addicts eat the whole bag, mostly on autopilot and not realizing that salt calls for more salt just as sugar calls for more sugar. And salt makes you thirsty and what you subsequently drink can increase your imbalances of the unhealthy kind. And if these mini reminders seem basic, I have learned from my websites and presentations, including television appearances and "makeover" spots, how often we are blind to the truth about what we're putting into our bodies. Hey, I used to put a lot of sugar in my coffee—now none.

Favour soups at lunch and dinner and at any season. They are easy and healthy additions to most menus. Many of us don't think about soup in the summertime, but almost any *soupe glacée* is delicious and our body loves their cool refreshment. In my case, whatever is left in my veggie bin—a few peppers, tomatoes, cucumber, whatever—is rinsed, roughly chopped, and with herbs, spices, water added, plus a few minutes in the blender, ready to be served with a drizzle of olive oil, fresh herbs, and a slice of whole wheat or any good bread.

For those who enjoy and are able to eat seafood, there are lots of healthy and pleasure bonuses, and as they are not readily gulped down fast, they force well-paced ingestion. Even peeling your prawns or cleaning your lobster takes time. Remember it takes 20 minutes for the satiety signal to kick in, so don't rush your meal or you may well overeat. Sit down, chew, and savour; all are necessary for assimilation and digestion. And you'll keep a flat stomach, too.

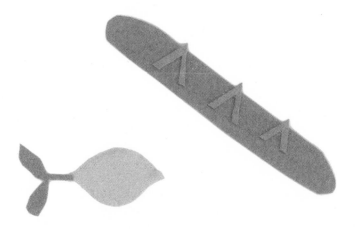

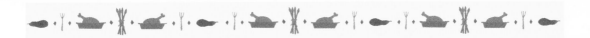

ORDINARY DAY

BREAKFAST

Glass of water

Grandma Louise's Oatmeal with Grated Apple

Slice of toasted whole wheat bread, buttered

Coffee or tea

LUNCH

Carrot and Orange Soup

Prawns and Fennel Salad

Yogurt and ½ grapefruit

Non-calorific beverage (or glass of white wine, but no wine at dinner)

DINNER

A few green olives (as an hors d'oeuvre and appetizer substitute)

Roasted Chicken with Endives

1 pear, 2 squares dark chocolate

Wine (optional): a glass of white (perhaps a New World Chardonnay)
or light or medium red (perhaps a Côtes-du-Rhône)

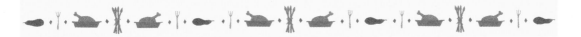

GRANDMA LOUISE'S OATMEAL
WITH GRATED APPLE

• SERVES 2 TO 4 •

My grandmother's oatmeal, which made its way into FWDGF, *is my idea of how to start the day with a yummy healthy breakfast, and it was heartily endorsed. I admit I've made the oatmeal for dinner now and then, particularly when I am alone and don't have much choice in the fridge.*

175 g old-fashioned oatmeal

525 ml water

Pinch of salt

1 medium apple, coarsely
   grated

½ teaspoon lemon juice

⅓ cup milk, whole or 2%

½ teaspoon butter

Brown sugar (or maple
   syrup) for serving

1. Combine the oatmeal, water, and salt. Bring to a boil.

2. Add the apple and lemon juice and cook for about 5 minutes, stirring occasionally.

3. Finish cooking by adding the milk and butter. Stir well. Serve immediately with a splash of brown sugar or a drizzle of maple syrup.

CARROT AND ORANGE SOUP

• SERVES 6 TO 8 •

4 tablespoons (½ stick)
unsalted butter

½ large onion, peeled and
chopped

450g carrots, peeled and
chopped

Zest of 1 orange

1 medium potato, peeled
and chopped

900ml chicken broth or
water

110ml milk, whole or 2%

Salt and freshly ground
pepper

1. Melt the butter in a large pot over medium-high heat. Add the onion and sauté until softened, 4 to 5 minutes.

2. Add the carrots, orange zest, potato, and chicken broth and bring to a boil. Cover, lower the heat, and simmer until the vegetables are tender, about 30 minutes.

3. Carefully transfer the mixture to a food mill or blender and purée until smooth. Add the milk and season to taste. This soup may be served hot or chilled.

PRAWN AND FENNEL SALAD

· SERVES 4 ·

1 shallot, chopped

2 tablespoons lemon juice

1 teaspoon fennel seeds

1 tablespoon sherry vinegar

4 tablespoons olive oil

Salt and freshly ground
  pepper

2 fennel bulbs, trimmed,
  cored, and thinly sliced

225 g medium prawns,
  cooked and peeled

1 apple, peeled, cored, and
  diced

1. In a small bowl, combine the shallot, lemon juice, fennel seeds, and sherry vinegar. Whisk in the olive oil and season to taste.

2. In a medium serving bowl, combine the fennel, prawns, and apple. Add the dressing and gently toss. Serve at once.

ROASTED CHICKEN
WITH ENDIVES

• SERVES 4 •

1 (1.8 kg) free-range
    chicken

2 lemons

1 tablespoon olive oil

Salt and freshly ground
    pepper

1 large red onion, peeled
    and thinly sliced

25 g peeled and coarsely
    chopped shallots

225 ml white wine (or dry
    vermouth)

2 tablespoons unsalted
    butter

4 endives, washed, dried,
    and quartered

1. Preheat the oven to 230°C/gas mark 8.

2. Rinse the chicken and pat dry. Slice 1 lemon and place inside the cavity. Rub the outside of the chicken with olive oil and season all over (including the cavity). Place the chicken in a roasting pan, place the pan in the oven, and cook for 30 minutes.

3. Reduce the temperature to 180°C/gas mark 4 and continue cooking for 15 minutes. Add the onion and shallots to the roasting pan and continue cooking for another 15 minutes.

4. Add the white wine to the roasting pan, reduce the temperature to 150°C/gas mark 2, and cook for an additional 30 minutes or until the juices run clear when the chicken is pierced with a fork. The total cooking time is about 1½ hours.

5. While the chicken roasts, melt 1 tablespoon butter in a frying pan over medium-high heat and brown the endives on both sides, about 5 minutes.

continued on next page

Press the juice of 1 lemon and add to the endives. Season to taste, reduce the heat to medium-low, and continue cooking until the endives are tender, about 10 minutes.

6. Remove the chicken from the oven and reserve the juices from both the chicken and endives. Strain the combined juices into a small saucepan. Skim the fat and simmer over medium-high heat until slightly reduced, 3 to 5 minutes. Stir in the remaining tablespoon of butter and season to taste.

7. Carve the chicken into pieces and arrange on a serving platter surrounded by the endives. Serve family style accompanied by sauce.

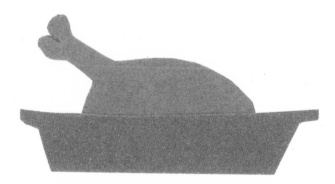

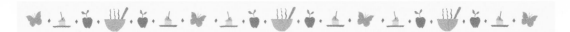

LIGHT WORK DAY

⌁ BREAKFAST ⌁

Glass of water

Granola with ½ banana and 2% milk

Slivers of 1 or 2 cheeses (such as Gruyère or Cantal or Parmesan)

Coffee or tea

⌁ LUNCH ⌁

Velouté of Haricots Verts with Peppers and Ham

Bruschetta with Endive

Yogurt with berries

Non-calorific beverage

⌁ DINNER ⌁

Leeks and Onion Parmesan

Roasted Daurade (Sea Bream) with Vegetables

Tarte au Chocolat

Wine: a glass of Chardonnay or in warm weather a still rosé

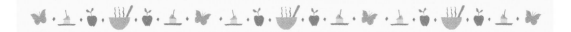

VELOUTÉ OF HARICOTS VERTS WITH PEPPERS AND HAM

· SERVES 4 TO 6 ·

1 tablespoon olive oil

2 medium shallots, peeled
and chopped

2 garlic cloves, peeled and
chopped

2 bell peppers (mix of red,
orange, or yellow),
seeded and chopped

2 medium potatoes, peeled
and diced

450g haricots verts (fresh or
frozen)

1.3 litres water

Salt and freshly ground
pepper

2 tablespoons crème fraîche

75g low-salt boiled ham,
cut into small dice

2 tablespoons finely chopped
fresh parsley

1. Heat the olive oil in a large pot over medium heat. Add the shallots and garlic and sauté until fragrant and softened, about 2 minutes. Add the peppers and sauté another minute. Add the potatoes, haricots verts, and water and bring to a boil. Cover, reduce the heat, and simmer for 20 minutes or until the vegetables are tender.

2. Carefully transfer the cooked vegetables to a blender and add just enough of the cooking liquid to blend to the desired consistency. Season to taste.

3. This soup may be served warm or chilled. Before serving, add the crème fraîche and stir well. Garnish with the ham and parsley and serve.

BRUSCHETTA WITH ENDIVES

• SERVES 4 •

1 head endive

3 tablespoons olive oil plus
additional for bread

2 tablespoons lemon juice

Salt and freshly ground
pepper

3 teaspoons white wine
vinegar

1 tablespoon golden raisins

4 slices country bread

1 garlic clove, peeled and
halved

1 teaspoon finely chopped
fresh rosemary

1 tablespoon pine nuts,
lightly toasted

1. Preheat the oven to 220°C/gas mark 7.

2. Trim the outer leaves of the endive and split into quarters. Rinse well and pat dry. Heat 1 tablespoon olive oil in a large frying pan over medium-high heat and add the endive. Cook, stirring, until it begins to wilt, about 5 minutes. Add the lemon juice and season to taste.

3. In a small bowl, combine the vinegar and raisins and set aside.

4. Lightly brush the bread with olive oil, rub with the cut side of the garlic, and lightly season with salt. Place directly on the oven rack and toast lightly, about 6 minutes.

5. Meanwhile, in a small bowl, whisk together the rosemary, vinegar and raisins, pine nuts, and the remaining 2 tablespoons olive oil. Season to taste.

6. To serve, place one quarter of the endive on each toast and spoon the vinaigrette on top.

LEEKS AND ONION PARMESAN

• SERVES 4 •

*6 leeks, white parts and
2–5 cm of green, washed*

2 tablespoons butter

2 tablespoons olive oil

*Salt and freshly ground
pepper*

*3 large red onions, peeled
and thinly sliced*

1 teaspoon lemon juice

¼ teaspoon fennel seeds

*Pinch of freshly grated
nutmeg*

50 g Parmesan

*2 tablespoons chopped fresh
parsley*

1. Cut each leek in half lengthwise and slice each half into thin strips. In a frying pan, heat 1 tablespoon of butter and 1 tablespoon of olive oil over medium-low heat and sauté the leeks until soft, 12 to 15 minutes. Season to taste.

2. Meanwhile, in a separate pan, heat the remaining tablespoon butter and olive oil and cook the onions until soft, about 10 minutes. Deglaze the pan with the lemon juice, stir in the fennel seeds and nutmeg, and season to taste.

3. To serve, place the warm leeks at the bottom of each plate. Cover with the sautéed onions and garnish with shavings of Parmesan (using a vegetable peeler) and chopped parsley.

ROASTED *DAURADE* (SEA BREAM) WITH VEGETABLES

• SERVES 4 •

3 onions, peeled and sliced

3 potatoes, peeled and sliced

2 yellow peppers, peeled and sliced

4 tomatoes, peeled and sliced

4 tablespoons olive oil

Salt and freshly ground pepper

4 (110–150g) sea bream fillets

Juice of 1 lemon

10g chopped fresh coriander

1 lemon, sliced

1. Preheat the oven to 200°C/gas mark 6.

2. Place the onions, potatoes, yellow peppers, and tomatoes in a baking dish. Add 2 tablespoons olive oil, toss to combine, and season to taste. Cover the dish with foil, place in the oven, and bake until the vegetables are tender and a bit caramelized, about 30 minutes.

3. Uncover the baking dish, add the fillets, and pour the remaining 2 tablespoons olive oil and lemon juice over the fish and vegetables. Season to taste and continue cooking, uncovered, until the vegetables are tender, about 8 minutes.

4. Remove from the oven and serve immediately, garnished with coriander and lemon slices.

TARTE AU CHOCOLAT

• MAKES ONE 20 cm TART •

. . . .

*1 recipe pâte brisée or pie
dough (store-bought or
homemade) for 9-inch
pie*

*175 g dark chocolate (70 to
80% cacao preferred),
chopped*

75 ml 2% or whole milk

75 ml double cream

4 tablespoons sugar

4 egg yolks

1. Preheat the oven to 200°C/gas mark 6.

2. Line a 20 cm tart pan with the pastry dough. Prick the bottom of the dough with a fork and cover the dough with foil, crimping the foil over the edges of the mould. Add dry beans or pellets and bake for 10 minutes. Remove the beans or pellets and foil and cook for another 5 minutes or until the tart shell is lightly golden. Remove from the oven and cool.

3. Lower the oven temperature to 140°C/gas mark 1. Place the chocolate in a double boiler insert set above simmering water over medium heat and melt, stirring occasionally.

4. Meanwhile, place the milk, cream, and sugar in a small heavy saucepan and bring to a simmer over low heat, whisking to dissolve the sugar. Remove from the heat and add the milk-cream mixture to the melted chocolate, stirring until smooth. Set aside and allow to cool a bit before whisking in the egg yolks.

5. Pour the chocolate mixture into the tart shell and bake for 20 minutes or until the filling is just set. Remove from the oven and cool before un-moulding and serving.

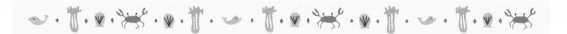

FISH DAY

⁓ BREAKFAST ⁓

Glass of water

Lemon Ricotta Pancakes

Coffee or tea

⁓ LUNCH ⁓

Avocado-Apple Salad with Gambas

Red snapper en Papillote

Yogurt with Crème Chocolat

⁓ DINNER ⁓

Scallop "Ceviche" with Mango and Parmesan

Skate à la Grenobloise

Cheese platter

Apricot Tart

Wine: a glass of Sancerre or other fruity but dry white

LEMON RICOTTA PANCAKES

• SERVES 4 TO 6 •

. . . .

*4 tablespoons unsalted
    butter, melted*

6 eggs, separated

335 g fresh ricotta

25 g white flour

25 g whole wheat flour

75 g sugar

Zest of 2 lemons

*1 tablespoon poppy seeds
    (optional)*

*Maple syrup (or honey) for
    serving*

1. Mix all the ingredients except the egg whites until just combined.

2. Beat the egg whites to soft peaks and gently fold into the mixture.

3. Heat a large nonstick frying pan over medium heat. Spoon the batter by tablespoonfuls (I prefer mini sizes—it feels like more when it is actually less) into the hot pan, and when holes appear in the pancakes, flip them and cook for another minute or two, until golden. Repeat until all the batter is used. Serve immediately with a drizzle of maple syrup or honey.

AVOCADO-APPLE SALAD
WITH GAMBAS

• SERVES 4 •

8 large prawns in the shell

Salt and freshly ground
    pepper

3 tablespoons olive oil

Juice of 2 limes

2 ripe avocados, peeled and
    sliced

2 Granny Smith apples,
    rinsed and cut into
    matchsticks

10 g fresh coriander,
    roughly chopped

1. Season the prawns to taste. Heat 1 tablespoon olive oil in a large frying pan over medium heat, add the prawns, reduce the heat, and cook over medium-low heat for 10 minutes. Remove from the heat and reserve.

2. In a large bowl, whisk together the lime juice with the remaining 2 tablespoons olive oil. Add the sliced avocados and apples, season to taste, and gently toss.

3. Peel the prawns, keeping the tails on. Add the prawns to the salad and garnish with the coriander. Serve immediately.

RED SNAPPER *EN PAPILLOTE*

1 teaspoon olive oil plus additional for greaseproof paper

2 medium tomatoes, rinsed and thinly sliced

1 lemon, rinsed and thinly sliced

1 courgette, rinsed and cut into matchsticks

Salt and freshly ground pepper

4 (110–150 g) red snapper fillets

1 cup fresh lemon verbena leaves

Fleur de sel

1. Preheat the oven to 190°C/gas mark 5.

2. Cut four pieces of greaseproof paper into 30 cm × 40 cm rectangles and brush the centres with olive oil. Place one quarter of the tomato and lemon slices and courgette matchsticks in the centre of the first piece of greaseproof paper and season to taste. Top with 1 red snapper fillet, a sprinkle of verbena leaves, and a drizzle of olive oil, and season to taste. Seal the packet by bringing up the sides to the centre and folding down tightly. Seal the ends by folding each in tightly. Repeat with the remaining ingredients, creating four packets.

3. Place the packets on a baking sheet and bake for 12 to 15 minutes. Open, sprinkle with fleur de sel, and serve immediately.

YOGURT WITH
CRÈME CHOCOLAT

• SERVES 4 •

55 ml double cream

110 g dark chocolate (70% to 80% cacao preferred), finely chopped

450 g plain Greek-style yogurt

1. Heat the cream in a small saucepan over low heat until it reaches a simmer. Place the chocolate in a medium bowl and pour the hot cream over the chocolate. Let stand for 2 minutes, then stir until smooth.

2. Divide the yogurt evenly among four small bowls and top with the chocolate cream. Serve immediately.

SCALLOP "CEVICHE" WITH MANGO AND PARMESAN

• SERVES 4 •

8 medium sea scallops, tough muscles removed and each cut horizontally into 4 slices

1 tablespoon lemon juice

Salt and freshly ground pepper

½ ripe mango, peeled and cut into matchsticks

25 g Parmesan, shaved using a vegetable peeler

1 teaspoon extra virgin olive oil

1. In a medium bowl, gently toss the sliced scallops with lemon juice and season to taste.

2. Slightly overlap 8 slices of scallops in a circle on each plate. Place a small amount of mango in the centre of the circle and top with a few shavings of Parmesan. Drizzle with olive oil and season to taste. Serve immediately.

SKATE *À LA GRENOBLOISE*

• SERVES 4 •

700g potatoes, peeled and
cut into 1 cm dice

Salt and freshly ground
pepper

4 (200g) boned skate wings

25g unbleached all-purpose
flour

6 tablespoons unsalted
butter

35g capers, drained

4 slices baguette or country
bread, cut into 5mm dice
and sautéed in butter
until golden

20g finely chopped fresh
parsley

1 lemon, sliced

1. Place the diced potatoes in a steamer insert set over a pot of boiling water and cook for 12 minutes or until soft. Season to taste and keep warm.

2. Season the skate wings with salt and pepper and dredge in the flour, shaking off any excess. Melt 2 tablespoons butter in a large nonstick frying pan over medium-high heat and cook the skate until golden brown and just cooked through, about 3 minutes per side.

3. Remove the skate from the pan and melt the remaining 4 tablespoons butter, swirling the pan, until the butter begins to brown and smell slightly nutty. Quickly remove the pan from the heat and add the capers (be careful; the butter may splatter).

4. Place one piece of skate and some steamed potatoes on each plate. Spoon the butter-caper sauce over the skate and sprinkle with the croûtons and chopped parsley. Garnish with lemon slices and serve immediately.

APRICOT TART

Marsha, an American friend who lives in our village in Provence, was proud to announce that she had learned a new word, chapelure, *from her French friends who love to bake. She was making lots of fruit tarts from the abundance of local fruits at our village market, but she felt her open-top pies were too juicy and messy. So her neighbours suggested she make a* chapelure, *which refers mostly to a coating for savoury dishes to prevent them from "falling apart," but anyone local knew what it meant with regard to making a tart. The trick with a fruit tart is to add a mix of ground almonds with a bit of sugar and spread it on the dough, thus providing a binding and structure for fruit that is then added on top. After baking the dough and apricots, just sprinkle a bit of sugar on top of the tart when it comes out of the oven. As the apricot season is one of the shortest of the fruit seasons, I always look forward to it and my annual apricot "cure" (a fruit-only diet orgy), which includes an apricot tart, to which I add some slivers of almond on top.*

1 recipe pâte brisée (store-bought or homemade) for a 9-inch tart

55 g blanched almonds, finely ground

55 g plus 2 teaspoons sugar

700–900 g fresh apricots, rinsed, cut in halves, and pitted

2 teaspoons honey

3 tablespoons slivered almonds, lightly toasted

Crème fraîche (optional)

1. Preheat the oven to 200°C/gas mark 6. On a lightly floured surface roll the dough to a 30 cm round. Transfer to a 20 cm fluted tart pan with a removable bottom. Prick the dough lining the bottom of the pan with a fork. Cover and chill for 10 minutes. Place the tart in the oven and par-bake for 10 minutes. Remove from the oven and reduce the temperature to 190°C/gas mark 5.

2. In a food processor, combine the blanched almonds and 55 g sugar and pulse just until the almonds are finely ground. Spread the mixture evenly over the bottom of the tart. Place the apricot

halves, cut side down, on top, slightly overlapping. Drizzle with honey, place in the oven, and bake for 40 minutes or until the crust is lightly browned.

3. Remove from the oven and sprinkle with the slivered almonds and 2 teaspoons sugar. Serve warm or at room temperature with slightly sweetened crème fraîche, if desired.

VARIATION: *Other wonderful fruit tart options include peaches (or a mix of peaches and nectarines) with pistachio nuts instead of almonds, plums with lemon zest and cherries, or Italian plums with a dash of cinnamon.*

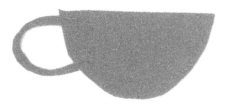

VALENTINE'S DAY DINNER

I always assumed that Valentine's Day was the biggest restaurant night for most couples. Sort of easy and still a rewarding way to celebrate—like guys buying girls flowers. It turns out Mother's Day is the big restaurant day, which makes sense—take Mom out of the kitchen for a day, no prepping, cooking, or cleaning for her at home (and easy on the kids and husband, plenty of food choices, and signing a credit card is the only hard labour involved). Valentine's Day is still a strong restaurant occasion, but as someone who ate in restaurants three hundred times a year during my Champagne career, dining at home was special, dining out was not (often it was plain work). And since for me cooking is an act of love, I like to stay home and celebrate Valentine's Day with a tête-à-tête dinner. I would cook up some of our special and not-everyday favourites and Edward would pick out a special bottle of wine. I appreciate that for some people, an assortment of children can get in the way sometimes, but surely there are occasional workarounds when, eventually or initially, there are no children around and Valentine's Day evening can be that very special romantic meal—corny to some but it remains a tradition, ritual, and renewal that is pleasurable, symbolic, and healthy. I recommend it. You might even consider the planning, preparation, and sharing that goes into making the meal a success a kind of gustatory foreplay.

HORS D'OEUVRE: *Caviar on toasts*

MAIN COURSE: *Duck Breasts* à la Gasconne *with Wild Rice*

SALAD COURSE À LA FRANÇAISE: *Salad of greens with lemon
and olive oil dressing (avoid vinegar when serving a good wine)*

CHEESE COURSE: *Slivers of three goat cheeses*

DESSERT: *Classic Chocolate Mousse*

WINE: *Champagne (or sparkling wine) to start, then a Pinot Noir
or a rosé Champagne throughout the meal*

DUCK BREASTS *À LA GASCONNE* WITH WILD RICE

Pinch of coarse salt

Pinch of crumbled bay leaves

Pinch of crumbled dried thyme leaves

½ teaspoon chopped fresh parsley

1 garlic clove, peeled and sliced

¼ teaspoon finely chopped shallots

4 peppercorns, coarsely crushed

2 (110g) duck magrets (breasts)

225 ml wild rice

1. In a large baking pan, mix the salt, bay leaves, thyme, parsley, garlic, shallots, and peppercorns. Roll the magrets in the mixture and spread them out, skin side up.

2. Cover with plastic and refrigerate the duck breasts for 24 hours, turning once.

3. Cook the wild rice according to the package directions. Drain and keep warm.

4. Remove the duck breasts from the marinade. Wipe or rinse to remove any excess seasoning; pat dry. Score the skin (so fat can render during cooking) diagonally at 1-inch intervals with a sharp knife to create a diamond pattern. (Discard the marinade.) Arrange the duck breasts, skin side down, on the grill rack (10 cm away from the heat). Grill for 1 to 2 minutes; turn over and grill for 3 to 4 minutes. The magrets should be medium-rare.

5. Place on a carving board and let rest for 2 to 3 minutes. Thinly slice the duck breast meat crosswise on the bias and serve on top of the wild rice.

CLASSIC CHOCOLATE MOUSSE

• SERVES 4 •

175g dark chocolate (70% to 80% cacao preferred), chopped

2 tablespoons unsalted butter, cut into small pieces

4 medium egg whites

Pinch of salt

2 tablespoons sugar

110ml double cream, chilled

1 teaspoon pure vanilla extract

Whipped cream and shaved chocolate (optional)

1. In a double boiler set over barely simmering water, melt the chocolate, stirring until smooth. Remove from the heat, stir in the butter, and let the chocolate cool until it's slightly warm but not hot to the touch.

2. In a mixing bowl, combine the egg whites and salt and beat until soft peaks form. Add the sugar and continue whisking until the egg whites form stiff, glossy peaks. Place the whipped egg whites in a large bowl and gently fold in a small amount of warm chocolate. Once incorporated, add the remaining chocolate, being careful not to overmix.

3. Place the chilled cream and vanilla in a clean mixing bowl and whip the cream until soft peaks form. Gently fold the whipped cream into the chocolate mixture in two batches. Divide the chocolate mousse among four dessert bowls and chill for 2 hours and up to 1 day. Remove from the refrigerator and let stand at room temperature for 20 minutes before serving. Chocolate mousse may be garnished with additional whipped cream and shaved chocolate, if desired.

NOTE: *Chocolate mousse for four on Valentine's Day? What kind of romance is that? The proper recipe calls for preparation of a portion larger than for two. So, compliments of the chef, eat the second portion the next day or two. Enjoy.*

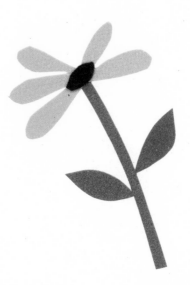

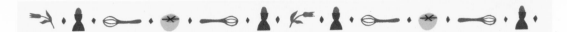

BRUNCH FOR 4 OR 8

(DOUBLE INGREDIENTS FOR 8)

Selection of cereal and fruit

Selection of breads and mini viennoiseries
(croissants, brioche, and pains au chocolat*)*

Scrambled Eggs with Herbs and Smoked Salmon–Bacon Toast

Crab Tartines *Avocado*

Coffee and tea

Sparkling wine or Champagne (optional)

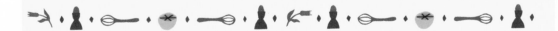

SCRAMBLED EGGS WITH HERBS AND SMOKED SALMON–BACON TOAST

• SERVES 4 •

8 eggs

Salt and freshly ground
  pepper

1 tablespoon butter

1 teaspoon water

1 tablespoon crème fraîche

2 tablespoons chopped fresh
  parsley

2 tablespoons chopped fresh
  chives

1 teaspoon chopped fresh
  dill

3 slices bacon

4 slices country whole wheat
  bread, toasted and
  buttered

4 slices smoked salmon

1. In a medium bowl, whisk the eggs together and season to taste. Melt the butter with 1 teaspoon water in a double boiler insert set over barely simmering water. Add the eggs and cook, stirring until thickened and just cooked through, about 6 minutes. Do not overcook, as you want the eggs to remain soft and creamy. Remove from the heat and stir in the crème fraîche and herbs. Keep warm.

2. In a sauté pan over medium-high heat, cook the bacon until crisp. Remove the bacon from the pan and drain on paper towels.

3. Place the buttered toasts horizontally on a cutting board and remove the crusts. Cover the top of each toast with 1 slice of salmon and cut each vertically into 3 *mouillettes* ("fingers"). Place 3 *mouillettes* on each plate and top with pieces of bacon, breaking the bacon to fit each *mouillette* as necessary. Spoon the eggs onto the plates and serve immediately.

CRAB *TARTINES* AVOCADO

• SERVES 4 •

1 ripe avocado, pitted and
   peeled

2 tablespoons lemon juice

½ teaspoon ground cumin

⅛ teaspoon hot sauce

1 garlic clove, peeled and
   chopped

1 small onion, peeled and
   chopped

½ medium tomato, diced

1 teaspoon chopped fresh
   coriander

Salt and freshly ground
   pepper

1 pink grapefruit

4 slices country bread,
   lightly toasted

225 g crabmeat, picked over
   for shells and cartilage,
   shredded

1. Place the avocado, lemon juice, cumin, hot sauce, garlic, and onion in a food processor and blend until smooth. Fold in the tomato and coriander, season to taste, and reserve in the refrigerator, covered, if not using immediately.

2. To prepare the grapefruit segments, cut slices off the top and bottom of the grapefruit and then slice away the peel and pith, top to bottom, following the curve of the fruit. Working over a bowl and using a small, sharp knife, cut between the membranes to release the segments.

3. To serve, spread toasted bread slices with the avocado mixture. Top with the shredded crabmeat, garnish with the grapefruit slices, and cut each *tartine* diagonally.

Chapter Seven

ONCE IN A WHILE A LITTLE CHAMPAGNE

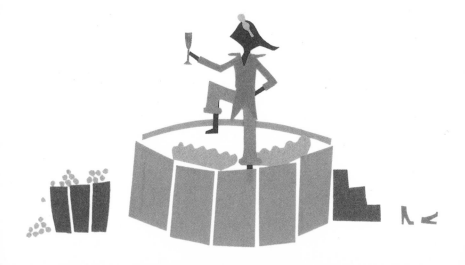

I recently had a couple from Brazil for lunch in Provence. After five years of living in Paris, they were getting ready to head back to São Paulo. While they had been to Provence before, they had not been to our corner of paradise, and I took them to the traditional Friday morning outdoor market (as in a centuries-old traditional village market) to shop for lunch. I was not surprised in the least when they chose a rotisserie chicken for their main dish. My guests often do, and so do I. There's a guy there (*c'est un phénomène,* as the French expression for a character goes) who roasts certified organic chickens in a specially built truck and rotisserie oven. Delicious. Typically French, he won't share the ingredients for the sauce, which definitely has olive oil, salt, herbes de Provence, and green olives. The secret ingredient is an enigma. We try to find out but to no avail.

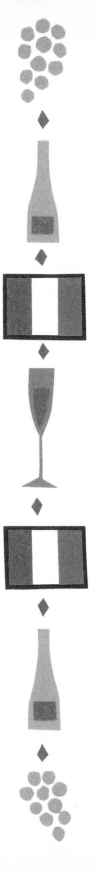

At home, I quickly made some ratatouille from the market vegetables to go with the chicken, offered some local olives and thin slices of *saucisson* as a nibble in the kitchen as I prepared things, and set the outdoor table. "What would you like to drink?" I asked. With this you can have a white, rosé, or red wine, or, of course, Champagne. The woman did not hesitate: Champagne.

Often in the spring in New York City, we throw a big cocktail party at our home and it goes on for hours inside the apartment and especially out on the terrace, with people coming and going. It is our chance to say hello to a lot of friends before people's summer plans take control of their lives, and for us that means less time in Manhattan to connect with friends. Each time we host the party, Edward insists we have bottles of a red wine on hand—usually a light Burgundy—along with sparkling and still waters and plenty of Champagne. Each year, no one drinks the red wine, but there are plenty of empty bottles of Champagne after the party. In my experience, it is indeed the rare person who shuns a glass of the foaming grape from Eastern France (Tennyson's term, not mine).

Champagne really is magic in a bottle. It is a great wine, tasty, refreshing, complex, but more than that: Champagne is a state of mind. It connotes at once carefree, celebratory, festive, and, yes, bubbly overtones. It is a great mood enhancer. To my ears, the pop of a Champagne (or sparkling wine) cork launches a festive mood of pleasure and celebration. No occasion is too small. And it is also a great and versatile food wine. In my profession, I was never shy about offering Champagne before, during, and after a meal. *Bien sûr,* I often offered a dinner *tout au Champagne,* only with the wines of Champagne served with each course. It is a recipe for success. So, I offer now two menus that marry well with Champagne and some additional tried and tested food ideas. And why in a book with not getting fat in its title? Champagne is a food that is both comparatively healthy and nonfattening, and that will become clearer. Also as Madame de Pompadour remarked, "Champagne is the only wine which leaves a woman beautiful after drinking it."

I've found two reasons why people are sometimes reluctant to offer Champagne or sparkling wine. They are uncomfortable or afraid to open a bottle, and they think Champagne gives you a headache (wrong, unless perhaps you over-indulge, but that's true of any alcoholic beverage). Before I address and hope-fully dismiss both those reservations, let's get on the same page with some Champagne basics.

Types and Styles

Here's a little primer to help you select and serve Champagne from France, which is a blended wine made of grapes from vineyards spread across a highly restricted and regulated region and only from Pinot Noir, Pinot Meunier, and Chardonnay grapes—mostly in combination but sometimes singly. There is *vintage* and *non-vintage* Champagne. When there is an exceptional harvest—perhaps three or four times in a decade—all wines used in the blend come from that harvest and its year appears on the bottle's label. The style and character of each vintage Champagne varies from vintage to vintage and from house to house (which, of course, source grapes from different vineyards and have differ-ent percentages of grape types in their blends). Most Champagne, however, is the less expensive non-vintage, which is made from a blend of wines from a given year plus reserve wines of various ages.

The blending maintains a consistently distinctive house "taste" from year to year, so that the style and character of a non-vintage Champagne does not vary from year to year, only from house to house. House styles vary from light to medium to full bodied, depending, among other things, upon the percentage of Chardonnay grape in the house blend. Generally, the more Chardonnay, the lighter the style wine. The House of Veuve Clicquot, for example, uses Char-donnay for only about a third of its blend, and thus the house style is full-bodied.

Most Champagnes are dry, indeed bone dry, and labeled *brut,* but to others more sugar is added and the resultant sweeter Champagne is, ironically, called extra dry. Even sweeter, it is called demi-sec (half dry). These sweeter styles of Champagne go well with some foods, but are generally reserved for desserts. Four other types and styles require a bit of quaffing to develop personal preferences and can be found in non-vintage and vintage versions but not from every house. A favourite "food wine" of mine is rosé Champagne, usually made by the addition of some still red wine during the blending process. Another type is *blanc de blancs* Champagne, a blend of only Chardonnay grapes, and the lightest of Champagnes. A *crémant* is a Champagne with slightly less effervescence, and not commonly produced; however, the word *crémant* is widely used to identify a great many sparkling wines from outside the Champagne region. Confused? Most Champagne houses also produce a "best we can make" Champagne, which they put in fancy bottles and charge more for than their other types and styles: They are the so-called prestige *cuvées* or *têtes de cuvée.* Again, these are a matter of personal preference (including price), and you sometimes have to bring a lot to the tasting experience to fully appreciate the taste nuances, subtleties, and rarities that help justify the prices, but they are certainly painstakingly made over many years before being released. Most, including Dom Pérignon, Cristal, and La Grande Dame, are only made in vintage years, but perhaps the most esteemed of all, Krug, is produced each year and is identified as MV for multi-vintage.

Opening the Bottle (or Two)

Opening a bottle is *très facile.* I learned to do it, and countless number of times I demonstrated to women and men in all sorts of settings—from restaurant staff sessions to cooking schools to live TV shows—the proper and safe way to open a bottle. Growing up with a mother whose favourite beverage was Champagne,

I saw lots and lots of cork popping in our home. My mother was a champion at opening bottles and toasting, so more often than not she was the one who did it all and then passed on the bottle to my father, who would do the pouring.

Chill the bottle properly before serving; the ideal temperature is 46 to 48 degrees. Twenty minutes in a bucket filled with ice and water or several hours in a refrigerator should cool the wine sufficiently.

If the bottle is wet, dry it off. To open, remove the cap foil and untwist the wire muzzle. You can completely remove the wire muzzle then or leave it draped over the cork. If you do take it off, beware—the cork can on occasion shoot out from the pressure in the bottle alone. Holding the cork (with loosened wire muzzle) firmly with one hand and generally with your thumb on top of the cork, point the bottle on a slight angle away from you or anyone else. Then with your other hand around the bottle's base or waist, slowly turn the bottle in one direction. The operative phase is "turn the bottle, not the cork." The cork will come out easily with a soft "pop" (or sigh) and without loss of froth, sparkle, or wine. Tulip or flute glasses should be filled about two thirds.

Once the cork is popped, it is hard to resist sharing the entire contents of the bottle, but if there's Champagne left, it can be maintained in the refrigerator for a day or two, depending on how much air versus wine is in the bottle *if* you recork the bottle in some fashion to keep the bubbles (CO_2) in and extra air (oxygen) out. Like most wines, exposure to oxygen causes oxidation in Champagne and the wine's flavours and complexity fade into oblivion, not instantly but gradually. So, the more air versus wine in a bottle, the less time it will survive at its peak flavour. Champagne, if kept under pressure, stays pretty well. And an inexpensive "Champagne recorker" (a plug with clasps to grab the neck of the bottle) is widely available and a good investment, though other stoppers work fine, even plastic wrap. I have a host of recorkers, mostly unused.

As for headaches, quality Champagne and sparkling wines are low in histamines and unless you have a special condition where alcoholic beverages of any kind trigger headaches including migraines, you should be fine. The same claim cannot be made for cheap sparklers made from different grapes and with different methods and having higher amounts of sugar. Champagne is a very dry (meaning not sweet) wine. Of course, it is bubbly, and that sometimes means it goes to your head a little quicker than a still wine, especially on an empty stomach, but lots of people enjoy the charms it brings to their head. It is, by the way, comparatively low in calories. A 125–150 ml serving is less than 90 calories, and usually a pour of Champagne is about 75 ml, perhaps 125 ml. It is bubbly, and some people do not like the aggressiveness of carbonated beverages. Champagne is not in the same class; it does not have big bubbles pumped into it as do fizzy drinks and some sparkling waters. Its bubbles are tiny and smooth and the result of a natural double fermentation process. And others claim they don't like the acidity of Champagne. It is acidic, but not more than most dry wines.

Once the bottle is open, it's meant to be drunk, and that means some food is de rigueur. If nothing else is available, bread is a wonderful accompaniment to Champagne. You probably know the French saying, *vivre d'amour, de pain et d'eau fraîche,* to live with love, bread, and water . . . well, I learned to replace the water with the bubbly. Not a bad combination, don't you think?

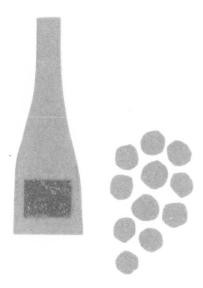

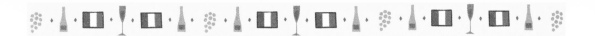

CHICKEN *TOUT AU CHAMPAGNE* MENU

I was amused though not surprised when one of the recipes from French Women Don't Get Fat *that received the most feedback and favourable attention from readers all over the world was and is the chicken au Champagne. So, I'm including it in this first menu sample because it is easy, foolproof, and most of all delicious. It is one of my safe bets that I have placed time and time again. You can try the same dish with white wine or dry vermouth and the chicken will have a different taste. Whenever possible I stick to the bubbly as the magic ingredient and with bottle open, I have no-excuse number 23,438,408 for a meal* tout au Champagne.

⌒ APPETIZER ⌒

Poêlée *of Mushrooms*

⌒ MAIN COURSE ⌒

Chicken au Champagne

⌒ SIDE DISH ⌒

Stuffed Courgette

⌒ DESSERT ⌒

Baked Apples with Lemon Cream

⌒ CHAMPAGNE ⌒

non-vintage brut or a non-vintage or vintage rosé throughout

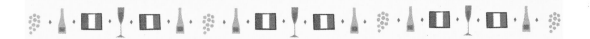

POÊLÉE OF MUSHROOMS

• SERVES 4 •

1 tablespoon olive oil

1 tablespoon unsalted butter

1 shallot, peeled and
    chopped

450g assorted mushrooms
    (use 3 varieties such as
    morels, crimini, shiitake,
    oyster, or portobello),
    cleaned and sliced

1 teaspoon lemon juice

Salt and freshly ground
    pepper

2 tablespoons chopped fresh
    parsley

1. In a large frying pan, heat the olive oil and butter over medium heat. Add the shallot and sauté until fragrant, about 1 minute.

2. Add the mushrooms and lemon juice, season to taste, and sauté for 8 to 10 minutes until cooked. Remove from the heat, sprinkle with fresh parsley, and serve.

CHICKEN *AU CHAMPAGNE*

• SERVES 4 •

4 chicken breasts (with skin and bone)

Salt and freshly ground pepper

Chervil, tarragon, or thyme (optional)

225 ml Champagne (Veuve Clicquot Yellow Label Brut recommended)

1 shallot, quartered

Cooked brown rice for serving

1. Place the chicken breasts in a roasting pan and season them. Pour half of the Champagne over the breasts. Make a slit in each breast and insert a piece of shallot.

2. Place the pan under the grill, skin side down, for 3 minutes, until the skin is nicely browned. Turn and grill the other side for 5 minutes.

3. Remove the chicken from the grill, baste with the pan juices, and add the remaining Champagne. Add additional herb, if using. Adjust the oven temperature to 190°C/gas mark 5 and bake the chicken for 30 minutes, basting once or twice.

4. Serve over brown rice. Pour the cooking juices from the chicken over the meat and rice. Serve the remainder of the bottle of Champagne (about 6 glasses) with the meal.

STUFFED COURGETTE

• SERVES 4 •

4 small round courgettes (if you can't find round, it's okay to use 4 small standard courgette)

Salt and freshly ground pepper

1 tablespoon olive oil

2 garlic cloves, peeled and chopped

1 large onion, peeled and finely chopped

350g minced beef

120g cooked rice

75g grated Parmesan

1 egg, beaten

400g tin chopped tomatoes

2 tablespoons chopped fresh parsley

225ml tomato sauce

1. Preheat the oven to 190°C/gas mark 5. Cut the stem and flower ends off the courgettes and cut each in half lengthwise. Using a grapefruit spoon or melon baller, scoop out and discard most of the courgette flesh and seeds, leaving an even 1 cm of flesh attached to the skin. Season inside with salt and pepper and set aside.

2. Heat the olive oil in a medium nonstick sauté pan over medium-high heat and sauté the garlic and onion until softened, about 4 minutes. Add the minced beef and cook until the meat is no longer pink and starts to brown. Remove from the heat, carefully drain, and place in a mixing bowl.

3. When the onion-beef mixture is cool, add the rice, half of the Parmesan, the egg, tomatoes, and parsley and mix to combine. Season to taste and fill the courgette halves with stuffing.

4. Pour the tomato sauce into a baking dish just large enough to hold the courgette and place the stuffed courgette on top. Sprinkle the courgette with the remaining Parmesan and bake for 40 minutes. Serve warm.

BAKED APPLES
WITH LEMON CREAM

2 firm baking apples, such as Golden Delicious

2 lemons

1½ tablespoons unsalted butter plus additional for baking dish

4 tablespoons sugar

75g crème fraîche

1. Preheat the oven to 190°C/gas mark 5. Rinse the apples and cut in half horizontally. Using a grapefruit spoon or melon baller, remove the core and seeds and sprinkle the cut sides with the juice of 1 lemon.

2. Lightly butter a baking dish and place the apple halves in it, cut side up. Sprinkle the apples with 1 tablespoon sugar, dot with butter, and bake for 20 to 25 minutes.

3. Wash the remaining lemon; grate the zest and press 3 tablespoons of juice. In a bowl, whip the crème fraîche with the remaining 3 tablespoons sugar, the lemon zest, and 3 tablespoons lemon juice. Cover and refrigerate until ready to serve.

4. Baked apples may be served warm or at room temperature. Garnish with a dollop of lemon cream.

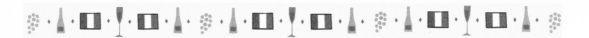

A CHAMPAGNE
MEDLEY DINNER

⌒ HORS D'OEUVRE ⌒

Prosciutto Wrapped Around Grissini

CHAMPAGNE: *A non-vintage brut, my first thought, but perhaps a crémant
or a blanc de blancs if you want to start off with a lighter, softer,
and more uncommon touch*

⌒ APPETIZER ⌒

Scallops Maison Blanche

CHAMPAGNE: *Vintage*

⌒ MAIN COURSE ⌒

Duck Breasts with Pears

CHAMPAGNE: *Vintage rosé, preferably a full-bodied style and
preferably 5 to 10 years old*

⌒ DESSERT ⌒

Strawberry Parfait

CHAMPAGNE: *Demi-sec*

⌒ NOTE ⌒

If you really want to splurge you can start with a prestige cuvée *Champagne,
the top of the line, and progress from a younger vintage to an older one.*

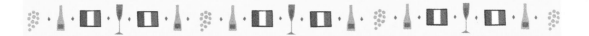

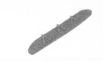

PROSCIUTTO WRAPPED
AROUND GRISSINI

This doesn't require a recipe, of course, just a little serving tip. While you can perhaps make your own grissini—those addictive thin breadsticks—most people and restaurants I know buy them. And unless you own a farm with pigs, I don't recommend you make your own prosciutto (not that I imagine you ever thought of doing so), just buy some paper-thin slices. One hundred or two hundred grams goes a very long way. Wrap a slice around one end of a breadstick so that a quarter to a half of the breadstick is covered and you have a great finger-food hors d'oeuvre, a bit like a lollipop or ice cream cone. I put the prosciutto end up, fanned out in a glass, and instead of finger food on a tray, I have a container in my hand to offer to guests. And sometimes, I simply strategically place a few of these around during aperitif time.

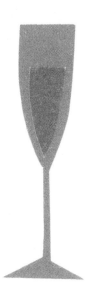

SCALLOPS *MAISON BLANCHE*

• SERVES 4 •

When the Obamas moved into the White House, like presidents and first ladies before them, their food and dining preferences got a good deal of attention, especially after Michelle Obama became a spokesperson for healthy eating and started a garden. The French ate this up and gave it a lot of media play. I also was in France during one of the Obamas' visit in the spring of 2009 and learned that the first lady loves spinach and the president loves scallops. I couldn't resist sharing one of my favourite marriages. So, voilà *scallops (on a bed of greens)* Maison Blanche. *Perhaps someday they may be served in the White House . . . you never know.*

2 teaspoons olive oil

900g fresh spinach, washed and drained

Sea salt

12 medium sea scallops

2 tablespoons lemon juice

1 tablespoon walnut oil

Fleur de sel

2 tablespoons chopped walnuts (optional)

1. Heat 1 teaspoon olive oil in a large, nonstick frying pan over medium heat. Add the spinach, a pinch of sea salt, and cover and cook over medium-low heat for 5 minutes or until the spinach is slightly wilted and just cooked. Transfer to a plate and keep warm.

2. Pat the scallops dry. Heat the remaining teaspoon olive oil in the same pan over medium-high heat and add the scallops. Add the lemon juice and sear 2 to 3 minutes on each side.

3. To serve, place one quarter of the spinach on each plate and top with three scallops. Drizzle with walnut oil and season with fleur de sel. Garnish with chopped walnuts, if using, and serve immediately.

DUCK BREASTS WITH PEARS

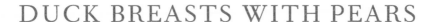

• SERVES 4 •

4 (175–200g) duck magrets (breasts)

Salt and freshly ground pepper

2 ripe Comice pears, rinsed, dried, cored, and cut lengthwise into 5mm slices

½ teaspoon Sichuan pepper

55ml balsamic vinegar

1. Pat the duck breasts dry and score the skin diagonally at 2cm intervals with a sharp knife to create a diamond pattern (be careful not to cut into the meat); season both sides with salt and pepper.

2. Heat a large sauté pan over medium-high heat and add the duck breasts, skin side down. Cook for 8 minutes, allowing the fat to render and the skin to become crisp. Turn over, and cook for an additional 4 to 5 minutes for medium rare. Remove from the pan, cover, and rest for 10 minutes.

3. Pour off all but 2 tablespoons of duck fat and add the pear slices. Season with the Sichuan pepper and cook over medium-high heat until golden brown and crisp-tender, about 1½ minutes per side. Remove the pears from the pan and keep warm.

4. Deglaze the pan with balsamic vinegar and reduce until syrupy, about 45 seconds. Slice each duck breast crosswise into 1cm-thick slices and fan on a plate. Drizzle with balsamic vinegar, garnish with pear slices, season to taste, and serve immediately.

NOTE: *If Sichuan pepper is difficult to find, a good substitution for this recipe is ½ teaspoon freshly ground pepper combined with a small pinch of crushed anise seed.*

STRAWBERRY PARFAIT

• SERVES 1 •

· ·

35 g fresh strawberries,
rinsed, hulled, and sliced

½ teaspoon lemon juice

110 g plain yogurt

Freshly ground pepper

1. In a small bowl, toss the strawberries with the lemon juice.

2. Using a parfait dish or other small glass dish, alternate layers of yogurt and strawberries, grinding a bit of fresh pepper on top of each layer of strawberries. Serve immediately.

More Food for Thought and Champagne

Bread and Champagne are for me a marriage made in Heaven, especially when the bread is a tad warm. Another similarly ambrosial combination is anything doughy, such as brioche, *gougères*, or puff pastry, served with Champagne, not indulgences you want to abuse but as a few bites as an aperitif, which should convince you Mae West was right when she said, "too much of a good thing . . . is wonderful." Alas, it is necessary portion control that proves that rule.

To me, however, seafood and fish are what I love best with my glass of bubbly. Oysters top my list, but really anything on the seafood platter from urchins to crabs to clams to scallops to mussels works for me. If going luxurious, without question lobster, that's a real treat, and I learned while living in New England that there is nothing better than just steaming the lobster, then serving it with some melted butter and a glass of bubbly. My American father of the day, a great seafood and bubbly lover, taught me that one. (I had never had fresh lobster before landing in New England and could have eaten it a few times a week.) And these days it's the special occasion treat I get going to the Union Square market in Manhattan and getting live lobster (females are best) trapped off Long Island.

Fish preparations, as long as they are not heavy on cream, are wonderful with Champagne and here my preferences are snapper, bass, *rouget* (red mullet), cod, skate, halibut, and turbot (the last only rarely ordered in restaurants), as well as local fish such as the river ones in Champagne called *sandre* (bream).

White meats are a great match with Champagne, whether the meat is chicken, poussin, turkey, or veal. Poussin stuffed with brown rice, nuts, and golden raisins served with Champagne is one of Edward's favourite dishes.

As for veggies, mushrooms are the ideal marriage. When in France in the autumn mushroom season, I love to sauté a few types of mushrooms with maybe an egg or omelette on the side, a slice of good sourdough bread, and a glass of bubbly. That's a perfect meal for me. In the spring, my all-time favourite fresh morels (but alas very expensive these days) would be my top choice. Cooked with a tiny bit of oil and butter, some shallots, and at the end a dash of cream and some fresh parsley very finely chopped is a dish I would probably order on a desert island or as one of the last meals of my life.

For asparagus, artichokes, salads, and most cheeses, especially the pungent ones, skip Champagne, since its complex, elegant flavours will be overpowered. Stick to fresh goat cheese or light but not too creamy cheese types; my favourite Champagne and cheese pairing is with Parmesan (the fat and oiliness that makes it a good marriage). Slivers of Parmesan make for a simple hors d'oeuvre served with Champagne.

For red meat, I enjoy a rosé Champagne combo with duck and even lamb. Either is always a conversation piece, as not many people think of Champagne with red meat. A full-bodied rosé Champagne is Pinot Noir, after all.

To go a step further, steak and pizza also marry well with the bubbly. The fat/oil works well with the acidity in the bubbly. So often while on the lecture tour, people would come to me after the Q & A to admit their favourite combo was pizza and bubbly or steak and bubbly (lucky them), but they were embarrassed to ask the question in public because they thought it was a poor combo. To this, I'd say nonsense. (I now bring up and ask the question myself.) I'd also add, there is no stupid question and personal preferences generally win in the end. Anyway, pizza and bubbly and steak and bubbly are two of my favourite combinations. I was privileged to have to drink Champagne with so many foods (and not to have to pay for the Champagne myself) to discover these special tastes—and a few more.

Popular perception to the contrary, Champagne is not the most dessert-friendly wine. What wines are? Mostly sweet wines, and a demi-sec Champagne works, but as with most sweet wines the sweetness alongside sweetness does not contrast or flatter either. (They are often better just by themselves.) And the dryness and comparatively sharp acidity of a brut Champagne is too strong a contrast for most, except with some fresh fruit, light fruit tarts, *crème anglaise*, or floating island. Indeed, not-too-sweet fruit pies with a great dough and crust work fine. Avoid chocolate with Champagne, since its strong and beguiling flavours destroy the taste and finesse of even an average bubbly: it is that simple, and for people like me who are both chocolate and Champagne lovers it may seem tempting, but sometime, just sometime, one must follow a sensible rule. Maybe a fruity rosé Champagne has a fighting chance, but I have never found chocolate or Champagne showing their best when served together. And at today's price of Champagne . . . and chocolate, don't unnecessarily reduce the tasting and savouring experience. Now, if you have some Champagne left in a bottle or glass, it is a wonderful palate cleanser ten or twenty minutes later, and thereafter. Enjoy.

Finally, if you are still deciding whether or not to pop a cork with your meal, here's a little expression that may help. It is a favourite of some of the people who sell Champagne: "Burgundy makes us think of naughty things, Bordeaux makes us discuss them, and Champagne makes us do them." As I said, enjoy.

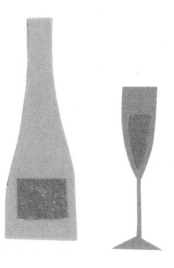

CHAPTER EIGHT

IN CASE YOU WERE ABOUT TO ASK

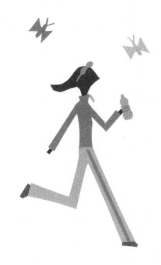

Read the Label

There was once an amusing American television commercial for a brand of spaghetti. It proclaimed it was the spaghetti harvesting season in Italy and showed a picturesque hillside of trees with spaghetti strands dangling from their many limbs. And if memory serves, there were peasants in centuries-old costumes, holding baskets, and filling them with freshly harvested pasta. Today we would call this artisanal pasta, or perhaps even "bio" or organic pasta, except, of course, for the fact that pasta does not grow on trees.

The humorous commercial played on the reality that most people neither connect what they eat, with what is in it, nor where it comes from. There is spaghetti and there is spaghetti, hundreds of brands plus homemade. There is, for example, whole wheat pasta that's touted today. Healthier? Less tasty? Pasta differences mostly have to do with the wheat that goes into the pasta, some of which are "enriched." What's that about? Do we need enriching? What are we putting into our bodies? But pasta is not a big offender loaded with added sugars or heavily salted or preserved with chemicals.

The list of common food items that have lost connection with their origins and genes is epidemic. I told the story in *French Women for All Seasons* of the boy who knew what apple pie was but not what an apple was. Just yesterday I was shopping in a gourmet speciality shop for fresh ricotta (now day-old homemade ricotta is a reason for a special detour), and I said to my husband, who was along for the walk, "Is there anything else we should get?" And he pointed to some dried sausages or *saucissons* as we call them in France, and said, "How about one or two of those?" (We occasionally nibble on a couple of slices while preparing dinner.) My response was to ask "How many times a week do you want to eat pork [the day before we had a pork roast]? Plus it is loaded with salt." A flash went off in his head and he said, "Gee [he really says gee], I know sausages are made from meat scraps and organs and body parts of animals we wouldn't eat if served on a plate, but I simply don't make a connection back to pigs—sausages are sausages." Yes, but unless they are labelled duck, venison, or turkey sausage or whatever, figure there's plenty of pork in them. It's implicit, but seemingly lost on the consumer.

I know reading labels: 1) is boring, 2) won't solve everything, 3) will scare you, but 4) is a lesson you will enjoy having learned, especially as it is a necessity in today's world of globalization with the ubiquitous availability of products created and "manufactured" far and wide, with new tastes regularly introduced from other cultures. I always look for two things as avoidance tips: 1) a long list of ingredients. I'd say five is fine—fifteen should set off alarms; and 2) corn syrup, high fructose corn syrup (yikes, an inexpensive sweetener and preservative that's low in nutritional value), words that sound like (and are) chemicals should be considered warnings. Plus I am alert to the quantity of salt and sugar contained in the labelled product. And let's recognize there are plenty of ambiguities on labels and ways for the food industry marketers both in the United States and abroad to mislead consumers.

Cereals and yogurts are two illustrative supermarket items that drive home the need to read labels and know what you are putting into your body. People with high blood pressure or water retention eat cereal without a clue that some are loaded with sodium. And they are sometimes eating cereal in order to lose weight to control their blood pressure and other health issues attributed to being overweight without knowing how much sugar and calories are in what they are eating. Almost the same thing can be said about yogurt.

A male friend of ours who was raised and lives outside the United States recently came to America to go to Canyon Ranch, a highly reputable spa, to lose weight, which also meant learning some things about nutrition for the first time. Over the years of busy life, busy travel, and busy entertainment he gained some pounds year after year. Then one day, as we say, he paid the price, which started with health issues that became more and more serious. He was told to lose weight and exercise but—you know the story. Finally he had reached the point when drugs, warnings, heart surgery, and the usual litany didn't work anymore, and it came to: you need to lose weight now, immediately, or you'll die soon. He needed help losing weight and regaining a healthy lifestyle and was able to afford the spa to start his "recovery."

When I saw him at a buffet brunch, I was not aware of the spa time but found him less heavy and, more important, looking different—let's say healthier and happier. So I said, "Wow," and congratulated him on the way he looked. He told me about his recent spa visit and how he had lost nine pounds (forty to go). He said he had learned a lot about nutrition, yet he was holding a bowl of cereal (looked like three portions to me—remember a cereal portion is 60 g, not 250 g or 350 g). I couldn't help asking if this was the breakfast he had at the spa. More or less, he said, even though there he ate granola. After five minutes more of "eating" conversation, I learned he had trouble with water retention, so I did ask if he was aware of the salt content in cereal. He was not.

Without going into the brand—read a major and well-known cornflakes name—here is what I found on the label of a popular box of cornflakes: over fifteen ingredients, including three that worry me: salt, sugar, and high fructose corn syrup. Any idea why we would need sugar *plus* high fructose syrup, which is more sugar, in our cereal? And the best line on that box was the little label on top that said "Diabetes Friendly." Who are they kidding? (Does "diabetes friendly" mean it introduces you to diabetes? Or welcomes diabetics? I doubt the company caught the irony.) Well, lots of people don't read labels and don't know what they are eating. The sodium content in this cornflake box is 220 mg (milligrams) per serving (and what they classify as a serving is 25 g) and servings are commonly, I expect, exceeded in practice by a factor of two or even three. My husband's favourite cereal has less than half that amount of sodium per equivalent serving, and I eat an original pecan granola that has zero sodium in it.

Of course, you have to know what X mg of sodium means in the context of knowing what you are putting into your body and making informed decisions. The current recommended daily intake is between 500 mg minimum and 2,400 mg maximum, which in visual and equivalent terms is a quarter teaspoon of salt minimum and a teaspoon maximum. Think about that the next time you pick up a saltshaker. So what I am pointing out is many of us are mindlessly overdosing on salt. Diet drinks? No calories, no cholesterol, but no salt? Wrong. The average diet drink has 28 mg of sodium. And, of course, since people think diet drinks are free of most "bad" stuff, they drink not one but two and even three a day. And remember the sodium content of that bowl of cornflakes—before adding milk and more sodium?

People think yogurt is a wonder food, and it is, if it is plain yogurt. But go to a big supermarket in America, in Brazil, anywhere, including France, and as I have done with reporters, you can stand in front of a huge wall covered with dozens, even hundreds of types and brands of yogurt. Read the labels. Most do not make the cut for my idea of plain yogurt (yogurt is yogurt is yogurt, and the recipe calls for milk and culture, period; beware of the additives, calories, and the rest). The worst kinds list fifteen ingredients. Pleazzze. Make your own, it takes no time. All it takes is 150 ml of milk, the culture (you can buy it in a health food store or use a tablespoon of a plain—real—yogurt), bring to a near boil, add the culture, mix, put into the pots and *voilà,* the yogurt maker—just a warmer and jar container—will do the rest and you'll have a week of freshly made yogurt, six to eight containers depending on the "yogurt maker" you select (Cuisipro Donvier, Salton, and Euro Cuisine are good brands) for the price of *one.* If you top the yogurt with a little fresh fruit or some honey or wheat germ, you'll know what you are putting into it—and you.

Going to a spa is great if you can afford it (I know people who go once a year to shed the few pounds they've gained during that year, better than nothing but a form of yo-yo diet to me), but anyone can and should learn a bit about nutrition and practice label reading. Plus I hope they will pass their knowledge on to our younger generation to help fight the obesity epidemic and its consequences. Hopefully, nutrition will increasingly be taught in schools as well.

Water and Walking

Two cornerstones of my own diet are water and walking, and they merit a gentle reminder. Are eight 220 ml glasses of water too much or not enough? It is sometimes difficult today to know what health advice to follow, since studies keep appearing that contradict past practices and wisdom and get their fifteen minutes of media attention only to be contradicted by new studies. When it comes to water, forget what you read, French women and most women know you cannot get enough water. And you don't just get it from a glass. Our bodies are 70 percent water; it makes sense that 70 percent of the food we eat should be high in water content. That's why mushrooms are a great diet food! Cucumbers, tomatoes, and melons are also high in water content.

Certainly drinking a large glass of water as I do each morning jump-starts our metabolism and rehydrates us after a dehydrating night of sleep. Water is good for our skin and hair. And water cuts our hunger and food cravings (with zero calories). It bears repeating that the next time you're hungry and feel like you need a snack during the middle of the day, try drinking a tall glass of water and see if the feeling subsides. Chances are, it will. Drinking water through the day should become automatic, and, if you can, a last glass before bedtime will complete the beneficial cycle.

Two other especially recommended times to drink your water are 30 minutes before and 90 minutes after meals. Bracketing meals with fluids helps you feel fuller for a longer period. But drinking a lot of water during meals slows down digestion and can distend the gastric pouch, which can result in discomfort.

A morning walk also kick-starts one's metabolism (some people use orange juice and coffee as morning stimulants), and moving well (regularity/consistency is key) before eating is as important to staying *bien dans sa peau* as eating well (balanced meals). They go together. As is notoriously known in most developed countries, a good third of the population doesn't move enough, and past age forty this increases risks for nasty conditions such as osteoporosis, atherosclerosis, high blood pressure, and, of course, more weight gain. Enough to give one more than a *frisson*. Not enough people know that all the organs of our body need to be involved to function properly and stay in good shape. (You've all heard the "use it or lose it" for memory and also lovemaking, but it's about the same for everything else.) Again, no need to go jogging for three hours a day, but a twenty- to thirty-minute daily walk and some other forms of movement of your choice two to three times a week for thirty to forty-five minutes will make a huge difference in your well-being.

To Detox or Not to Detox

So much has been and is currently being said about detox, but no one, including doctors, agrees on how important it is to consciously detox. If you are drinking enough water, you are enabling your body to flush out toxins (including vitamin and mineral overdoses, things that up to a point are good for you), as well as those that accumulate while you sleep. Or if you are lucky enough to get a massage, you are practicing detox. So, detoxing can be a pleasurable way of achieving balance. But what about all the products available out there from liquid fasts to herbal supplements and more? I'd agree that most are a scam.

My notion of detox is to flush out some toxins and give my body a little rest and reawaken my taste buds, which in turn will make me feel good and help reduce the amount I eat without much effort.

What works for me and worked for my mother and grandmother is the Magical Leek Broth 36-hour detox. So does a soup day or simply a light food day. In my book that does not mean artificially reduced low-calorie "light" foods, but whole foods in small portions, limited amounts of fresh and well-selected food high in fibre, omega-3, and all the good things we need. I like a few prunes and yogurt with half a piece of toasted seven-grain bread, a soup and/or salad with some veggies and lemon vinaigrette versus oil, and fruit on a relatively light food day. Detox does not mean deprivation or starvation; it should not last more than a few days and can be as short as a day. The best short detox is a day of ever so lightly salted vegetable soups or bouillons for lunch and dinner.

My friend Nicole likes to do a three- to five-day light meal detox after the holiday season or at the end of winter. Her breakfast is lemon juice with luke-warm water followed with fruit salad or compote and a cup of green tea. For lunch: 75 g of canned tuna in olive oil with fennel, tomatoes, and olives, and 55 g of whole grain brown rice. For dinner: soup and fruit compote. The last two days she adds 75 g of fish or white chicken meat or tofu. She claims that after this, she feels reborn.

Our complex body knows how to manage excesses, but in the twenty-first century, excesses tend to be too often and too extreme for many people. We do, after all, absorb all kinds of chemicals through food, air, and water, so a short detox can't hurt. Listen to and watch your body.

I also like to think of my kind of detox as an easy, fast, and yummy way to a 3/5/7-pound loss in 3/5/7 days. In addition to the leek broth jump-start, when I want to shed a few pounds, I follow a Magical Breakfast Cream detox scenario for three days to a week. (It is important to stick to the basic yogurt/flaxseed oil/lemon juice *Tante* Berthe recipe, see page 15.) It is a nice and delicious way to reset one's body and take a break. The weight loss is more a side effect than a goal, unless you use it to change your relationship with food so that you do not return to the eating pattern that put the weight on in the first place. No yo-yo. A periodic recalibration, yes. Again, don't think about extending this beyond a few days or a week. Think about a quarterly refresher.

For three mornings in a row, I have the MBC and coffee for breakfast. For lunch and dinner, I eat steamed vegetables plus fish or white meat chicken for protein. And I cut out bread and wine for three days or more. (Or, say, cakes, cookies, and pastries if they are your offenders.) Try it, a lot of people felt better, shed a few pounds, did not feel hungry, gave their body all the necessary nutrients, and came back with added energy, well-being, and differences in skin, hair, mood, and much more after three to five days.

My Husband Eats Like a Pig!

I've borrowed the words of Brillat-Savarin many times that you are what you eat. If you are surrounded by a husband or a family that guzzles down junk and rushes through dinner without the simplest care or respect for the food and the meal, even the strongest-willed French lady would become frustrated and frequently fall off track.

"My husband eats like a pig" is a complaint I've read and heard many times. One woman wrote to me that she was fed up with her husband inhaling his dinner in less than five minutes and was concerned for her sons, who were following in his bad example, wolfing down their food like there was no tomorrow. I immediately felt sorry for her. That was no way to "enjoy" dinner: night after night of being left at the table to finish her dinner alone, the men in her life polishing off their food before she even had a chance to sit down. Sound familiar? I even heard complaints about children and husbands who refused to eat new, better quality food being presented, opting instead for frozen TV dinners and junk food without a single "thank you" to the budding new chef (aka Mom) in the kitchen. And it doesn't stop there. I've been questioned continuously by women wanting to know how to overcome food obstacles between them and their spouses, boyfriends, stubborn relatives, and children. Many women feel that they cannot live the French lifestyle without the cooperation of their spouses and family. And I understand their frustration, but where there's a will, there's a way. After all, we French women can be stubborn, too.

Teach Them a Lesson

"My big kid of a hubby grew up on junk and a fridge filled with fizzy drinks available any time. He still comes home from work many nights with a Coke can in his hand and a chocolate bar before dinner!" Alice vented on my website's message board.

A chocolate bar *and* fizzy drink before dinner? You've got to be kidding. Could Alice's husband really be that reckless and irresponsible about his health? Maybe not. In my experience, most men are often unaware of what they are putting into their bodies. Ditto for children. They don't cook. They don't read ingredients, and, even if they did, they usually don't have a frame of reference for what is healthy versus unhealthy, a proper portion size, or nutritional data. I am singing an old song in a new verse. If you want to coax them into eating better, you must make them understand what they are putting into their bodies (and what it does once inside). Take Joyce, a fwdgf.com member who shared her story about a friend who taught her children a life-changing math problem.

"A friend tried to cajole, rant, and nag her children into cutting their fizzy drink addiction. Though she never kept it in the house, they'd buy it at school, or drink it at friends' houses. What finally did work was a little math problem and science experiment. She had them help her calculate how much sugar (in teaspoons) is in a typical can of fizzy drink. Then she had them measure out the teaspoons into a clean glass and fill the glass with 350 ml of water from a drinks can. 'Now drink it,' she said. The kids were horrified and refused to drink it! They considerably cut their consumption when they were able to see what they were really drinking. Her words meant nothing to her teens, but the reality was hard to ignore!"

Fantastique idea, I must admit. Try it with your own fizzy drink addicts. And if your husband or teenagers still don't want to listen to reason, try Michelle's solution, who told me she demanded her husband keep his twelve-packs of drinks, Ding Dongs, and other poison snacks in his car after he refused to stop bringing them in the house! Hey, if you can't convey the harm he's doing to his own body, at least you can keep the junk out of sight of you and your children. Don't be afraid to put your foot down like Michelle; this is your family's health you're talking about!

Peu à Peu . . . and Patience

Let's face it, men are creatures of habit, and one of the hardest things to break is a bad habit. Chances are your husband comes from a long history of unhealthy, old-fashioned American-style eating. As Cathy said, "My husband grew up with very bland, oversalted frozen food, and beef nightly. No fresh anything, nothing even remotely different or tasty." So how do you get them to step out of the frozen food box, and into the French lifestyle? Remember, *peu à peu*. (If I say it three times it is true!) You must introduce new and different things little by little. Almost every woman who has had success with a stubborn family or husband has given the same advice. Fwdgf.com members Jan and Lisa suggest, "Offer a 'weird' thing with more familiar things. I insist everyone take two bites' worth of everything made. My teens are often surprised that they like something new," and "My best suggestion is to start small—the resistance is already built, so go slow. Start by adding an extra veggie to your regular recipes, weaning them off white bread, adding in whole grains, explaining gently every day how health and foods are important. You'll get there!"

In *French Women Don't Get Fat*, I wrote about learning to spot your personal offenders. But what if eating with your husband or significant other *is* an offender? Marcy realized it was one of hers: "If there is an offender, it is eating with my husband. Not only do we differ greatly when it comes to eating healthy but when we do eat together, I feel as if I'm galloping away trying to catch up with him. I don't know if he even chews his food, but our dinner is usually a stressful event for me."

And I can't tell you how many times I've heard women say that by the time their husbands and children are finished with dinner, they've barely touched their salad. Cope by telling your family that even after they've finished their dinner, you'd like them to stay at the table until everyone is done. Lead by example, pausing to put down your fork while asking family members a question about their day. Little by little you may see the pace of your meals start to slow down.

Next, subtly change the way you and/or your family thinks about the dinner itself. Dinner can be an aesthetic event, not just a forum for refuelling. Elevate the experience of your meals with a tablecloth, nice plates, and a presentation that makes your family say, "Wow!" Little touches such as chopped parsley or a dollop of crème fraîche in a bowl of soup can transform a boring dish into a conversation piece. Malcolm Gladwell noted in *The Tipping Point* that the most effective way to reduce street crime in a community is to change the appearance of the neighbourhood. The same principle applies here: change the appearance, change the entire mind-set. Sometimes big changes require only small initiatives. This is a bit like the art of seduction. Eating well can be lovely—from biting into really fresh fruit, to the time it takes to make a delicious salad, to learning how to roast a chicken properly, to buying really good Parmigiano-Reggiano. It's yummy.

When it comes specifically to husbands, try to explain to them your reasoning. One reader suggested, "When I am embracing a new idea/lifestyle/mind-set, I talk with my hubby about it, sharing my enthusiasm. I try not to insist that he copy me, just listen to my ideas and energy. Inevitably he starts buying into it along the way."

And if he really won't listen? Be stubborn, stay on the course you've charted for yourself. In fact, the same woman who complained "my husband eats like a pig" applied this very principle. "I used to get caught in eating and drinking faster, just to keep up and get my share! No longer! I use their eating habits to my advantage. While they're on their second or third helping of a dish, I can still be grazing on my first. There is no temptation for a snip of seconds when the food is already gone! Dinner is not a competitive sport!"

Men's Health, Women's Health, Children's Health

Have you and your husband, boyfriend, brother, or male friend ever dieted together, only to find that he was outpacing you in the weight-loss race, despite the fact that you were eating the same thing? (You may have even been eating less.) Men have more natural muscle mass than women. Since the number of calories you burn is proportionate to the amount of muscle you have, men naturally burn more calories than women, even when eating the same foods, similar portions, and exercising together. So the next time you succumb to sharing that Twix with your hubby, remember he's going to burn it off much quicker than you. It's a harsh reality: Women cannot eat, and in some ways cook, like men.

But there's another reason to get your husband and children involved in the French lifestyle, beyond just wanting to stay within the confines of your own new meal plans: their health.

Women tend to gain weight in their hips and behinds; men are more likely to put on weight around the waist. Doctors are not sure why, but the risk factors of developing heart disease and other complications such as high blood pressure, diabetes, sleep apnea, and even cancer increase dramatically in those who store fat around their waists, especially those with a waist size over forty inches. So, those few extra inches on his waistline may be more harmful than you think. Thankfully, men tend to lose weight rather quickly when they cut out their offenders (we women are not as lucky in this department!). After a couple of weeks of the new French lifestyle in her home, an ecstatic member commented about her husband, "He didn't really need to lose weight, but he'd been concerned about his little belly that showed up in his early forties. It's now gone!"

As for children, it's vital to get them started on the right track as early as possible: lifetime eating habits begin at a very young age. The USDA has reported that only 36 percent of United States children eat the recommended three to five servings of daily vegetables, and only 26 percent eat the two to four recommended servings of fruit. These numbers are abysmal. Many mothers have complained that they receive major resistance from their kids on eating healthy food. But for little kids, there should be no choice. You do the food shopping, you make the rules. Feel free to get creative, too. If your child has an insatiable sweet tooth, learn to reframe their notion of dessert as did Monica, a very resourceful woman, who turned her kids' obsession with ice cream sundaes into a healthy fix by creating a yogurt parfait station in the kitchen after dinner. She realized a small bowl of yogurt and a station of healthy toppings such as granola, chopped fruits, and honey gave her children the illusion they were indulging in a decadent treat. Other mothers have found that fresh fruit over a little ice cream instead of packaged cookies and candy was happily accepted by their children. Be realistic, though, do not strive for perfection. They will always find junk at a friend's house, or find something to complain about. Do try to instill awareness and a few values in them for what they are putting into their body, and help cultivate a taste for fruits and veggies.

Head to the Kitchen

The lack of connection to food and cooking is what prevents many of us from finding balance, harmony, and pleasure. Of all the reader mail/email I have received over the years, those who reported the most success with changing to the healthy holistic lifestyle I describe in my writings are the ones who started to cook or cooked more, or more often. Makes sense to me. Cooking means connection and is a key to changing your relationship with food and pleasure, and until you understand and control what you are putting in your body, you are merely following a plan without a master: you.

Each of us is responsible for our own body. And it all starts with respect for one's body, as we only have one, right? Respect may not always mean love, but if one respects one's body, that respect surely will grow into taming it, then loving it, and once you love it, you'll take care of it and be responsible for it. Common sense. It's the basic story of the little prince and the fox about making friends. Changing your relationship with food means just that. Make food (and your body) not your enemy but your friend and head for the kitchen instead of the television set or whatever else you pick to do to avoid cooking.

It goes without saying that homemade food, where one can control fat, salt, and sugar, helps us lose weight or at least control our weight. Plus, let's be honest: today with all the gadgets to help us cook, making a meal is not such a big deal. In many cases, it takes just a bit longer than getting canned or prepared food ready. So, *pas d'excuses*. A bit of planning and organizing and soon one can learn to make dinner in 20 to 30 minutes daily.

Globalization has its side effects in both cooking and the kitchen. Today, in France, depending which statistics one reads, over 60 percent of people in their twenties have no culinary knowledge. Starting from scratch, we must teach them (they usually start panicking when they have kids to feed) how to shop at the market (including recognizing products) so they can pick the right products and ways of cooking vegetables in a simple, quick, and flavourful way following the seasons. Many people are getting tired of poor eating (read prepared dishes and fast food), and cooking classes are growing like mushrooms. This is something totally new in France, where nine out of ten French people have never taken a cooking class. Now it's more like a hobby and gone are the long, expensive and complicated ones.

Today, one of the most successful cooking courses/programmes in France is L'atelier des Chefs, created by two young men passionate about cooking. The key word is casual and their classes are short—one hour. Their principle during lunchtime is cooking for thirty minutes and then eating lunch—fun, inexpensive, and a way to be with people (not a small aspect at a time where so many tech gadgets isolate human beings in many ways). What one learns is to make one dish per class, an ideal way for most "students" who have zero knowledge. In hard economic times, what these students learn is that home cooking not only means better quality (less salt, sugar, and fat) but also huge savings, as it's not that difficult to prepare a meal for a family of four. The key is to go to schools linked with real chefs, since some are managed by amateurs who are not automatically feeding people's needs, let alone have the appropriate knowledge. People need a basic savoir faire, tips and tricks, and what chefs call *le bon geste* (the right technique). People need reassurance that they can go home and duplicate the meal, and in a relaxed environment everyone comes out with self-confidence. The proof is men are discovering that women love men who know how to cook, so it's time to change the famous French saying *l'amour de l'homme passe par l'estomac*. With a few classes and good basics, it's then easy to go home and practice and make one's own innovations and improvisations soon enough.

The French Call It *BIO* . . .
Eating Organic

I get asked a lot about my take on organic foods. Not all organic food is automatically of the greatest quality, and, as far as nutrients are concerned, there's not much difference between most organic foods and their nonorganic commercial counterparts. If you buy most of your food locally and seasonally, and minimize processed foods in your diet, you are already doing well.

When I can, however, I eat organic produce for two reasons. The first is taste. Most of the organic food I buy at the Greenmarket tastes a lot better than what I find in supermarkets. Part of that is the little extra concentration and purity of flavour I find in organic produce, but I suspect an added flavour booster is the freshness of Greenmarket produce over supermarket produce. Many but not all organic foods from a Greenmarket taste better to me than organic items from a supermarket, and I attribute that to relative freshness more than the particular origin and cultivation of the food. In terms of price, yes, organic is a bit more expensive (think about all the additional cultivation work required, the lower yields, and other "uncommercial" practices and be thankful there are people who care to raise these foods to feed us), but remember taste first. Here my theory of "it's all in the first few bites" applies, so I buy a bit less, enjoy it more, and it works out affordably and healthily.

The second reason I prefer organic is more important. I prefer eating food raised without pesticides, chemical fertilizers, and supplements. I don't want to put those things in my body with any regularity. The potential for side effects such as allergies and diseases these chemicals cause is more than I want to risk. There are certain items such as eggs and chickens—you've all heard about those zillion chickens that never see the light, look anorexic, are fed garbage and pills, taste artificial, and literally produce "rotten" eggs. I would rather not eat them. Amen.

Dans ma cuisine or In My Kitchen

Alors, if cooking with fresh, high-quality ingredients is the most important part of making a good meal (it is), then having a kitchen stocked with the right staples, spices, and tools to pull it all together is the second most important. Many people find it tricky to keep a well-stocked pantry, but knowing which spices to have on hand and which kitchen tools to invest in is actually quite simple—and can save you money in the long run. (And learn that dried parsley, basil, and a few other spices are a waste of money—their flavours are real and explosive only when fresh, so buy or grow them fresh.) I own a wok and a *tajine,* but I never use them. They were given to me as gifts. I eat Chinese and Middle Eastern cuisine, but don't make it at home. That's not me. I cook French, Italian, Mediterranean, and American. I cook food that reflects my travels and experiences, the recipes and tips I've picked up from friends and family along the way. So, what follows is what I have in my kitchen based on what I like to eat, and what will more than cover what is needed for the recipes in this book.

DANS LES PLACARDS OR IN THE PANTRY

Anchovies (canned)	Dried fruits (golden raisins, cranberries)
Baking powder	Flour
Baking soda	Garlic
Beans	Honey
Capers	Mustard (Dijon or grainy)
Dark chocolate (does not stay prime for	Nuts (walnuts, almonds particularly)
long)	Oatmeal/rolled oats

Oil (olive, safflower, walnut, vegetable)

Onions

Pasta (spaghetti, linguine, ziti, farfalle)

Peanut butter

Potatoes

Quinoa

Red wine, sherry, and balsamic vinegar

Rice (brown, basmati)

Sardines (canned)

Shallots

Spirits (Pernod, Calvados)

Sugar (brown and white)

Tomatoes (canned)

Tomato paste

Tuna (canned in oil or water)

Vanilla beans and/or premium pure vanilla extract

Whole wheat pasta

DANS LE FRIGO OR IN THE FRIDGE

Bacon

Butter (unsalted)

Carrots

Celery

Champagne

Cheese (Parmesan, pecorino, goat cheese, and a semi-hard cow's cheese)

Cornichons

Crème fraîche

Dry white wine or vermouth

Eggs

Fennel

Fresh herbs (parsley, basil, rosemary, thyme—or in a window box)

Fromage blanc

Jam (once opened)

Leeks

Lemons

Maple syrup (once opened)

Milk, 2%

Mustard (grainy and/or Dijon once opened)

Olives (black and green)

Onions

Oranges

Prunes (once opened)

Yogurt

DANS LE CONGÉLATEUR OR IN THE FREEZER

Blueberries

Bread

Chicken, skinless and boneless breasts

Chicken and beef stock, frozen in
    250–450 ml servings

Edamame

Peas

Pesto (pesto freezes very nicely—I like
    to store mine in ice cube–size servings)

Puff pastry

Raspberries

ÉPICES OR SPICES

Cardamom

Cayenne pepper

Cinnamon

Cumin

Curry powder

Nutmeg

Paprika or piment d'Espelette

Pepper, black

Peppercorns

Red pepper flakes

Salt (kosher, sea, and fleur de sel)

Star anise

Tarragon

SUR LE COMPTOIR OR ON THE COUNTERTOP

Bowl for fruits and vegetables that
    should not be refrigerated (tomatoes,
    peaches, bananas)

Coffee maker

Salt and pepper grinder

Slotted spoon, spatulas, whisks in a
    ceramic container

Small food processor

Teakettle

Toaster

IN CASE YOU WERE ABOUT TO ASK

I've omitted the tools that every kitchen must have: a pot with a tight-fitting lid, at least two or three sharp, high-quality knives for cutting meat and produce, a frying pan or sauté pan, and oven-safe dishes for baking. Once you've invested in these, you can move on to the following:

Apple corer	Meat thermometer
Baking sheet	Nonstick baking mat
Blender	Offset spatula/fish spatula
Cheese grater	Ring moulds
Colander	Scales (electronic or mechanical)
Double grill	Springform pan
Food mill	Stand mixer
Greaseproof paper	Steamer insert
Knife sharpener/stone	Tongs
Lemon juicer	Vegetable peeler
Mandoline (the inexpensive one)	Wine corkscrew
Measuring cups and spoons	Zester

AU MARCHÉ OR AT THE MARKET

Now that you've stocked your kitchen with every French woman's and chef's essentials, it's off to the market for the really important stuff: fresh, local produce. Of course, you'll have to tailor your list to the time of year, as seasonality is still the guiding force of the French palate. With the staples I mentioned and a few of the suggestions here, you will have a balanced meal.

SPRING/SUMMER

Apricots	Berries
Artichokes	Broad beans
Asparagus	Corn
Aubergine	Leeks
	Lemons

Peas
Rhubarb
Spinach
Tomatoes

FALL/WINTER
Apples
Broccoli
Mushrooms (locally foraged)
Pears
Pumpkin
Quince
Squash varieties

AVAILABLE YEAR-ROUND
Bananas
Citrus
Courgettes
Cucumbers
Endives
Garlic
Grapes
Kiwi
Onions
Potatoes
Root vegetables (carrots, parsnips,
    turnips)
Salad greens
Shallots

CUISINER DANS LA CUISINE, OR COOKING IN THE KITCHEN

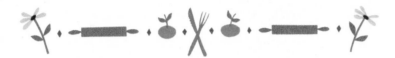

*I*n the end, this is a cookbook, after all; this is a recipe book. So, head to the kitchen and cook a few things. It is the best way to understand what you put into your body and is an act filled with pleasures. With due appreciation for the ambiguity and caginess of generalizations, I conclude by observing that:

- Cooking is an *act of love,* for sure, as those of us who've cooked all our lives know that to spoil others is a great source of pleasure, even though for some who cook dinner every night it may sometimes seem like a chore.

- Cooking is *self-expression,* a way of finding the aromas, colours, and flavours that define your personality.

- Cooking is *nourishment* of the body and soul.

- Cooking is *sensibility:* think about the art of making a sauce no matter how simple.

- Cooking is a *contemplative* experience reaching and probing deep in our thoughts and emotions.

- Cooking is *seduction,* from creating the atmosphere and setting, to the giving of what is loved and shared, to the cumulative engagement of the senses and being.

- Cooking is *memory,* as it links to a person's culture and values. Whenever we eat something, the taste and memory of all the times we have eaten that dish live in the present.

- Cooking is *conviviality* and *sharing,* especially when cooking with others—a spouse, a friend, or children.

- Cooking is *fun,* from picking the produce to preparing the dishes to serving the final preparation, and sharing the results with others.

- Cooking is *relaxing,* and focusing on your preparation can be a getaway from daily stress.

- Cooking is *sexy*—like a kiss, a physical emotion, a union between human beings, and an experience that is sensual, engaging all of one's senses.

- Cooking is *le goût* or *taste,* a heightening awareness and refinement of the senses in conflict, in harmony, and in combination and celebration with one another.

- Cooking is *improvisational;* recipes are a guide not a formula for intimidation. Make do with what you have and how you like it.

- Cooking is good for the mind, *good for mental health,* using your hands to craft a delicious and complete finished dish or meal.

- Cooking is *conversation,* as a meal gathers values, tastes, rituals, and words that are passed on for generations and play an extremely important social role not only over holiday seasons.

- Cooking is *respecting the seasons* and appreciating the fleeting moment of the short availability of cherries, apricots, asparagus, clementines, and much more.

- Cooking is *time:* like writing, it demands that impalpable seasoning. It takes time, but then time is something we can control. It is an investment, a brilliant use of time to feed and nurture ourselves and those we care about.

- Cooking is *reading* from a recipe in a cookbook or on the Internet, thus absorption *and learning.*

- Cooking is an *art form* and obliges us to be creative while involving smelling, touching, tasting, savouring at a given time and place and then it's gone, until the next time.

- Cooking is *humour*—let us not take ourselves seriously and make dishes with thirty ingredients, a *batterie de cuisine* with two days of preparation. If a chicken falls off the worktop, pick it up; if the cake cracks, ice it.

- Cooking is a *social act* that reveals ourselves, our attitudes and behaviours, and telltale characteristics.

- Cooking is *education* and eating at the table is a good way to teach kids about respecting food, learning to be responsible for their own bodies, and teaching them the art of conversation, manners, and pleasure.

- Cooking is *transportive.* It helps us relive our childhoods through favourite foods and people, say Grandma's coffee cake, and brings us to places where we've eaten memorable dishes, perhaps a pastry in Paris or a grilled fish along a lake.

- Cooking is *playing jazz;* one can never cook the same dish twice or have the same experience or pleasure.

- Cooking is both *finite* and *infinite* along life's continuum.

- Cooking is *pleasure* and an integral part of what is called *l'équilibre alimentaire,* a *balanced* approach to eating.

- Cooking is the *reward* for shopping.

- Cooking is *healthy.*

- Cooking is *slimming.*

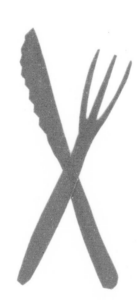

REMERCIEMENTS

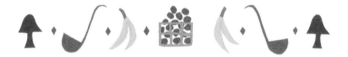

Once upon a time I was cooking lunch for a journalist who was interviewing me for a women's magazine. As I was about to put the main-course fish in the oven, the oven seemingly died. After an attempt to restart it, I realized I was out of my depth and quickly switched to a stovetop preparation, talking the entire time to the journalist, who was busily taking notes. Stuff happens. I took it in stride, but the journalist was impressed and published the story of the snafu and saving grace. I thank her and all of my guests in America and France who have good-naturedly eaten my food. Sometimes it wasn't up to my standards and sometimes it wasn't up to their tastes, but this book is a result of what I learned. Generally, things worked out fine.

Several people stand out as noble contributors in their roles of testers, testees, and collaborators in support of this book: my mother, though no longer with me save in spirit, certainly gave me my love for food and good cooking, and prepared for me many of the dishes included here. My husband, Edward, has eaten all of the dishes in this cookbook; indeed, sometimes three days in a row as I played with the recipe. He maintained his sense of humour and weight throughout. He is very much part of the story told in these pages.

Erin Jones once again provided me with valuable help with a manuscript and in this case with some additional recipe testing and research. Sarah Hearn used her substantial food and cooking expertise to make this a stronger offering, including by retesting the recipes for taste, proportions, and consistency in the Boston air and on her apartment stove. I welcome and appreciate Erin and Sarah's contributions, which more than saved me from a fallen soufflé or two. Similarly, I thank a long list of French and primarily Provence friends who shared and fussed over recipes with me over the years.

My editor, Peter Borland, has as a result of our continuing collaboration acquired an early addiction to MBC (Magical Breakfast Cream), and with this effort has notched his first cookbook during a distinguished career as an editor. Once again, it was an easy and rewarding experience working with Peter, who in many ways made this a better book than I was capable of doing on my own. Thanks also go to Judith Curr and the entire Atria team of publishing professionals for their support, enthusiasm, and expertise.

In one of those pleasant surprises in life, it seems I have acquired an official MG illustrator. My friend R. "Nick" Nichols has again used his wit and wondrous powers for illustration to make my prosaic efforts attractive beyond my imagination. Thank you. I hope readers appreciate your talent as much as I do.

My agent, Kathy Robbins, has been a major collaborator and conspirator throughout my encore career as an "author." Without her, there would be no *French Women Don't Get Fat* to follow up with this cookbook. And without her and Rachelle Bergstein from The Robbins Office reading and worrying about this book, it would be a vastly inferior effort. It's great to have the entire Robbins Office behind what I have done and do.

I recognize I am blessed with such a consistent and gifted team of people noted here as well as a few other guest members along the way. I appreciate that daily. But I am most blessed with readers who encouraged me to write this and my other books and whose lives touch mine in so many ways. Thank you, dear readers. *Merci.* Now do go and cook something.

INDEX

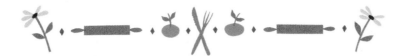

ALSO BY MIREILLE GUILIANO

Women, Work & the Art of Savoir Faire

French Women for All Seasons

French Women Don't Get Fat

THE
FRENCH
WOMEN
DON'T GET FAT
COOKBOOK